D1560254

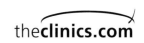

VETERINARY CLINICS
OF NORTH AMERICA

Small Animal Practice

Rehabilitation and Physical Therapy

GUEST EDITORS
David Levine, PT, PhD, CCRP
Darryl L. Millis, MS, DVM, CCRP
Denis J. Marcellin-Little, DEDV, CCRP
Robert Taylor, MS, DVM, CCRP

November 2005 • Volume 35 • Number 6

SAUNDERS

An Imprint of Elsevier, Inc.
PHILADELPHIA   LONDON   TORONTO   MONTREAL   SYDNEY   TOKYO

W.B. SAUNDERS COMPANY
A Division of Elsevier Inc.

Elsevier, Inc., 1600 John F. Kennedy Blvd., Suite 1800, Philadelphia, PA 19103-2899

http://www.vetsmall.theclinics.com

VETERINARY CLINICS OF NORTH AMERICA:	**Volume 35, Number 6**
SMALL ANIMAL PRACTICE	**ISSN 0195-5616**
November 2005	**ISBN 1-4160-2848-X**
Editor: John Vassallo	

The ideas and opinions expressed in *Veterinary Clinics of North America: Small Animal Practice* do not necessarily reflect those of the Publisher. The Publisher does not assume any responsibility for any injury and/or damage to persons or property arising out of or related to any use of the material contained in this periodical. The reader is advised to check the appropriate medical literature and the product information currently provided by the manufacturer of each drug to be administered to verify the dosage, the method and duration of administration, or contraindications. It is the responsibility of the treating physician or other health care professional, relying on independent experience and knowledge of the patient, to determine drug dosages and the best treatment for the patient. Mention of any product in this issue should not be construed as endorsement by the contributors, editors, or the Publisher of the product or manufacturers' claims.

Veterinary Clinics of North America: Small Animal Practice (ISSN 0195-5616) is published bimonthly (For Post Office use only: volume 35 issue 6 of 6) by Elsevier, Inc. Corporate and editorial offices: Elsevier, Inc., 1600 John F. Kennedy Blvd., Suite 1800, Philadelphia, PA 19103-2899. Accounting and circulation offices: 6277 Sea Harbor Drive, Orlando, FL 32887-4800. Periodicals postage paid at Orlando, FL 32862, and additional mailing offices. Subscription prices are $170.00 per year for US individuals, $275.00 per year for US institutions, $85.00 per year for US students and residents, $225.00 per year for Canadian individuals, $345.00 per year for Canadian institutions, $235.00 per year for international individuals, $345.00 per year for international institutions and $115.00 per year for Canadian and foreign students/residents. To receive student/resident rate, orders must be accompanied by name of affiliated institution, date of term, and the *signature* of program/residency coordinator on institution letterhead. Orders will be billed at individual rate until proof of status is received. Foreign air speed delivery is included in all *Clinics* subscription prices. All prices are subject to change without notice. POSTMASTER: Send address changes to *Veterinary Clinics of North America: Small Animal Practice*, Elsevier, Customer Service Department, 6277 Sea Harbor Drive, Orlando, FL 32887-4800, USA; phone: (+1)(877) 839-7126 [toll free number for US customers], or (+1)(407) 345-4020 [customers outside US]; fax: (+1)(407) 363-1354; email: usjcs@elsevier.com.

Veterinary Clinics of North America: Small Animal Practice is also published in Japanese by Gakusosha Company Ltd., 2-16-28 Nishikata, Bunkyo-ku, Tokyo 113, Japan.

Reprints: For copies of 100 or more, of articles in this publication, please contact the Commercial Reprints Department, Elsevier Inc., 360 Park Avenue South, New York, New York 10010-1710. Tel. (212) 633-3813 Fax: (212) 462-1935, email: reprints@elsevier.com

Veterinary Clinics of North America: Small Animal Practice is covered in *Current Contents/Agriculture, Biology and Environmental Sciences, Science Citation Index, ASCA, Index Medicus, Excerpta Medica, and BIOSIS.*

Printed in the United States of America.

ELSEVIER
SAUNDERS

VETERINARY CLINICS
SMALL ANIMAL PRACTICE

Rehabilitation and Physical Therapy

GUEST EDITORS

DAVID LEVINE, PT, PhD, CCRP, Diplomate, American Board of Physical Therapy Specialists (Orthopaedic Certified Specialist); UC Foundation Professor of Physical Therapy, University of Tennessee at Chattanooga, Chattanooga, Tennessee; Adjunct Associate Professor, Department of Small Animal Clinical Sciences, University of Tennessee College of Veterinary Medicine, Knoxville, Tennessee; Adjunct Professor, Department of Clinical Sciences, North Carolina State University College of Veterinary Medicine, Raleigh, North Carolina

DARRYL L. MILLIS, MS, DVM, CCRP, Diplomate, American College of Veterinary Surgeons; Professor of Orthopedic Surgery and Director of Surgical Services, Department of Small Animal Clinical Sciences, University of Tennessee College of Veterinary Medicine, Knoxville, Tennessee

DENIS J. MARCELLIN-LITTLE, DEDV, CCRP, Diplomate, American College of Veterinary Surgeons; Diplomate, European College of Veterinary Surgeons; Associate Professor, Orthopedic Surgery, North Carolina State University College of Veterinary Medicine; Chief Medical Officer, Animal Rehabilitation and Wellness Hospital, Raleigh, North Carolina; Clinical Faculty, Department of Physical Therapy, University of Tennessee at Chattanooga, Chattanooga, Tennessee

ROBERT TAYLOR, MS, DVM, CCRP, Diplomate, American College of Veterinary Surgeons; Alameda East Veterinary Hospital, Denver, Colorado

CONTRIBUTORS

CAROLINE ADAMSON, MSPT, CCRP, Director, Rehabilitation Services, Alameda East Veterinary Hospital Sports Medicine and Rehabilitation, Denver, Colorado

GREG ARNOLD, DVM, Department of Small Animal Clinical Sciences, University of Tennessee College of Veterinary Medicine, Knoxville, Tennessee

KIM DANOFF, DVM, CCRP, Veterinary Holistic and Rehabilitation Center, Vienna, Virginia

JACQUELINE R. DAVIDSON, DVM, MS, CCRP, CVA, Diplomate, American College of Veterinary Surgeons; Associate Professor of Companion Animal Surgery, Veterinary Clinical Sciences, School of Veterinary Medicine, Louisiana State University, Baton Rouge, Louisiana

DIANNE DUNNING, MS, DVM, Diplomate, American College of Veterinary Surgeons; North Carolina State University College of Veterinary Medicine, Raleigh, North Carolina; Formerly, Assistant Professor, Veterinary Clinical Medicine, University of Illinois at Urbana-Champaign, Urbana, Illinois

NICOLE EHRHART, VMD, MS, Diplomate, American College of Veterinary Surgeons; Associate Professor Surgical Oncology, Animal Cancer Center, Department of Clinical Sciences, Colorado State University College of Veterinary Medicine and Biomedical Sciences, Fort Collins, Colorado

DAVID FRANCIS, MS, DVM, Vancouver, Canada

TERESA R. GLICK, PT, Department of Small Animal Clinical Sciences, University of Tennessee College of Veterinary Medicine, Knoxville, Tennessee

KRISTA B. HALLING, DVM, Diplomate, American College of Veterinary Surgeons; Clinical Associate Professor, North Carolina State University College of Veterinary Medicine, Raleigh, North Carolina; Formerly, Assistant Professor Small Animal Surgery, Department of Clinical Studies, Ontario Veterinary College, University of Guelph, Guelph, Ontario, Canada

JUNE HANKS, PhD, PT, UC Foundation Associate Professor, Department of Physical Therapy, The University of Tennessee at Chattanooga, Chattanooga, Tennessee

DAVID A. HICKS, DVM, Department of Small Animal Clinical Sciences, University of Tennessee College of Veterinary Medicine, Knoxville, Tennessee

MARTIN KAUFMANN, AT, Orthopets, Thornton, Colorado

SHARON C. KERWIN, DVM, MS, Diplomate, American College of Veterinary Surgeons; Associate Professor of Small Animal Surgery, Small Animal Clinical Sciences, College of Veterinary Medicine, Texas A&M University, College Station, Texas

DAVID LEVINE, PT, PhD, CCRP, Diplomate, American Board of Physical Therapy Specialists (Orthopaedic Certified Specialist); UC Foundation Professor of Physical Therapy, University of Tennessee at Chattanooga, Chattanooga, Tennessee; Adjunct Associate Professor, Department of Small Animal Clinical Sciences, University of Tennessee College of Veterinary Medicine, Knoxville, Tennessee; Adjunct Professor, Department of Clinical Sciences, North Carolina State University College of Veterinary Medicine, Raleigh, North Carolina

DENIS J. MARCELLIN-LITTLE, DEDV, CCRP, Diplomate, American College of Veterinary Surgeons; Diplomate, European College of Veterinary Surgeons; Associate Professor, Orthopedic Surgery, North Carolina State University College of Veterinary Medicine; Chief Medical Officer, Animal Rehabilitation and Wellness Hospital, Raleigh, North Carolina; Clinical Faculty, Department of Physical Therapy, University of Tennessee at Chattanooga, Chattanooga, Tennessee

DARRYL L. MILLIS, MS, DVM, CCRP, Diplomate, American College of Veterinary Surgeons; Professor of Orthopedic Surgery and Director of Surgical Services, Department of Small Animal Clinical Sciences, University of Tennessee College of Veterinary Medicine, Knoxville, Tennessee

NATASHA OLBY, Vet MB, PhD, Diplomate, American College of Veterinary Internal Medicine (Neurology); Associate Professor of Neurology, Department of Clinical Sciences, College of Veterinary Medicine, North Carolina State University, Raleigh, North Carolina

DEBORAH GROSS SAUNDERS, MSPT, CCRP, Diplomate, American Board of Physical Therapy Specialists (Orthopaedic Certified Specialist); Private practice, Middletown, Connecticut

GARY SPODNICK, DVM, Diplomate, American College of Veterinary Surgeons; Veterinary Specialty Hospital of the Carolinas, Cary, North Carolina

JANET E. STEISS, DVM, PhD, PT, Associate Professor, Department of Anatomy, Physiology, and Pharmacology, College of Veterinary Medicine, Auburn University, Auburn, Alabama

ROBERT TAYLOR, MS, DVM, CCRP, Diplomate, American College of Veterinary Surgeons; Alameda East Veterinary Hospital, Denver, Colorado

J. RANDY WALKER, PT, PhD, UC Foundation Associate Professor of Physical Therapy, University of Tennessee at Chattanooga, Chattanooga, Tennessee

JOSEPH P. WEIGEL, DVM, MS, Diplomate, American College of Veterinary Surgeons; Department of Small Animal Clinical Sciences, University of Tennessee College of Veterinary Medicine, Knoxville, Tennessee

ELSEVIER
SAUNDERS

VETERINARY CLINICS
SMALL ANIMAL PRACTICE

Rehabilitation and Physical Therapy

CONTENTS   VOLUME 35 • NUMBER 6 • NOVEMBER 2005

Preface   xiii
David Levine, Darryl L. Millis, Denis J. Marcellin-Little, and
Robert Taylor

Introduction to Veterinary Physical Rehabilitation   1247
David Levine, Darryl L. Millis, and Denis J. Marcellin-Little

> Physical therapy is a profession with an established scientific basis in hu-
> man beings and companion animals. It has a large number of clinical
> applications in the restoration, maintenance, and promotion of optimal
> physical function. In providing physical therapy, the goal is to restore,
> maintain, and promote optimal function, optimal fitness, wellness, and
> quality of life as they relate to movement disorders and health. A major
> emphasis is to prevent or minimize the onset, clinical signs, and progres-
> sion of impairments, functional limitations, and disabilities that may re-
> sult from diseases, disorders, conditions, and injuries.

Biomechanics of Rehabilitation   1255
Joseph P. Weigel, Greg Arnold, David A. Hicks, and
Darryl L. Millis

> The biomechanics of motion and rehabilitation are complex, with many
> tissue types and structures involved. In addition, consideration must be
> given to the stage of tissue healing with some injuries, such as fractures.
> A more thorough knowledge of some of the infrequently discussed bio-
> mechanical aspects of musculoskeletal tissues and motion during reha-
> bilitation, combined with known features of tissue recovery, should
> enhance the development of rehabilitation programs for patients.

Joint Mobilization   1287
Deborah Gross Saunders, J. Randy Walker, and David Levine

> Therapeutic touch has been used in human beings to soothe aches and
> pains. Most dogs also seem to enjoy being touched. Manual therapy
> techniques are skilled hand movements intended to improve tissue ex-
> tensibility; increase range of motion; induce relaxation; mobilize or ma-
> nipulate soft tissue and joints; modulate pain; and reduce soft tissue
> swelling, inflammation, or restriction. The intent of this article is to pro-
> vide an overview of the principles of manual therapy, followed by se-
> lected treatment techniques for the hip, stifle, elbow, shoulder, carpus,
> and thoracic and lumbar spine. The techniques of G.D. Maitland, an

Australian physical therapist who developed a clinically based approach in the 1960s and 1970s, are emphasized.

Physical Agent Modalities   1317
Janet E. Steiss and David Levine

The purpose of this article is to review the use of cold, heat, therapeutic ultrasound, and electrical stimulation in small animal rehabilitation. The material in this article is a compilation from the veterinary and human literature. Additional information is needed on how to adapt the techniques used in human beings to small animals and then to establish the efficacy of these techniques in animals.

Emerging Modalities in Veterinary Rehabilitation   1335
Darryl L. Millis, David Francis, and Caroline Adamson

Many new modalities have been introduced in human and veterinary physical rehabilitation. In many instances, there is sound theory of how they may impact the physiology of various cells, tissues, or organs. This article reviews some of the modalities that have been introduced recently in human and veterinary rehabilitation. Topics include low-level laser, phototherapy, and extracorporeal shock wave treatment.

Rehabilitation for the Orthopedic Patient   1357
Jacqueline R. Davidson, Sharon C. Kerwin, and Darryl L. Millis

An understanding of orthopedic conditions and their medical and surgical treatment is important to help the therapist develop a treatment plan that will help the patient return to function quickly with minimal complications. The therapist must constantly assess the patient for improvement or complications and adjust the therapy plan accordingly. Knowledge of the stages of tissue healing and of the strength of tissues is critical to avoid placing too much stress on the surgical site, yet some challenge to tissues must be provided to optimize the return to function.

Rehabilitation for the Neurologic Patient   1389
Natasha Olby, Krista B. Halling, and Teresa R. Glick

A properly designed rehabilitation program should be an important component of the treatment plan of animals with neurologic disease. Such a program should be designed in conjunction with appropriate treatment of the underlying problem and after special consideration of the origin of the neurologic problem, the severity of the signs, the cause of the signs, their anticipated progression, and the needs of the owner and the pet. This article describes the pathophysiology of injury and recovery in the central and peripheral nervous systems, assessment of the neurologic patient, data on the prognosis and expected course of recovery for a variety of different diseases, and rehabilitation exercises appropriate for neurologic patients.

Rehabilitation of Medical and Acute Care Patients   1411
Dianne Dunning, Krista B. Halling, and Nicole Ehrhart

Cancer and serious systemic illness result in several physiologic changes that involve multiple body systems. While the primary conditions are addressed with traditional modalities of medicine, the side effects, secondary changes, and complications can be ameliorated or even prevented with rehabilitation and supportive care. This article reviews problems facing the oncologic and critically ill animal, discusses basic techniques in the management of these animals, and highlights the essential role of rehabilitation in obtaining maximal functional capacity in the critically ill patient.

Rehabilitation and Conditioning of Sporting Dogs   1427
Denis J. Marcellin-Little, David Levine, and Robert Taylor

Owners and trainers exercise sporting dogs to increase their fitness and optimize their conditioning and performance. Training is designed to increase strength, endurance, and agility and is sport-specific. Sporting dogs are susceptible to specific musculoskeletal injuries. The rehabilitation of sporting dogs after these injuries follows specific principles during the acute, subacute, and reconditioning periods.

Assistive Devices, Orthotics, and Prosthetics   1441
Caroline Adamson, Martin Kaufmann, David Levine,
Darryl L. Millis, and Denis J. Marcellin-Little

Deciding on which supportive device, orthotic, or prosthetic is best suited for a given patient is a complex process involving many different factors. The ability to manage biomechanical abnormalities successfully may be enhanced by an understanding of the properties of the various materials that comprise these devices, their effect on functional performance, and other associated patient factors. Veterinary health care providers are faced with the challenge of effectively addressing the physiologic and fiscal needs of the patient in a rapidly changing patient care environment.

Wound Healing in the Veterinary Rehabilitation Patient 1453
June Hanks and Gary Spodnick

Wound healing is a biologically complex cascade of predictable overlapping events and is a natural restorative response to tissue injury. The biologic process for wound healing is the same for all wounds, although the specific mechanisms may vary. This article reviews the wound healing process, discussing factors that may delay normal healing progression and potential modalities and treatments to aid healing.

Logistics of Companion Animal Rehabilitation 1473
Denis J. Marcellin-Little, Kim Danoff, Robert Taylor, and
Caroline Adamson

Setting up rehabilitation services presents several challenges to the veterinary practitioner. Members of the rehabilitation team need to have a solid knowledge base of acute and chronic orthopedic and neurologic disorders and a knowledge of rehabilitation principles and applications. The working environment has to be adapted to patients with limited mobility, specific equipment and supplies are to be used, and a fee structure should be implemented. This article reviews these logistic aspects of companion animal rehabilitation.

Cumulative Index 2005 1485

GOAL STATEMENT

The goal of the *Veterinary Clinics of North America: Small Animal Practice* is to keep practicing veterinarians up to date with current clinical practice in small animal medicine by providing timely articles reviewing the state of the art in small animal care.

ACCREDITATION

The *Veterinary Clinics of North America: Small Animal Practice* offers continuing education credits, awarded by Cummings School of Veterinary Medicine at Tufts University, Office of Continuing Education.

Cummings School of Veterinary Medicine at Tufts University is a designated provider of continuing veterinary medical education. Veterinarians participating in this learning activity may earn up to 6 credits per issue up to a maximum of 36 credits per year. Credits awarded may not apply toward license renewal in all states. It is the responsibility of each participant to verify the requirements of their state licensing board.

Credit can be earned by reading the text material, taking the examination online at *http://www.theclinics.com/home/cme*, and completing the program evaluation. Following your completion of the test and program evaluation, and review of any and all incorrect answers, you may print your certificate.

TO ENROLL

To enroll in the *Veterinary Clinics of North America: Small Animal Practice* Continuing Veterinary Medical Education Program, call customer service at 1-800-654-2452 or sign up online at *http://www.theclinics.com/home/cme*. The CVME program is now available at a special introductory rate of $99.95 for a year's subscription.

VETERINARY CLINICS
SMALL ANIMAL PRACTICE

FORTHCOMING ISSUES

January 2006

Dermatology
Karen L. Campbell, DVM, MS
Guest Editor

March 2006

Practice Management
David E. Lee, DVM, MBA
Guest Editor

May 2006

Pediatrics
Autumn P. Davidson, DVM
Guest Editor

RECENT ISSUES

September 2005

General Orthopedics
Walter C. Renberg, DVM, MS
Guest Editor

July 2005

Dentistry
Steven E. Holmstrom, DVM
Guest Editor

May 2005

Geriatrics
William D. Fortney, DVM
Guest Editor

Vet Clin Small Anim 35 (2005) xiii–xiv

VETERINARY CLINICS
SMALL ANIMAL PRACTICE

PREFACE

Rehabilitation and Physical Therapy

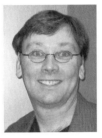 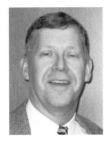 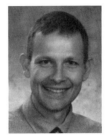 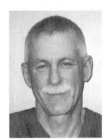

David Levine, PT, PhD, CCRP,
Darryl L. Millis, MS, DVM, CCRP,
Denis J. Marcellin-Little, DEDV, CCRP,
Robert Taylor, MS, DVM, CCRP

Guest Editors

R ehabilitation and physical therapy for humans is a well-known discipline, and its positive effects have been well documented. Historically, little attention has been given to veterinary patients needing these services. Rehabilitation and physical therapy in veterinary medicine, however, is rapidly becoming a recognized discipline and is being sought after as a service by veterinary professionals and owners. There is a tremendous interest on the part of veterinary caregivers to investigate and provide rehabilitation and therapy following injury, surgery, and illness. Techniques used in human physical therapy are being adapted for use in small animal patients, and their effectiveness is being studied.

The intent of this issue is to present a practical approach to rehabilitation of small animals as well as the science and research behind it. After an article introducing the principles of rehabilitation, the biomechanics of physical therapy, manual therapy, physical modalities, and emerging modalities are presented. Information on rehabilitation and physical therapy of specific patients follows, including sporting dogs, orthopedic, neurologic, and medically compromised patients and patients that have wounds. The issue concludes with an article on the logistics of companion animal rehabilitation in small animal practice.

We would like to thank the authors who have contributed their time, expertise, and experience to this issue. Particular credit goes to John Vassallo

0195-5616/05/$ – see front matter
doi:10.1016/j.cvsm.2005.09.016

at Saunders for his help and patience in assembling the issue. We would also like to express our gratitude to our families and colleagues for their support.

David Levine, PT, PhD, CCRP
Department of Physical Therapy
University of Tennessee at Chattanooga
615 McCallie Avenue
Chattanooga, TN 37403-2598, USA

E-mail address: david-levine@utc.edu

Darryl L. Millis, MS, DVM, CCRP
Department of Small Animal Clinical Sciences
University of Tennessee
College of Veterinary Medicine
2407 River Drive
Knoxville, TN 37996, USA

E-mail address: boneplate@aol.com

Denis J. Marcellin-Little, DEDV, CCRP
Department of Clinical Sciences
North Carolina State University
College of Veterinary Medicine
4700 Hillsborough Street
Raleigh, NC 27606, USA

E-mail address: denis_marcellin@ncsu.edu

Robert Taylor, MS, DVM, CCRP
Alameda East Veterinary Hospital
9770 East Alameda Avenue
Denver, CO 80247, USA

E-mail address: rtdvm@aevh.com

Vet Clin Small Anim 35 (2005) 1247–1254

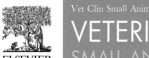

VETERINARY CLINICS
SMALL ANIMAL PRACTICE

Introduction to Veterinary Physical Rehabilitation

David Levine, PT, PhD, CCRP[a,b,c,*],
Darryl L. Millis, MS, DVM, CCRP[a,b],
Denis J. Marcellin-Little, DEDV, CCRP[c]

[a]Department of Physical Therapy, Dept. 3253, University of Tennessee at Chattanooga, 615 McCallie Avenue, Chattanooga, TN 37403–2598, USA
[b]Department of Small Animal Clinical Sciences, University of Tennessee College of Veterinary Medicine, 2407 River Drive, Knoxville, TN 37996, USA
[c]Department of Clinical Sciences, North Carolina State University College of Veterinary Medicine, 4700 Hillsborough Street, Raleigh, NC 27606, USA

Physical therapy is a profession with an established scientific basis in human beings and companion animals. It has a large number of clinical applications in the restoration, maintenance, and promotion of optimal physical function [1]. It is beneficial in helping people to recover from anterior cruciate ligament reconstruction, fracture stabilization, joint arthroplasty, spinal surgery, and many other injuries or diseases [2–5]. It also improves function in a variety of patients with osteoarthritis, total joint arthroplasty, and chronic lower back pain throughout their lives [6–8]. It also helps athletes to individualize their training and optimize their fitness [9,10]. Similar applications exist in animals.

In providing physical therapy, the goal is to restore, maintain, and promote optimal function, optimal fitness, wellness, and quality of life as they relate to movement disorders and health. In dogs, this may include treating patients during their recovery from orthopedic surgical procedures (eg, femoral head ostectomy), monitoring weight loss programs, strengthening specific muscle groups, and helping to manage chronic conditions (eg, osteoarthritis) or progressive conditions (eg, degenerative myelopathy). A major emphasis is to prevent or minimize the onset, clinical signs, and progression of impairments, functional limitations, and disabilities that may result from diseases, disorders, conditions, and injuries. Examples in people include designing and delivering treatment programs for patients with problems like pneumonia, multiple

*Corresponding author. Department of Physical Therapy, Dept. 3253, University of Tennessee at Chattanooga, 615 McCallie Avenue, Chattanooga, TN 37403–2598, USA.
E-mail address: david-levine@utc.edu (D. Levine).

0195-5616/05/$ – see front matter
doi:10.1016/j.cvsm.2005.07.002

sclerosis, diabetes, cerebral palsy, lower back pain, or frozen shoulders [1,11–14].

TREATMENT PHILOSOPHY

Physical therapists use a variety of treatment interventions, such as manual therapy, including stretching, targeted massage, passive range of motion, and joint mobilization. They also use electrical and thermal modalities and therapeutic exercises to help patients reach their goals. These treatments work synergistically to achieve the therapeutic goals. When designing a treatment plan, the therapist should be aware of the scientific evidence supporting the use of each modality and exercise for the problems being treated. For example, when treating postoperative edema, ice has been proven to be beneficial and low-level laser treatment is relatively unproven. The therapist should integrate the individual treatment plan with established perioperative and postoperative pain management protocols. Although the clinical signs present in many dogs with orthopedic or neurologic problems may improve over time, such as after fracture repair, a well-designed physical rehabilitation program may accelerate the recovery, prevent permanent disability, and help to prevent future reinjury.

Patients with movement disorders, weakness, pain, and limited endurance are candidates for physical rehabilitation. Examples of conditions include dogs recovering from orthopedic or other surgery and dogs with osteoarthritis, tendonitis, or other soft tissue injuries. After a medical diagnosis is available, the therapist evaluates several aspects of the patient's health, particularly the health of the cardiopulmonary, neurologic, orthopedic, and integumentary systems. The more specific the medical diagnosis, the more directed the care can be. For example, the medical diagnosis for a patient may be osteoarthritis of the elbow, and the physical rehabilitation diagnosis for that patient may be limited flexion and extension with cranial and caudal joint capsule tightness. These factors may be limiting function in terms of gait; improving elbow range of motion through specific treatment interventions may improve the functional status of the patient. In the practice of physical therapy for human beings, the areas evaluated include aerobic capacity, balance, arousal, cognition, environmental barriers, ergonomics, posture, gait, pain, range of motion, prosthetic requirements, and assistive and supportive devices. Most of these parameters may be evaluated in dogs.

Physical rehabilitation in veterinary medicine follows the same principles. The therapist collects functional information by evaluating the dog's physical fitness as well as its orthopedic and neurologic health. This may be done in conjunction with or after the veterinarian's orthopedic and neurologic evaluations. There is overlap in these evaluations; whereas the veterinarian evaluates the patient to obtain a diagnosis and to prescribe medical or surgical treatment plans, the therapist evaluates the patient to create a physical rehabilitation treatment plan. This evaluation includes the assessment of muscle mass, joint motion, joint stability, and pain. For example, loss of range of motion may be present with elbow dysplasia, whereas loss of sensation and muscle atrophy may be observed with radial nerve injuries.

Physical rehabilitation plays an important role in the prevention of and recovery from injury. Educating owners in proper warm-up and cool-down techniques, for example, may help to prevent orthopedic injuries during training or competition. Owners may have a substantial emotional and financial investment in their dogs and are generally willing to assist in carrying out rehabilitation programs when properly instructed.

EVALUATION FOR PHYSICAL REHABILITATION

The physical rehabilitation evaluation involves the assessment of active motion during various gaits and while performing specific activities, such as stair climbing. The dog should be evaluated at a walk, trot, and gallop if the patient is able and it is safe to do so. The evaluation also includes the assessment of function at rest, including posture, balance, and strength. Balance may be assessed by performing various perturbation maneuvers, such as pushing the dog off balance and evaluating the dog's response. Balance is further tested by evaluating overall coordination, gait, and the presence of falls. Proprioception during ambulation is tested by evaluating toe dragging, knuckling, awkward stepping, and limb carriage and placement. Strength is tested by evaluating muscle mass and the ability to perform normal activities. For example, hip extensor strength may be assessed by observing the dog when it rises. The evaluation continues with assessment of pain and motion of joints. The therapist evaluates discomfort and the condition of injured and abnormal tissues, such as excessive laxity or restriction of motion as a result of scar formation (Table 1). The therapist collects this information to understand how these limitations affect function and how they may be targeted during therapy.

To help determine the cause of articular, muscle, or connective tissue restrictions in motion, the examiner assesses the end feel. The end feel is the sensation imparted to the examiner's hands at the end of the range of motion of the tissue being examined (Fig. 1) [15]. The normal end feel for most joints is imparted by the joint capsule and is a reflection of the slight elasticity of that capsule. Abnormal end feels are described in Table 2.

REHABILITATION CANDIDATES

All dogs who have neurologic or orthopedic problems are candidates for rehabilitation, particularly hunting and working dogs and those dogs that perform strenuous physical activities, such as agility, racing, field trials, and Schutzhund. Rehabilitation also applies to dogs recovering from surgery. For example, range-of-motion exercises may be used after repair of a fracture of the distal femur in a puppy to prevent quadriceps tie-down. Also, a reconditioning program may be instituted after major abdominal surgery to help return the patient to its previous status.

DEVELOPING A PHYSICAL REHABILITATION PLAN OF CARE

Based on the results of the medical history and diagnosis and the physical rehabilitation evaluation, a clear evidenced-based plan of care is developed and

Table 1
Specific tissue assessments during the physical rehabilitation evaluation

Tissue	Parameters	Anomalies	Potential causes
Muscle	Mass/size	Atrophy	Denervation, disuse, contractures
		Hypertrophy	Edema, hematomas, neoplasia
	Tone	Increase	Spasm, guarding, denervation (upper motor neuron)
		Decrease	Denervation (lower motor neuron)
	Pain	Acute pain	Tear, myositis, spasm
		Chronic pain	Tear, contracture, spasm, referred neurogenic pain
Tendon	Pain	Acute pain	Tendonitis, strain
		Chronic pain	Tendonitis
	Tension	Increase	Adhesion, contracture
Joints	Motion	Loss	Contracture, periarticular fibrosis or adhesions, effusion
		Abnormal	Subluxation, luxation
	Pain	Acute pain	Subluxation, infection
		Chronic pain	Osteoarthritis
Ligaments	Stability	Decrease	Sprain, rupture
		Increase	Adhesion, contracture
	Pain	Acute pain	Sprain
		Chronic pain	Adhesion

implemented. In some instances, the plan of care is designed using evidence-based conclusions from human studies and having knowledge of the anticipated tissue responses to therapy in dogs. The therapist chooses the treatment plan that is likely to have the fastest and most predictable positive outcome for the patient. Acute postoperative edema, for example, may be treated using ice, bandaging, and pain-free passive range of motion. As the acute inflammation subsides, gradual resumption of activity may be combined with hot packs or ultrasound therapy. The plan of care is subsequently modified based on frequent reassessments, which are generally made weekly. Patients may be treated as inpatients in the hospital or as outpatients in rehabilitation centers (Fig. 2). The plan of care must be unique to the patient and must take into account all abnormal findings and other factors, including the severity of the anomalies, the age and disposition of the dog, the expectations for future performance, the urgency of the recovery, the available equipment and technical skills of the clinicians, and the cost of treatment. A typical plan of care may include a choice of thermal and electrical modalities as well as specific exercises aimed at strengthening with gradual reintroduction of specific physical activities. The therapist chooses the specific type, intensity, duration, frequency, and progression of these exercises. Exercises are generally initiated with a low intensity and duration that increases progressively as healing progresses and tissue strength increases. It is also important to have established treatment goals or end points to guide progress.

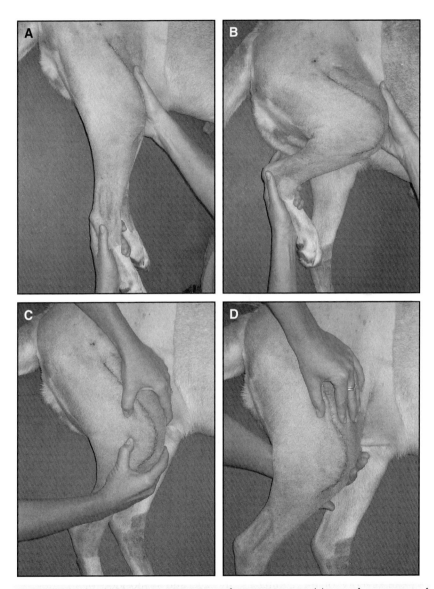

Fig. 1. This Labrador Retriever is recovering from open surgical lavage for treatment of a large hematoma and infection after extracapsular stabilization of a torn cranial cruciate ligament. A physical therapist evaluates range and end feel with stifle extension (A) and flexion (B), the presence of cranial drawer (C), and swelling and adhesions of tissue planes (D) in the operated area.

Table 2
Anomalies in end feel assessed during the physical rehabilitation evaluation

Type of end feel	Definition	Potential causes	Example
Capsular	Slight elasticity	Normal joint	Normal shoulder extension
Firm capsular	Decreased elasticity	Periarticular fibrosis, adhesions	Loss of stifle extension after cranial cruciate ligament rupture
Springy	Increased bounce	Joint effusion, joint mouse	Torn meniscus
Soft tissue approximation	Motion limited by soft tissues	May be normal or caused by swelling	Normal hip flexion
Empty	End of motion cannot be reached	Pain	Intra-articular fracture
Hard	Abrupt stop	Bone on bone contact, mature contractures	Chronic quadriceps contracture after distal femoral physeal fracture

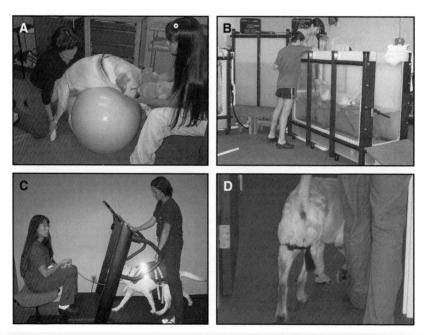

Fig. 2. A 6-month-old Labrador Retriever is recovering from extracapsular stabilization of the left stifle joint after avulsion of the cranial cruciate ligament. The dog is undergoing static weight-shifting exercises (A), walking on an underwater treadmill (B), trotting on a treadmill (C), and walking with an elastic band eliminating the external rotation present in the right pelvic limb during the recovery period (D).

The therapist may also develop preventive strategies. These include monitoring the dog's weight, monitoring floor surfaces at home, having a pre-season training period in athletic dogs, developing proper warm-up and cool-down periods, recommendations for adequate rest between strenuous exercise sessions, and monitoring transportation between locations. For example, a dog with osteoarthritis of the stifle joint may benefit from weight loss; a judicious exercise plan with frequent exercise of short duration on soft surfaces; a padded surface on which to sleep; and a careful strategy of pharmacologic management, including analgesic medications and disease-modifying osteo-arthritic agents.

DELIVERY OF CARE

The owner, trainer, therapist, therapist assistant, and others may deliver aspects of the physical rehabilitation plan of care. Some tasks may be delegated to the owner. Other more technical tasks should be performed by the therapist. Specifically, owners may exercise their dogs and may apply cold packs. Some owners may have the ability to perform neuromuscular electrical stimulation or therapeutic ultrasound. The care must be supervised and coordinated by one or two clinicians who assess the patient; decide who is going to perform the treatments; and determine how the treatment plan should be modified over time, including increases or decreases in exercise duration and frequency and initiating or discontinuing modalities. Feedback (ie, the severity of current clinical signs and the presence or absence of new clinical signs) must be collected from all involved in the dog's care, and adjustments in the patient care plan must be communicated to all involved.

References

[1] Guide to physical therapy practice [2nd edition]. Phys Ther 2001;81:9–21.
[2] Shelbourne KD, Nitz P. Accelerated rehabilitation after anterior cruciate ligament reconstruction. Am J Sport Med 1990;18:292–9.
[3] Sherrington C, Lord SR. Home exercise to improve strength and walking velocity after hip fracture: a randomized controlled trial. Arch Phys Med Rehabil 1997;78:208–12.
[4] Moffet H, Collet JP, Shapiro SH, et al. Effectiveness of intensive rehabilitation on functional ability and quality of life after first total knee arthroplasty: a single blind randomized controlled study. Arch Phys Med Rehabil 2004;85:546–56.
[5] Ostelo RWJG, de Vet HCW, Waddell G, et al. Rehabilitation after lumbar disc surgery. Cochrane Database Syst Rev 2002;2:CD003007.
[6] Dias RC, Dias JM, Ramos LR. Impact of an exercise and walking protocol on the quality of life for elderly people with OA of the knee. Physiother Res Int 2003;8:121–30.
[7] Munin MC, Rudy TE, Glynn NW, et al. Early inpatient rehabilitation after elective hip and knee arthroplasty. JAMA 1998;279:847–52.
[8] Aure OF, Hoel Nilsen J, Vasseljen O. Manual therapy and exercise therapy in patients with chronic low back pain: a randomized, controlled trial with 1-year follow up. Spine 2003; 28:525–32.
[9] Yeung EW, Yeung SS. A systematic review of interventions to prevent lower limb soft tissue running injuries. Br J Sport Med 2001;35:383–9.
[10] Chu KS, Eng JJ, Dawson AS, et al. Water-based exercise for cardiovascular fitness in people with chronic stroke: a randomized controlled trial. Arch Phys Med Rehabil 2004;85:870–4.

[11] Ntoumenopoulos G, Presneill JJ, McElholum M, et al. Chest physiotherapy for the prevention of ventilator-associated pneumonia. Intensive Care Med 2002;28:850–6.

[12] Di Fabio RP, Choi T, Soderberg J, et al. Health-related quality of life for patient with progressive multiple sclerosis: influence of rehabilitation. Phys Ther 1997;77:1704–16.

[13] Baker LL, Chambers TR, DeMuth SK, et al. Effects of electrical stimulation on wound healing in patients with diabetic ulcers. Diabetes Care 1997;20:405–12.

[14] Engsberg JR, Ross SA, Park TS. Changes in ankle spasticity and strength following selective dorsal rhizotomy and physical therapy for spastic cerebral palsy. J Neurosurg 1999; 91:727–32.

[15] Cyriax JH. Textbook of orthopaedic medicine, vol. I. Diagnosis of soft tissue lesions. 8th edition. London: Ballière Tindall; 1982.

ELSEVIER
SAUNDERS

Vet Clin Small Anim 35 (2005) 1255–1285

VETERINARY CLINICS
SMALL ANIMAL PRACTICE

Biomechanics of Rehabilitation

Joseph P. Weigel, DVM, MS, Greg Arnold, DVM,
David A. Hicks, DVM, Darryl L. Millis, MS, DVM, CCRP*

Department of Small Animal Clinical Science, University of Tennessee College of Veterinary
Medicine, 2407 River Drive, Knoxville, TN 37996, USA

Biomechanics may be defined as the application of the discipline of mechanics to biologic systems. Rehabilitation is a practice dedicated to the restoration of function to a body impaired by injury or disease. Because rehabilitation is focused on the form and motion of a system of interrelated parts, an appreciation for biomechanical theory and application is appropriate. This application provides a basis for understanding diagnostic and evaluation methods, treatment modalities, and pathologic effects of the affected musculoskeletal system. This article presents applicable mechanical theory, including the concepts of moment and lever systems; linear kinetics of ground reaction forces (GRFs), linear momentum and impulse determination; and angular kinematics of displacement, velocity, acceleration, momentum and impulse, work, energy, and power (Box 1). A description of muscle biomechanics, gait and motion analysis, and the mechanics of various therapeutic exercises is also presented.

APPLICABLE MECHANICAL THEORY
Moments and Levers
Understanding force mechanisms aids the rehabilitation specialist in the formulation of protocols to improve function of the muscles, joints, and bones. In biologic systems, forces seldom act directly along central axes and through centers of motion, and therefore result in a tendency toward rotation. Such tendencies are referred to as moments and are important to the understanding of how force influences the capacity for function in the body.

The moment of a force involves an axis of rotation, a force with magnitude and direction, and a moment arm, which is the perpendicular distance from the force vector to the axis of rotation. Mathematically, the moment (M) is directly related to the force (F) and the length of the moment arm (d):

$$M = Fd$$

*Corresponding author. *E-mail address*: dmillis@utk.edu (D.L. Millis).

0195-5616/05/$ – see front matter
doi:10.1016/j.cvsm.2005.08.003

Box 1: Summary of common terms and formulas used in biomechanics

Linear Kinetics

Moment = force × length of the moment arm

$$M = Fd$$

Sum of the forces on the body = mass of the body × acceleration of the body

$$\Sigma F = ma$$

Because acceleration = change in velocity/change in time

$$a = \frac{dv}{dt}$$

The sum of the forces on the body = mass of the body
× change in velocity/change in time

$$\Sigma F = m \times \frac{dv}{dt}$$

Linear momentum = mass × velocity

$$G = mv$$

Change in momentum over a change in time = mass
× change in velocity over time

$$\frac{dG}{dt} = M \times \frac{dv}{dt}$$

This may be rewritten as

$$\frac{dG}{dt} = \Sigma F \text{ or as } \Sigma Fdt = dG$$

Linear impulse is the integration of the change in momentum over a period of time, t1 to t2:

$$\int_{t1}^{t2} \Sigma Fdt = G_2 - G_1$$

Angular Kinematics

Angular displacement is movement between two points measured in angles

$$\Delta\theta = \theta_2 - \theta_1$$

Angular velocity is the change in angle over time

$$\omega = \frac{d\theta}{dt}$$

Angular acceleration is the change in velocity over time

$$\alpha = \frac{d\omega}{dt}$$

Angular momentum is the body's mass moment of inertia × angular velocity

$$L = I\omega$$

Angular impulse is the integration of moments causing rotation/time = change in angular momentum/time:

$$\int_{t1}^{t2} \Sigma Mdt = L_2 - L_1$$

Work, Energy, and Power

Work = force × displacement

$$W = Fx$$

If the force varies over time, work is an integral of force and displacement over a distance:

$$\int_{x1}^{x2} W = Fxdx$$

Kinetic energy is related to work and is $1/2$ mass × velocity^2:

$$E_K = \frac{1}{2}mv^2$$

Total work to move a body from one place to another is related to the difference in kinetic energy of the body:

$$W = E_{K2} - E_{K1}$$

Power is the change in work over a period of time:

$$P = \frac{dW}{dt}$$

This relation states that the tendency to rotate can be influenced not only by the magnitude of the force but by the length of the moment arm. For example, in quadruped animals, the force of the triceps muscle acts on the ulna to create a moment about the elbow that is sufficiently large to bear the weight of the forequarter. The magnitude of this moment is not only related to the magnitude of the triceps force but to the perpendicular distance from the axis of rotation in the humeral condyle to the line of action of the triceps muscle. The longer the olecranon is for a given force of the triceps muscle, the greater is the moment. In a biped, such as a human being, the forearm is non-weight bearing; therefore, less moment is required, so the olecranon is short when compared with the olecranon of a quadruped (Fig. 1).

Structural alterations from congenital deformities, joint luxations, or malunion fractures can compromise the capacity of muscles to generate appropriate moments by shortening the moment arm. For example, in the stifle, the patella establishes a significant moment arm that the quadriceps muscle uses to produce a large enough moment to resist weight-bearing forces [1]. In cases of patella luxation, the length of this moment arm is reduced, severely compromising the ability of the quadriceps to generate a sufficient moment to resist weight bearing (Fig. 2). This may be one reason why dogs with this condition are unable or less able to jump up on furniture or up into a vehicle.

Moments can also be altered by changing the magnitude of the force generating the moment. For example, the strength of the quadriceps muscle is decreased after cranial cruciate injury and surgical repair [2]. Efforts in rehabilitation should be focused on strength recovery of the quadriceps muscle so that the extension moment about the stifle becomes more capable of stabilizing the stifle in weight bearing.

Lever systems in mechanics are based on the generation of moment (load force) by the application of force (effort force) to a lever operating on a fulcrum (center of rotation) There are three classes of lever systems in mechanics, and each is determined by the relative locations of the effort force, load force,

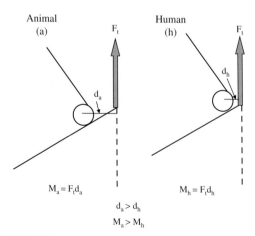

Fig. 1. The extended length of the olecranon (d_a) in the quadriped animal generates a larger moment (M_a) per unit of force (F_t) generated by the triceps brachii. In such animals, larger moments are necessary for weight bearing as opposed to the human being, who bears no weight on the forearm.

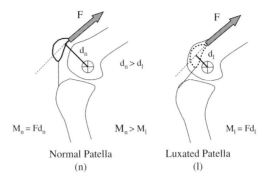

Fig. 2. Luxation of the patella compromises weight bearing by lessening the moment (M_l) generated by quadriceps contraction through shortening of the moment arm (d_l).

and fulcrum [3]. A class I lever has the fulcrum situated between the effort force and the load force. A class II lever has the load force between the effort force and the fulcrum. A class III lever has the effort force between the fulcrum and the load force. Different classes of lever systems are operational in biologic systems. For example, extension of the elbow operates as a class I lever system (Fig. 3), whereas flexion of the elbow operates as a class III lever system (Fig. 4) [4].

Linear Kinetics

Fundamental to the assessment of function is the evaluation of the animal in motion. Force plate analysis quantifies weight-bearing forces and is principally a kinetic analysis. The principle values that are useful are the GRFs, momentum, and impulse. Analysis of GRFs is based on Newton's third law of motion, which states that every action force on a body has an equal, collinear, and opposite reaction force. Testing by force plate methods involves quantification of the equal, collinear, and opposite reaction forces to the three vector force components of the resultant force causing the motion. The reaction force along the vertical (Z) axis represents the weight-bearing component of the resultant force. The reaction force along the horizontal (Y) axis represents the propulsive component in the positive direction and the braking component in the negative

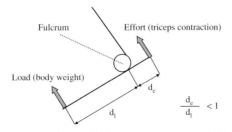

Fig. 3. The mechanical advantage for this class II lever system is less than 1, because the moment arm of the load force (d_l) is greater than the moment arm of the effort force (d_e).

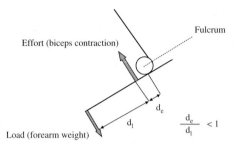

Fig. 4. In flexion, the elbow switches to a class III lever system, but the mechanical advantage is still less than 1.

direction of the resultant force. The reaction force along the transverse (X) axis is small and has been considered largely insignificant for most gait studies in dogs. Because these are all reaction forces occurring at the point of contact with the ground, they are referred to as GRFs.

The term *peak force* represents the maximum value of the GRF occurring at an instantaneous moment of time, whereas impulse represents the generation or dissipation of reaction force occurring over a period of time. Impulse reflects a change in motion or momentum and is derived from Newton's second law of motion, which states that the sum of the forces (F) acting on the body is equal to the mass (m) of the body times the acceleration (a) of the body:

$$\Sigma F = ma$$

Velocity is related to acceleration because acceleration is the change in velocity over time. Observing motion in terms of mass and velocity introduces the concept of momentum. For example, the momentum of a large mass, such as a fully loaded transport truck at 60 mph, is much greater than that of a subcompact car moving at the same speed. Linear momentum (G) is defined as the mass (m) times the velocity (v):

$$G = mv$$

As the velocity changes over time, the momentum also changes. Change in momentum over time leads to the concept of impulse. Impulse is a quantity of force delivered over time. The force over a specified time may be graphed; the total amount of force generated in that period is the impulse and is found by determining the area under the curve. Mathematically, this is done by integrating the function of force versus time over a specified time. The concepts of momentum and impulse can be tied together in the following expression [5]:

$$\int_{t1}^{t2} \Sigma F dt = G_2 - G_1$$

Impulse, the area under the force versus the time curve, is equal to the change in momentum over time. When comparing only peak vertical GRFs between individuals, how rapidly the limb is loaded and how long the limb bears the load are overlooked. These factors affect the impulse value and are not reflected in the peak force. In the case in which the load versus the time curve shifts to the left, the limb is loaded rapidly and generates more vertical impulse, even though the peak force is unchanged. Also, if the limb bears load longer, for a similar peak load, the impulse is significantly greater (Fig. 5). In general, the greater the velocity, the greater is the peak vertical force in normal dogs. For example, the peak vertical force (Z_{Peak}) on a rear limb is greater while trotting than while walking. Because the stance time is longer at a walk, however, the impulse is greater while walking than while trotting, because the limb is bearing weight over a longer time, even though the peak vertical force is less. Therefore, changes in peak reaction force and impulse should be evaluated when rating gait performance, and repeated evaluations may only be compared if the dog is ambulating at the same gait, velocity, and acceleration.

Angular Kinematics

Displacements of the limb and limb segments about the joints involve rotational motion. Flexion, extension, circumduction, adduction, and abduction are rotary in nature; therefore, angular displacement, velocity, and acceleration are important to quantify the motion. Rotary motion is movement in a circular path and is described in terms of angles. Angular displacement can be simply described as a change in angle.

The analysis of angular motion during gait, such as flexion and extension movements, is normally symmetric and repetitive, similar to harmonic motion. Consider the movement of the femur during flexion and extension of the hip joint while trotting; if a tracing were made at the distal femur, it would represent a harmonic wave pattern (Fig. 6). From this plot, several values, such as amplitude, range of motion (ROM), period, and frequency, can be derived

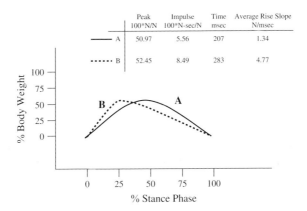

Fig. 5. Force plate data were obtained from the lame right rear limb in case A and the left rear limb in case B, which had a history of a shifting rear leg lameness. This isolated example illustrates the value of comparing multiple sources of data.

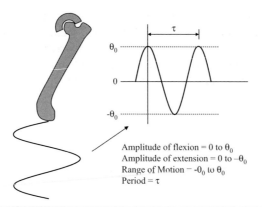

Fig. 6. Angular displacements associated with flexion and extension can be analyzed on the basis of harmonic motion.

[6]. Similar to linear velocity, angular velocity is expressed as angular displacement with respect to the change in time. Likewise, angular acceleration is found by expressing the change in angular velocity with respect to the change in time.

Sophisticated motion analysis systems have the capability to detect and record angular displacements in three dimensions. When such data are synchronized with force plate data, the analysis can be expanded to include angular momentum and impulse. Although linear momentum (G) is the product of the body's mass and its velocity, angular momentum (L) is the product of the body's mass moment of inertia (I) and its angular velocity (ω):

$$L = I\omega$$

Just as for linear impulse, angular impulse is the integration of the all the moments causing the rotation over a specified period and is equal to the change in angular momentum over that same time [7]:

$$\int_{t1}^{t2} \Sigma M dt = L_2 - L_1$$

Work, Energy, and Power

Other methods of analyzing motion include the concepts of work, energy, and power [8]. Work is the relation between force and displacement and is expressed as the product of the force and displacement. If the force varies, work (W) takes the form of an integral of the force function (Fx) and the displacement (dx) over a specified distance ($x_2 - x_1$):

$$\int_{x1}^{x2} W = Fxdx$$

Even though work is a scalar value with magnitude only and not direction, convention has defined positive work as that in which the direction of the force is the same as the displacement and negative work as that in which the direction of the force is opposite to that of the displacement. Work performed by a propulsive force is positive, whereas that done by a braking force is negative. The dissipation of kinetic energy, or energy attributable to motion, is directly related to work done. Kinetic energy (E_K) is directly and exponentially related to the velocity of the body:

$$E_K = \frac{1}{2}mv^2$$

The total work done on a body to move it from one point to another is directly related to the difference in the kinetic energy of the body:

$$W = E_{K2} - E_{K1}$$

Power (P) is the change in work (dW) with respect to the corresponding change in time (dt):

$$P = \frac{dW}{dt}$$

A powerful muscle, for example, is one that can deliver energy in a short period.

KINETIC ASSESSMENT OF GAIT

Lameness may result from painful conditions, such as trauma or osteoarthritis, or from mechanical dysfunction, such as quadriceps contracture or patella luxation. Although subjective evaluation of gait is commonly used to assess lameness, a subtle lameness poses a diagnostic challenge. Also, changes attributable to medical or surgical intervention may be difficult to quantify from one visit to the next based on subjective analysis alone. Therefore, the desire for more objective methods of gait analysis has led to the implementation of kinetic or force plate analysis of gait. Kinetic assessment quantifies the forces that are responsible for or exerted by the movements of a body [9,10]. Kinetic gait analysis can be used to evaluate normal weight bearing; identify alterations in weight bearing; aid in the diagnosis of disorders of locomotion; and evaluate treatment effects, such as rehabilitation, weight loss, and medications.

Because of their symmetry and convenient speed, the walk and trot are the conventional gaits that are evaluated for lameness. A force plate or platform measures weight-bearing forces while a limb is in contact with the ground (Fig. 7). The force plate is usually embedded in the floor for the subject to pass over. A handler walks or trots the animal on a leash over the force plate at a specific velocity range, being certain that there are no extraneous or sudden movements. The force plate is connected to a computer that acquires the data for analysis. A software program then converts the information obtained from the force plate to the three planes of GRFs. The trot is usually the easier gait at which to obtain data. At a walk, dogs are more likely to be distracted and have a less consistent gait.

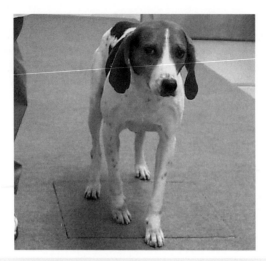

Fig. 7. The dog is trotting over the force platform, which is connected to a computer for the measurement of GRFs. (*From* Millis DL, Levine D, Taylor RA, editors. Canine rehabilitation and physical therapy. St. Louis (MO): WB Saunders; 2004. p. 212; with permission.)

Walking generates a biphasic Z force curve similar to that in people, resulting in a classic "M-shaped" graph, where the initial peak represents the vertical force component associated with the initial paw strike in the early stance phase and the second peak represents the increase in vertical force at the time of toe-off or propulsion (Fig. 8) [9]. The Y plane is biphasic, with the initial negative deflection indicating the braking force and the subsequent positive force

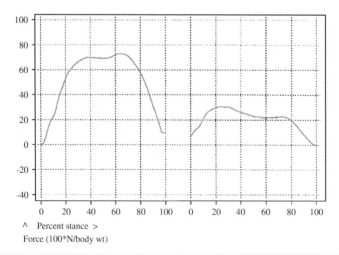

Fig. 8. Vertical forces of a forelimb and hind limb while walking. Note the biphasic nature of the force curves.

signifying propulsion [9]. The forelimbs generally have greater braking than propulsive forces, whereas the hind limbs have greater propulsive than braking forces when ambulating on level ground. At the trot, the Z force demonstrates a single peak, because the individual events during the stance phase occur more rapidly (Fig. 9) [9]. The negative braking and positive propulsive forces in the forelimbs and rear limbs are illustrated in Fig. 10.

The stance time of the gait cycle is the time when the limb is in contact with the ground and depends largely on the velocity of the subject. As the velocity increases, the stance time decreases [11,12]. In addition, a lame limb typically has a shorter stance time compared with an unaffected limb [12–14]. Peak vertical force is affected by the gait; the velocity and acceleration of the dog; and the dog's body weight, conformation, and musculoskeletal structure [14,15]. At the walk and trot, Z_{Peak} increases as the forward velocity of the animal increases [11,15]. Also, as velocity increases at a trot, the vertical impulse increases as a result of the increased force [11,12,15]. The animal's center of gravity (COG) is particularly important in weight distribution at a stance or while in motion. For example, animals with painful conditions, such as bilateral cruciate ligament disease, may shift most of their weight to the forelimbs in an attempt to decrease pain. Traveling uphill tends to shift the balance of forces toward the hind limbs, and moving downhill shifts the forces to the forelimbs. These factors may affect the forces during muscle contraction and can be used advantageously during strengthening programs.

KINEMATIC ASSESSMENT OF GAIT

Kinematic gait analysis evaluates the characteristics of motion and examines gait from a spatial and temporal perspective without reference to the forces

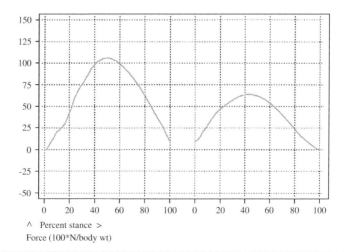

Fig. 9. Vertical forces of a forelimb and hind limb while trotting. Note that there is only a single smooth curve for the forelimb and rear limb, with the greater force placed on the forelimb.

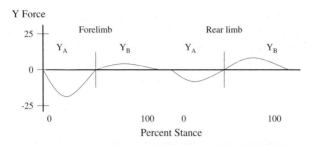

Fig. 10. Braking and propulsion forces of a forelimb and hind limb while trotting. Note the biphasic nature of the force curves, with the negative deflections representing braking and the positive deflection representing propulsion. (*From* Millis DL, Levine D, Taylor RA, editors. Canine rehabilitation and physical therapy. St. Louis (MO): WB Saunders; 2004. p. 213; with permission.)

causing the motion [9,10]. Position, velocity, and acceleration of the body, limbs, and joints are commonly assessed. The most valuable systems assess motion in three dimensions, and these are the current standard. Two-dimensional systems are commercially available, and although they are relatively inexpensive, they are less useful than three-dimensional systems.

Kinematic gait evaluation is currently performed using a series of cameras and reflective targets placed on the dog's skin over specific anatomic landmarks. The landmarks typically reflect centers of joint motion or bony prominences used for reference points [16,17]. In addition, these landmarks define linear segments that can be used to calculate various moments, linear, and angular measurements. A calibration frame or wand is used to calibrate a spatial three-dimensional space, typically to a level of accuracy within 2 mm. After calibration, two or more cameras emit infrared light that reflects from the reflective targets, and computer software records their positions. The kinematic data can also be synchronized with kinetic data from a force plate, allowing for a detailed analysis of forces and motion. Typical data acquired include stride length, stance and swing times, joint angles in all planes of motion, and linear and angular joint velocity and acceleration.

The stance phase of gait is the period when the foot is in contact with the ground, whereas the swing phase occurs when the foot is off the ground between stance phases. The swing phase has three distinct movements. The limb initially swings caudally after propulsion. The limb is then pulled cranially and finally travels caudally toward the ground in preparation for the next stance phase [9,10,17]. The distance from initial contact of one limb to the point of second contact of the same limb is termed *stride length*, whereas a gait cycle is a series of events that includes one stride for each of the four limbs [9,10,17].

OTHER METHODS OF LAMENESS EVALUATION
Force plate and motion analysis systems are costly and require a relatively large dedicated workspace. Therefore, their use in private practice is limited.

Subjective lameness scales have traditionally been used but have significant limitations. Weight bearing at a stance may be one method to obtain quantitative data regarding the relative amount of force placed on each limb while standing. A computerized force pad system to evaluate weight bearing objectively at a stance in dogs may be useful for this purpose (Fig. 11). Preliminary studies indicate that there is good correlation between peak vertical force at a trot determined by force plate analysis and static weight-bearing pressures in dogs with rear limb lameness [18].

Pressure pads or mats have also been developed and have the advantage of being able to evaluate patients too small to participate in force platform analysis and to collect data from multiple limb strikes. This may allow the objective evaluation of small dogs and cats with conditions like avascular necrosis of the femoral head and medial patellar luxation [19].

KINETIC AND KINEMATIC GAIT ANALYSIS RESEARCH
Normal Gait

Knowledge of typical weight-bearing patterns in normal dogs and those with orthopedic conditions provides information that may be valuable in the rehabilitation of patients. In a normal standing patient, each forelimb bears approximately 30% of the dog's body weight and each rear limb bears 20% of the dog's body weight. The relative proportion of weight bearing on the forelimbs and rear limbs is relatively consistent at the walk and trot, which are symmetric gaits. Because of the relation of velocity and acceleration to the forces placed on the limbs during the stance phase of gait, however, significant increases in absolute forces during weight bearing occur with increasing speed at various gaits. For example, a dog may have peak vertical forces of 55% and 40% of body weight at a walk in

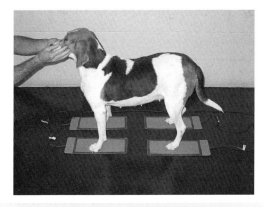

Fig. 11. A computerized force pad system may be used to measure weight bearing on each limb while standing. In addition, the distribution of weight to various limbs may be assessed during therapeutic exercises, such as weight shifting.

each forelimb and rear limb, respectively. The forces may increase to 100%, 118%, and 125% in the forelimbs and to 70%, 80%, and 85% in the rear limbs while trotting at 1.5 to 1.8, 2.1 to 2.4, and 2.7 to 3.0 m/s, respectively.

Several studies have evaluated normal GRFs and kinematic motion of dogs at the walk and trot [10,12–17,20–30]. Studies in normal dogs indicate that each joint has a characteristic and consistent pattern of flexion and extension during the walk but that complex joint movements may occur during the swing phase [17,30]. Two additional studies described kinematic motion of the joints of normal dogs at a trot [16,21]. The coxofemoral and carpal joints were characterized by a single peak of maximal extension, and the femorotibial, tarsal, scapulohumeral, and cubital joints had two peaks of extension, with one peak occurring before the stance phase and a second peak occurring during the stance phase. Motion in the shoulder, elbow, and carpus at a walk is approximately 30°, 45°, and 90°, respectively [17,30]. Increasing the speed to a trot increases joint excursions by approximately 5° [16]. In the rear limb, motion in the hip, stifle, and hock is approximately 35°, 35°, 30°, respectively, at a walk. At a trot, hip and hock motion is similar to that at the walk but motion in the stifle increases to 55°. There were insignificant differences between trials and few differences among dogs of similar body type. It was concluded that kinematic gait analysis may provide a reliable description of joint motion in dogs of similar size and conformation. A recent study has not only evaluated the joint angle excursions at a walk but has defined angular velocity and acceleration rates of those movements. This study indicated that these parameters are consistent and repeatable and helps to characterize the normal walking gait of hound type dogs further [30]. Additional studies are warranted to determine the sensitivity and specificity of alterations in these parameters as markers for specific causes of lameness.

The interrelation of kinematics and kinetics in dogs is not completely understood, and it is only through continued investigation that additional information is likely to become available to evaluate and help in treatment planning for patients with orthopedic and neurologic conditions. Through the use of this technology, clinicians may be able to differentiate between subtle muscle, ligament, skeletal, and neurologic causes affecting gait. In addition, results of therapeutic and rehabilitative treatments may be evaluated.

Cranial Cruciate Ligament Disease

After cranial cruciate ligament rupture (CCLR), peak vertical force may be only 50% of normal at a walk, and dogs may be non-weight bearing at a trot [31]. By 7 months after surgical repair, weight bearing is usually equal in both rear limbs at a walk. Experimentally, peak vertical force at the trot with an extracapsular repair technique was normal by 20 weeks after surgery [32]. Interestingly, weight bearing in the contralateral rear limb initially increases, likely as a result of redistribution of weight from the affected limb to normal limbs, and then returns to normal as weight bearing improves on the affected limb.

Dogs with CCLR have variable degrees of lameness and demonstrate altered movement in the coxofemoral, femorotibial, and tarsal joints [33]. The femorotibial joint angle in the cruciate-deficient state was more flexed throughout the stance and early swing phase of stride and failed to extend fully in late stance, when limb propulsion is typically developed. In addition, extension velocity is negligible. The coxofemoral and tarsal joint angles, in contrast, were extended more during the stance phase, perhaps as a result of compensatory changes [33]. This objective information further defines the pathologic gait of CCLR patients and provides a basis for evaluation of surgical and rehabilitation treatments for this disease.

Hip Dysplasia

Dogs with hip dysplasia also have reduced weight bearing on the affected limbs. In addition, hind limb propulsion is reduced in dysplastic limbs. These differences persist 1 month after total hip replacement, and in many instances, weight bearing is initially lower after surgery in the operated limb as compared with presurgical values [34]. By 3 to 6 months after surgery, weight bearing is improved at a trot. In most dogs, hip dysplasia is bilateral and weight may actually be transferred from the unoperated side to the side with the total hip replacement. In addition, young dogs having triple pelvic osteotomy for treatment of hip dysplasia have weight bearing while walking on the operated side that is similar to preoperative levels by 10 weeks and have significantly greater weight bearing on the operated side by 28 weeks after surgery as compared with preoperative values [35].

A recent study reported that dogs with hip dysplasia have complex gait alterations that may not be manifested as overt clinical lameness, making subjective evaluation of lameness difficult [36]. Dynamic flexion and extension angles and angular velocities have been calculated for the coxofemoral, femorotibial, and tarsal joints [29,36]. In the late-stance phase of the gait cycle, the hind limb gait of dogs with hip dysplasia was characterized by a more extended coxofemoral joint and by more flexed femorotibial and tarsal joints throughout the stance and early swing phases of the stride. All joints flexed more rapidly in the early swing phase. These changes may be the result of pain in the hip joint early in the stance phase when maximum muscle contraction and limb propulsion would be expected, with the increased extension at the end of the stance phase being the result of a relatively passive sudden extension of the hip to complete the gait cycle. Other characteristic changes in the swing phase of the gait cycle, such as an increased stride length and decreased peak vertical forces, were also evident in dogs with hip dysplasia. A subsequent study identified additional kinematic variables describing the abnormal gait in dogs with hip dysplasia [29]. Dogs with hip dysplasia had a greater degree of coxofemoral joint adduction, greater range of abduction-adduction, and greater lateral pelvic movement compared with controls. These differences were thought to be indicative of compensation in the gait of affected dogs as a result of discomfort or biomechanical effects attributable to hip dysplasia and degenerative joint disease.

BIOMECHANICS OF JOINT MOTION

Whereas the force of muscle contraction acting on the long bones causes motion at a particular joint, the shape of the articular surfaces of bones helps to define the motions available for a joint. Soft tissue structures may limit or prevent motions that would be possible based on joint surface shape or geometry alone. Articular surfaces of two bones forming a joint are usually concave on one bone and convex on the other. Intra-articular structures, such as a meniscus, may modify the relation of the joint surfaces. Understanding the joint surfaces helps to determine the possible joint motions based on articular surface shape. This knowledge helps to ensure that appropriate intervention, such as passive ROM and joint mobilization, may be correctly instituted.

The primary motion of a joint is the movement of bones as a whole, such as occurs with stifle flexion and extension, and is termed *physiologic* or *osteokinematic* motion. The joint motion is named by movement of the distal bone relative to the proximal bone.

The second type of joint motion occurs at the surface of the joint and is much more subtle. This motion is termed *accessory* or *arthrokinematic* motion. Examples of these motions are glide (slide), roll, spin, distraction or traction, and compression or approximation. Glides are shear or sliding motions of opposing articular surfaces. A normal amount of glide occurs in normal functioning joints. Glides at joint surfaces often are imposed interventions using joint mobilization to regain normal motion in a joint with pathologic change. Joint surface geometry, soft tissue resistance, and external forces all affect glide. Rolls involve one bone rolling on another. Gliding motion in combination with rolling is needed for normal joint motion. Spins are joint surface motions that result in continual contact of a single area of articular cartilage on adjacent articular cartilage within a joint. Distraction or traction accessory motions are tensile (pulling apart) movements between bones. Compressive or approximation accessory motions are compressive (pushing together) movements between bones.

Normal joint motion involves a combination of physiologic and accessory motions. Physiologic motion in joints with a concave articular surface and a convex articular surface involves roll and glide for most joint motions. For example, canine elbow flexion involving the ulna and the humerus is a cranial glide of the ulna on the humerus and a roll of the humerus on the ulna. Accessory motions are undoubtedly important in animals and are likely necessary for full pain-free ROM, but they have not been adequately studied.

It is also noteworthy that intra-articular pressure may change during passive movement of joints because of alterations in the physical shape of the joint capsule. Continuous passive motion of the canine stifle joint results in maximal intra-articular pressure during flexion (50°–70°) and minimum pressure during extension (70°–130°) [37]. The magnitude of this effect depends on the volume of joint effusion. The velocity of joint movement has little effect on the maximum and minimum intra-articular pressures, but the initial rise in pressure with flexion occurs later, at a more flexed angle, with a higher velocity of movement. The increased intra-articular pressure may result in increased pain and affect rehabilitation, and the therapist should be aware of the potential of joint pressure increases during exercises and joint motion activities.

BIOMECHANICS OF SKELETAL MUSCLE

Skeletal muscles are the primary organ system responsible for force generation and movement. It is important to understand the biomechanics of muscles so that strategies may be designed to restore function in animals with decreased muscle force or joint movement attributable to disease. A brief review of basic muscle contraction is necessary to understand more completely the biomechanics of skeletal muscle. Muscle fibers are composed of smaller subunit myofibrils. The sarcomere is the unit of the contractile system of muscles found in the myofibrils and consists of actin and myosin in an orderly arrangement of transverse banding. The myosin filaments have cross-bridges that attach to the actin filaments. During muscle contraction, it is the relation of the cross-bridges to the actin that results in shortening of the myofibrils, similar to an oar that is rowing to advance a boat through the water. This is also known as the sliding filament theory [38]. The force of muscle contraction depends on the relative number of cross-bridges formed by the interaction of the actin and myosin filaments. A larger muscle, for example, is able to generate a greater amount of force or tension because it forms more cross-bridges than a smaller muscle.

Although the interaction of actin and myosin is responsible for muscle contraction, the interaction of the tendon with its muscle acts as a spring-like elastic unit [38]. The connective tissue of the muscle, including the epimysium, perimysium, and endomysium, acts as an additional elastic component. When these elastic components are passively stretched beyond normal resting length, tension is produced and potential energy is stored. When the stretch is released, elastic recoil occurs, energy is released, and the muscle returns to its resting length [38]. These properties of muscle-tendon units result in the generation of muscle tension in a smooth fashion during contraction and ensure that the muscle returns to its resting state to prevent overstretching and possible damage.

Motor nerves stimulate their muscle units and create a muscle contraction, or twitch. The contraction and relaxation time depend on the nerve and muscle fiber type. If the motor nerve initiates a number of action potentials before the twitch is completed, the stimuli are added to the initial twitch; this phenomenon is known as summation [38]. The greater the frequency of muscle fiber stimulation, the stronger is the muscle contraction. When the frequency of stimulation increases to a rapid enough rate, a tetanic or smooth muscle contraction occurs. At this point, there is little or no relaxation time before the next contraction occurs. In the whole muscle, individual motor units contribute to the contraction of the entire muscle. Although it seems that the muscle is undergoing a smooth contraction, individual subunits are recruited with repetitive twitching in an asynchronous manner.

The types of muscle contractions may be classified by the relation between the muscle tension (muscle force) generated and the resistive force (load) to be overcome. There are two main forms of muscle contraction. Isometric muscle contraction occurs when the muscle is not allowed to change length during contraction. An example of this form of contraction is the muscle tension that is generated to maintain the joints in position to overcome gravity while standing. With isotonic contractions, the muscle is stimulated and allowed to shorten (or lengthen) against a constant load. The associated joint also moves to some degree. Contractions that permit the muscle to shorten (the load is less than the maximum muscle contraction, and the muscle shortens) are known as concentric contractions. With this type of contraction, the force generated by the muscle is less than the muscle's maximum force. As the load decreases, the contraction velocity increases. Conversely, as the load imposed on the muscle increases, the load eventually becomes greater than the tension the muscle can generate. Thus, the muscle is forced to elongate. This is referred to as an eccentric contraction [39]. Unlike concentric contractions, the absolute tension is largely independent of lengthening velocity, suggesting that skeletal muscle is resistant to lengthening. This property allows muscles to function as brakes to decelerate a limb or to absorb the momentum of the body during stance. Muscle injury and soreness are thought to be associated with eccentric contractions. A common example of this phenomenon is quadriceps action during downhill running in people or "negatives" done by slowly lowering a weight, such as in a bench press. In reality, normal movement consists of a combination of concentric, eccentric, and isometric contractions.

The force generated by the muscle varies with the muscle's length. Muscles generate relatively little tension when a muscle is maintained in an extremely long or extremely shortened state. Muscles generate greater force with the muscle at intermediate, or optimal, lengths. For example, the biceps muscle generates the greatest force in human beings at an angle of approximately 90°. The tension generated in muscle is a function of the overlap between the actin and myosin filaments. This phenomenon is known as the sarcomere length-tension relation [39]. With a long muscle length (full extension), there is little overlap between actin and myosin filaments, and because there are few cross-bridges, little tension is generated. As muscle length decreases, there is overlap of actin and myosin and greater tension may be generated. This reaches its maximum effect when the muscle is at its optimal length. As the muscle shortens, a point is reached when further decreases in muscle length do not result in greater tension, because there is much actin-myosin overlap and additional cross-bridges cannot be formed. With even further shortening of the muscle, actin filaments begin overlapping with other filaments on the opposite side of the sarcomere and there is interference with cross-bridge formation, resulting in decreased muscle tension.

The length-tension situation is altered when a muscle is stretched to various lengths without stimulation, or with passive movement. Near the optimal length of muscle, passive tension in the muscle is almost zero. As the muscle is stretched to longer lengths, however, passive tension increases dramatically. Therefore, passive tension by stretching the muscle can play a role in providing resistive force, even in the absence of muscle activity. The phenomenon of passive muscle tension may be attributable to titin, a large protein within the myofibrils, which connects the thick myosin filaments end to end [40]. This protein may also stabilize the myosin lattice so that high muscle forces do not disrupt the sarcomeres [41].

The effect of passive tension is greater in muscles that cross two joints, such as the hamstring or caudal thigh muscles. In this situation, it is difficult to extend the stifle joint fully while the hip is flexed maximally, because the passive tension of the stretched hamstring muscles prevents further stifle extension. This is important clinically when performing activities like as ROM, goniometry, and even an orthopedic examination.

In contrast to the length-tension relation, the force-velocity relation seen with muscle contractions does not have a precise anatomically identified basis. The force-velocity relation establishes that the velocity of muscle contraction is inversely proportional to the load applied to the muscle [39]. For example, as the load applied to a muscle increases, the muscle shortens more slowly. If the external load equals the maximal force of muscle contraction, the muscle contraction velocity is zero. If the load is further increased, eccentric muscle contraction and muscle lengthening occur.

The force of muscle contraction is also proportional to the contraction time [38]. The longer the contraction time, the greater is the force of contraction. Although maximum force may be developed relatively quickly in the contracting muscle, longer contraction times generate additional forces in the elastic components of the muscle-tendon unit.

The arrangement of the sarcomeres affects muscle contractile properties. Muscle velocity and excursion are proportional to the number of sarcomeres in series, whereas muscle force is proportional to the total cross-sectional area of sarcomeres [39]. Muscles designed for generation of high forces often have muscle fibers slanted at an angle, an arrangement called pennated muscles. Various muscle groups seem to be designed for the production of high forces or velocity and high excursions. The quadriceps muscles seem to be designed more for the production of force, whereas the sartorius muscles, with their longer length and lower cross-sectional areas, are more adapted to high excursions. The caudal thigh muscles are also designed for large excursions.

Muscles generate force and transmit this force via tendons to the bones. If the muscles generate adequate force, the bones rotate about joint axes. This activity can be defined as torque, which clinically represents strength. Torque is a mathematic relation between force and the length of the moment. Torque is measured in newton-meters or foot-pounds. Torque, or strength, may be changed by changing the magnitude of force (tension-producing capability of muscles); changing the length of the moment (changing the location of the muscle insertion site); or changing the angle between a force, such as a loading force, and the magnitude of the moment generated by a muscle. When a joint is fully extended, there is an unfavorable mechanical advantage to the muscle, because the moment is relatively small [39]. Much of the force generated by muscles in this situation compresses the joint surface rather than rotating the joint. The maximum moment of most joints, and therefore maximal strength, occurs with the joint flexed to 90°. Studies of torque generation have demonstrated that the joint angle at which the muscle generates maximal force is not the same angle at which the moment arm is maximum, however. During normal joint motion, the moment arm and muscle force are constantly changing, making the measurement of torque complex. A thorough understanding of the principles regarding generation of force by muscles may allow development of treatments for specific muscle groups that have a rational physiologic basis and result in measurable improvements.

BIOMECHANICS OF EXERCISE MODIFICATION

Knowledge of the alterations in body posture or positioning that patients undergo while recovering from surgery or during rehabilitation of chronic conditions helps the therapist to appreciate and take advantage of these factors to improve the effectiveness of therapeutic exercises. In patients with proprioceptive disorders, the size of the base of support affects stability. For example, it is more difficult to balance with the feet close together than it is with the feet spaced wide apart. Similarly, the stability of the ground surface may progress from a static or stable surface, such as the floor, to a more mobile base, such as a balance board or trampoline. The tactile and proprioceptive input may also be varied by standing and walking on surfaces like foam rubber.

Increasing the external load that a limb experiences is important for muscle strengthening. Although it is obvious that increasing the weight a limb carries (eg, by using weights) increases the magnitude of resistance, there may also be increased feedback from muscle and joint receptors enhancing the response. The length of the moment arm undergoing an increased load also affects the resistance that a limb undergoes. Placing the weight distally on the limb increases the length of the moment arm and increases the force necessary to move the limb. Therefore, if a muscle is relatively weak and a limb is not able to withstand a high load, a leg weight should be placed relatively proximal on the limb. As muscle strength improves and additional strengthening is desired, the weight may be moved further distally. The speed of the exercise should also be considered. It is usually easier to perform an exercise at a medium rate of speed than at an extremely slow or rapid rate.

Consideration of limb position is also important when targeting muscles that cross two joints. The tension exerted by a muscle spanning more than one joint depends on the position of the second joint over which it passes, because this determines the total length of the muscle. The semitendinosus and semimembranosus muscles are more effective flexors of the stifle when the hip is also flexed as compared with the limb with the hip joint extended. If hip joint extension is desired (with concurrent shortening of the gluteal muscles), the contribution of the hamstring muscles to resistance may be minimized if the stifle is kept flexed during hip extension as compared with extending the stifle because of the influence of the lengthened hamstring muscles on hip extension (Fig. 12). The increased resistance of the rectus femoris muscle, the only portion of the quadriceps muscle group that spans the hip and stifle joints, may prevent full hip extension while the stifle is flexed, however, because of the increased tension of this muscle. In reality, the relative "tightness" of the various muscle groups determines the amount of hip extension that may be achieved with the stifle in various degrees of flexion and extension.

Likewise, hip flexion is limited if the stifle is concurrently extended, but hip flexion increases if the stifle is simultaneously flexed (Fig. 13). Similarly, hock flexion is greater when the stifle is concurrently flexed but is limited if the stifle is kept extended (Fig. 14). These considerations are particularly important when planning and performing stretching and ROM exercises. When performing passive ROM exercises, it is also important to consider the hand placement of the therapist from a biomechanical perspective. If the joint is somewhat

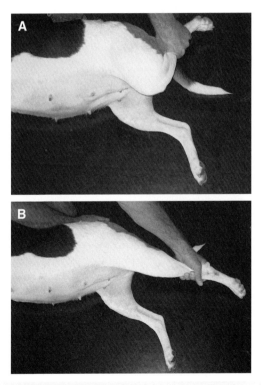

Fig. 12. If hip joint extension is desired (with concurrent shortening of the gluteal muscles), the contribution of the hamstring muscles to resistance may be minimized if the stifle is kept flexed during hip extension (A) as compared with extending the stifle (B), because of the influence of the lengthened hamstring muscles on hip extension. The increased resistance of the rectus femoris muscle, which spans the hip and stifle joints, may prevent full hip extension while the stifle is flexed, however, because of the increased tension of this muscle.

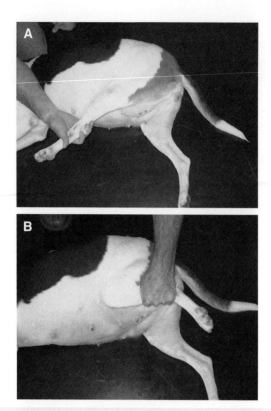

Fig. 13. Hip flexion is limited if the stifle is concurrently extended (*A*), but hip flexion increases if the stifle is simultaneously flexed (*B*).

unstable, the ROM exercise should be performed with the hands on either side of the joint but close to the joint. For example, in the stifle, one hand should be placed on the distal femur and one hand on the proximal tibia. By keeping the hands closer together, the forces acting on the stifle are minimized by keeping the lever arm short. If the repair is strong, the hands can be moved further apart, providing a longer lever arm and a stronger ROM force at the joint.

Sensory facilitation or inhibition may be used to alter muscle responses. For example, compression of a joint may stimulate the joint receptors and facilitate extensor muscle activity and stability around a joint. One method of increasing extensor muscle activity with joint compression is rhythmic stabilization. This activity may be accomplished by placing the dog in a standing position on a compressible surface, such as an air mattress or exercise ball. Weak dogs may be supported with a sling or hand to be certain that they do not collapse. While keeping the dog in a standing position, the dog is gently and rhythmically pushed down (Fig. 15). As the joints become compressed, the extensor

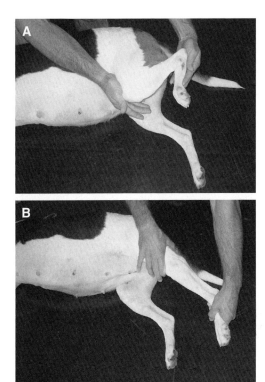

Fig. 14. Hock flexion is greater when the stifle is concurrently flexed (A) but is limited if the stifle is kept extended (B).

muscles responsible for maintaining posture are stimulated to prevent collapse. Conversely, traction separates joint surfaces and is useful if increased ROM is desired.

BIOMECHANICS OF THERAPEUTIC EXERCISES
Treadmill Walking

Walking on a ground treadmill is a commonly performed exercise for conditioning and to encourage limb use after surgery. One study determined that dogs have an increased stance time and greater stride length when walking on a ground treadmill as compared with walking over ground, but there were no differences in swing time [42]. Furthermore, maximum extension, flexion, and ROM angles are similar for the front and hind limb joints between the ground and treadmill walking (Table 1). Maximum joint flexion velocity tended to be lower in dogs walking on ground treadmills, perhaps because of the active assisted nature of walking on a treadmill. Therefore, if increased weight bearing on an affected limb is desired with similar joint angle excursions but less rapid joint motion, walking on a ground treadmill should be considered.

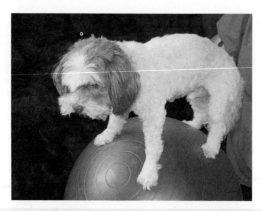

Fig. 15. Rhythmic stabilization may be accomplished by supporting the dog in a standing position on an exercise ball and gently pushing the dog down in a rhythmic fashion to stimulate the extensor muscles to contract so as to maintain body posture.

Walking on a treadmill with a 10% incline results in joint motion similar to walking on a level treadmill [43]. The mean maximum hip extension was 3° and maximum hip flexion was 4° greater with incline treadmill walking, and the mean maximum hock extension and flexion were 3° greater with incline treadmill walking.

Wheelbarrowing

Raising the rear limbs off the ground and walking the dog forward is a therapeutic exercise known as wheelbarrowing (Fig. 16). The main objective is to increase the use of the forelimbs and increase weight bearing on them. Several specific events occur during wheelbarrowing. The forelimb is a complex structure, with multiple joints continuously undergoing joint angular acceleration and deceleration, with the limb held at changing angles to the ground during the stance phase. During wheelbarrowing, the dog must move its forelimbs

Table 1
Joint motion during selected therapeutic exercises

Joint	Walking	Ground treadmill	10% incline ground treadmill	Wheelbarrowing	Dancing forward	Dancing backward
Shoulder	120[a]–148	121–146	—	131–162[b]	—	—
Elbow	94–144	93–146[b]	—	80[a]–130	—	—
Carpus	99[a]–192	100–194	—	112–198[b]	—	—
Hip	103[a]–136	107–138	103[a]–141	—	120–140	135–164[b]
Stifle	106–154	111–156[b]	109–153	—	110–155	88[a]–129
Hock	125–162	128–163	125–166[b]	—	134–163	115[a]–157

Values represent mean flexion and extension angles, respectively.
    For each joint, the minimum joint flexion[a] and maximum joint extension[b] are indicated.

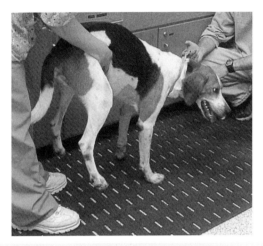

Fig. 16. Wheelbarrowing exercise is performed by supporting the rear limbs of the dog and walking forward on the forelimbs. (*From* Millis DL, Levine D, Taylor RA, editors. Canine rehabilitation and physical therapy. St. Louis (MO): WB Saunders; 2004. p. 257; with permission.)

to keep from falling; in doing so, the stride length changes as the dog attempts to keep its balance. In one study of hound type dogs, wheelbarrowing resulted in a significantly shorter stride length (0.66 versus 0.86 m), stance time (0.27 versus 0.37 second), and swing time (0.22 versus 0.27 second) as compared with walking at the same speed [44]. Dogs had a mean peak vertical force of 91% of body weight, which is intermediate between that expected of walking (approximately 50%) and that of trotting (approximately 100%–110%) (Table 2). Mean vertical impulse was 17% of body weight, which is similar to walking and trotting (approximately 20%). Although some of the dog's body weight is shifted to the forelimbs, the forces placed on the forelimbs are only intermediate between walking and trotting, likely because of the shorter stride length and stance time. In addition, some of the weight is also transferred to the handler.

Regarding joint kinematics, dogs that wheelbarrowed had significantly more shoulder extension (162° versus 148°), elbow flexion (80° versus 94°), and carpal extension (189° versus 182°) and less shoulder flexion (131° versus 120°),

Table 2
Kinetic characteristics of therapeutic exercises

	Walking forelimb	Walking hind limb	Trotting forelimb	Trotting hind limb	Wheelbarrowing	Dancing forward
Peak vertical force	54%	40%	111%	66%	91%	76%
Vertical impulse	21%	15.2%	20%	12%	17%	16%

Values are expressed as a percentage of body weight.

elbow extension (130° versus 144°), and carpal flexion (112° versus 99°) as compared with walking [44]. These differences are approximately 10° to 15°. Therefore, wheelbarrowing may be used to help increase motion in a particular joint, such as elbow flexion, to a greater degree than walking.

Dancing

Raising the forelimbs off the ground and walking the dog forward and backward is known as dancing (Fig. 17). The main goal is to increase weight bearing on the rear limbs. A comparison of peak vertical forces and vertical impulse of nine hound type dogs that danced forward and were trotted across a force plate indicated that dancing resulted in greater peak vertical forces than trotting (75.6% versus 65.4% body weight) and greater vertical impulse (16.1% versus 12%) [44].

Dancing forward may result in different kinematic characteristics compared with walking over ground and dancing backward. There was significantly less hip flexion (120° versus 103°), total hip ROM (20° versus 33°), hock flexion (134° versus 125°), and hock total ROM (28° versus 37°) with forward dancing compared with walking [44]. The stride length (0.56 versus 0.84 m, respectively) and swing time (0.18 versus 0.26 second, respectively) were shorter with forward dancing as compared with walking, but the stance times were

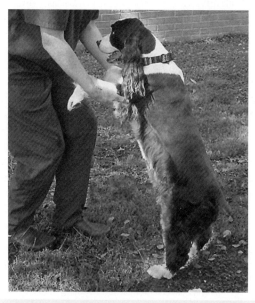

Fig. 17. Dancing exercise is performed by supporting the front limbs of the dog and moving the dog in a forward or backward direction. A muzzle is recommended if the dog is in pain or resists the exercise in any way. (*From* Millis DL, Levine D, Taylor RA, editors. Canine rehabilitation and physical therapy. St. Louis (MO): WB Saunders; 2004. p. 256; with permission.)

similar (0.32 second). Dancing backward also differed from walking over ground. Hip extension (164° versus 136°) and stifle flexion (88° versus 106°) were greater with backward dancing as compared with walking, whereas hip flexion (135° versus 103°), hip ROM (29° versus 33°), stifle extension (129° versus 154°), and stifle ROM (41° versus 47°) were less. This information may be useful in rehabilitating dogs with various conditions. For example, in the early phases of a therapeutic exercise program for a dog with hip dysplasia that is painful with hip extension, gluteal muscle strengthening may be more comfortable by dancing the dog forward rather than backward.

Aquatic Biomechanics and Exercises

One of the principle advantages of exercising in water is the buoyancy that the water exerts, resulting in less force on limbs. Buoyancy can be defined as the resultant force exerted by the water on a submerged or floating body equal to the weight of the water displaced by the body. It is an important force in aquatic therapy because animals in water are lifted upward so that the effect of gravity is partially canceled. Therefore, the need for antigravity muscle action is greatly reduced. The amount of unloading is related to the height of the water in relation to the height of the individual. One study evaluated the changes in body weight on ground compared with different water levels while standing [45]. Dogs standing in water to the level of the tarsus, stifle, and greater trochanter weighed 91%, 85%, and 38% of body weight, respectively, as compared with standing on dry ground, indicating that buoyancy can be a significant factor in reducing loads placed on limbs. This may be of particular advantage in animals with lower motor neuron conditions that have difficulty in supporting their weight or in patients with arthritic joints to help reduce the weight-bearing forces on painful joints.

Movement of a body through water is complex and involves forces generated by the individual and counterforces to the movement by the water [46]. Thrust refers to the forces in the direction of velocity of movement and may be thought of as the force that the body generates to push the water backward. This helps to accelerate the body and keep it moving forward.

Drag is a force that is opposite to the velocity of movement and opposes the motion between the body and the fluid:

$$\text{Drag Force} = (\text{Constant})(\text{Area})(\text{Drag Coefficient})(\text{Velocity})^2$$

The constant is determined by the density of water, and area is the cross-sectional area of the body in the direction of the motion. The drag coefficient is affected by the shape of the body and the surface of the body. Of particular importance is the velocity of the body, which is an exponential function. Therefore, if the velocity of the dog moving in water doubles, the amount of drag quadruples. The major resistance to moving through water is the turbulent drag, with formation of eddies and currents behind the body.

Another important source of drag exists at the surface of the water at the water-air interface. There is high surface tension of the water here, and movement just under the surface tends to create waves. The energy loss with this motion results in an increase in forces that resist movement close to the cube of the velocity rather than the square. Therefore, with movement just beneath the surface of the water, nearly eight times as much energy must be expended to double the velocity of the body.

One study determined stifle joint ROM and angular velocities during swimming and walking in healthy dogs and in dogs that had undergone surgical treatment of a ruptured cranial cruciate ligament [47]. For dogs in both groups, swimming resulted in significantly greater overall ROM of the stifle joint than did walking, primarily because of greater joint flexion. Dogs had significantly less stifle extension while swimming compared with walking, however. This study provides some clinical insights that may be useful in rehabilitation. For example, if a dog is recovering from cruciate repair and has lost stifle extension, walking on a land or underwater treadmill is likely to help regain stifle extension more effectively than swimming.

Two-dimensional kinematic analysis of gait has been used to evaluate joint motion in dogs walking on ground and underwater treadmills. In addition, the effect of different water levels on active joint ROM was evaluated when patients walk underwater [48]. Hip, stifle, hock, shoulder, and elbow flexion are greater in dogs walking in water compared with walking on land. Joint flexion is generally greatest with water levels at or higher than the joint of interest. Maximum joint extension is similar for underwater and ground treadmill walking. Maximum and minimum joint flexion and extension are related to the level of water; these effects are likely a result of the sudden action of a limb to break the surface tension of the water at different water heights.

SUMMARY

The biomechanics of motion and rehabilitation are complex, with many tissue types and structures involved. In addition, consideration must be given to the stage of tissue healing with some injuries, such as fractures. A more thorough knowledge of some of the infrequently discussed biomechanical aspects of musculoskeletal tissues and motion during rehabilitation, combined with well-known features of tissue recovery, should enhance the development of rehabilitation programs for patients.

References

[1] LeVeau B. Williams and Lissner. Biomechanics of human motion. 2nd edition. Philadelphia: WB Saunders; 1977. p. 70.

[2] Millis DL. Responses of musculoskeletal tissues to disuse and remobilization. In: Millis DL, Levine D, Taylor RA, editors. Canine rehabilitation and physical therapy. St. Louis (MO): WB Saunders; 2004. p. 113–59.

[3] Low J, Reed A. Basic biomechanics explained. Boston: Butterworth-Heinemann; 1996. p. 82–5.

[4] Rasch PJ, Burke RK. The body as a lever system. In: Kinesiology and applied anatomy. The science of human movement. 6th edition. Philadelphia: Lea & Febiger; 1978. p. 127–41.

[5] Meriam JL, Kraige LG. Kinetics of particles. In: Engineering mechanics, vol. 2. Dynamics. 2nd edition. New York: John Wiley and Sons; 1986. p. 109–232.

[6] Ozkaya N, Nordin M. Angular kinematics. In: Fundamentals of biomechanics equilibrium, motion, and deformation. 2nd edition. New York: Springer-Verlag; 1991. p. 275–94.

[7] Ozkaya N, Nordin M. Impulse and momentum. In: Fundamentals of biomechanics equilibrium, motion, and deformation. 2nd edition. New York: Springer-Verlag; 1991. p. 317–36.

[8] Ozkaya N, Nordin M. Linear kinematics. In: Fundamentals of biomechanics equilibrium, motion, and deformation. 2nd edition. New York: Springer-Verlag; 1991. p. 255–72.

[9] DeCamp CE. Kinetic and kinematic gait analysis and the assessment of lameness in the dog. Vet Clin North Am Small Anim Pract 1997;27(4):825–40.

[10] McLaughlin RM. Kinetic and kinematic gait analysis in dogs. Vet Clin North Am Small Anim Pract 2001;31(1):193–201.

[11] Riggs CM, DeCamp CE, Soutas-Little RW, et al. Effects of subject velocity on force plate-measured ground reaction forces in healthy greyhounds at the trot. Am J Vet Res 1993;54:1523–6.

[12] Renberg WC, Johnston SA, Ye K, et al. Comparison of stance time and velocity as control variables in force plate analysis of dogs. Am J Vet Res 1999;60:814–9.

[13] McLaughlin RM Jr, Roush JK. Effects of subject stance time and velocity on ground reaction forces in clinically normal Greyhounds at the trot. Am J Vet Res 1994;55:1666–71.

[14] Roush JK, McLaughlin RM Jr. Effects of subject stance time and velocity on ground reaction forces in clinically normal Greyhounds at the walk. Am J Vet Res 1994;55:1672–6.

[15] Budsberg SC, Verstraete MC, Soutas Little RW. Force plate analysis of the walking gait in healthy dogs. Am J Vet Res 1987;48:915–8.

[16] DeCamp CE, Soutas-Little RW, Hauptman J, et al. Kinematic gait analysis of the trot in healthy Greyhounds. Am J Vet Res 1993;54:627–34.

[17] Hottinger HA, DeCamp CE, Olivier NB, et al. Noninvasive kinematic analysis of the walk in healthy large-breed dogs. Am J Vet Res 1996;57:381–8.

[18] Hicks DA, Millis D, Arnold GA, et al. Comparison of weightbearing at a stance vs. trotting in dogs with rear limb lameness. In: Proceedings of the 32nd Annual Conference Veterinary Orthopedic Society. Okemos (MI): Veterinary Orthopedic Society; 2005. p.12.

[19] Romans CW, Conzemius MG, Horstman CL, et al. Use of pressure platform gait analysis in cats with and without bilateral onychectomy. Am J Vet Res 2004;65:1276–8.

[20] Jevens DJ, Hauptman JG, DeCamp CE, et al. Contributions to variance in force-plate analysis of gait in dogs. Am J Vet Res 1993;54:612–5.

[21] Allen K, DeCamp CE, Braden TD, et al. Kinematic gait analysis of the trot in healthy mixed breed dogs. Vet Comp Orthop Traumatol 1994;7:148–53.

[22] Rumph PF, Lander JE, Kincaid SA, et al. Ground reaction force profiles from force platform gait analyses of clinically normal mesomorphic dogs at the trot. Am J Vet Res 1994;55: 756–61.

[23] Budsberg SC, Verstraete MC, Brown J, et al. Vertical loading rates in clinically normal dogs at a trot. Am J Vet Res 1995;56:1275–80.

[24] McLaughlin R Jr, Roush JK. Effects of increasing velocity on braking and propulsion times during force plate gait analysis in Greyhounds. Am J Vet Res 1995;56:159–61.

[25] Bertram JEA, Lee DV, Todhunter RJ, et al. Multiple force platform analysis of the canine trot: a new approach to assessing basic characteristics of locomotion. Vet Comp Orthop Traumatol 1997;10:160–9.

[26] Schaefer SL, DeCamp CE, Hauptman JG, et al. Kinematic gait analysis of hind limb symmetry in dogs at the trot. Am J Vet Res 1998;59(6):680–5.

[27] Rumph PF, Steiss JE, West MS. Interday variation in vertical ground reaction force in clinically normal Greyhounds at the trot. Am J Vet Res 1999;60:679–83.

[28] Bertram JE, Lee DV, Case HN, et al. Comparison of the trotting gaits of Labrador Retrievers and Greyhounds. Am J Vet Res 2000;61:832–8.

[29] Poy NSJ, DeCamp CE, Bennett RL, et al. Additional kinematic variables to describe differences in the trot between clinically normal dogs and dogs with hip dysplasia. Am J Vet Res 2000;61(8):974–8.

[30] Arnold GA, Millis DL, Schwartz P, et al. Three dimensional kinematic motion analysis of the dog at a walk. In: Proceedings of the 32nd Annual Conference Veterinary Orthopedic Society. Okemos (MI): Veterinary Orthopedic Society; 2005. p. 47.

[31] Budsberg SC, Verstraete MC, Soutas-Little RW, et al. Force plate analyses before and after stabilization of canine stifles for cruciate injury. Am J Vet Res 1988;49(9):1522–4.

[32] Jevens DJ, DeCamp CE, Hauptman J, et al. Use of force-plate analysis of gait to compare two surgical techniques for treatment of cranial cruciate ligament rupture in dogs. Am J Vet Res 1996;57:389–93.

[33] DeCamp CE, Riggs CM, Olivier NB, et al. Kinematic evaluation of gait in dogs with cranial cruciate ligament rupture. Am J Vet Res 1996;57(1):120–6.

[34] Budsberg SC, Chambers JN, Van Lue SL, et al. Prospective evaluation of ground reaction forces in dogs undergoing unilateral total hip replacement. Am J Vet Res 1996;57(12):1781–5.

[35] McLaughlin RM, Miller CW, Taves CL, et al. Force plate analysis of triple pelvic osteotomy for the treatment of canine hip dysplasia. Vet Surg 1991;20(5):291–7.

[36] Bennett RL, DeCamp CE, Flo GL, et al. Kinematic gait analysis in dogs with hip dysplasia. Am J Vet Res 1996;57(7):966–71.

[37] Straface SF, Newbold PJ, Nade S. The effects of direction and velocity of movement, and intra-articular fluid volume and intra-articular pressure. Vet Comp Orthop Traumatol 1988;3:113–21.

[38] Pitman MI, Peterson L. Biomechanics of skeletal muscle. In: Nordin M, Frankel VH, editors. Basic biomechanics of the musculoskeletal system. 2nd edition. Philadelphia: Lea & Febiger; 1989. p. 89–111.

[39] Lieber RL, Bodine-Fowler SC. Skeletal muscle mechanics: implications for rehabilitation. Phys Ther 1993;73(12):844–56.

[40] Funatsu T, Higuchi H, Ishiwata S. Elastic filaments in skeletal muscle revealed by selective removal of thin filaments with plasma gelsolin. J Cell Biol 1990;110:53–62.

[41] Horowitz R, Podolsky RJ. The positional stability of thick filaments in activated skeletal muscle depends on sarcomere length: evidence for the role of titin filaments. J Cell Biol 1987;105:2217–23.

[42] Schwartz P, Millis D, Hicks DA, et al. A kinematic comparison of over ground vs. treadmill walking in dogs. In: Proceedings of the 31st Annual Conference Veterinary Orthopedic Society. Okemos (MI): Veterinary Orthopedic Society; 2004. p. 7.

[43] Gassel AG, Millis DL, Schwartz P, et al. Kinematic gait analysis of the pelvic limb; comparison of overground versus incline walking in 10 dogs. In: Proceedings of the 32nd Annual Conference Veterinary Orthopedic Society. Okemos (MI): Veterinary Orthopedic Society; 2005. p. 29.

[44] Millis DL, Schwartz P, Hicks DA, et al, Kinematic assessment of selected therapeutic exercises in dogs. In: Proceedings of the Third International Symposium on Physical Therapy and Rehabilitation in Veterinary Medicine. Raleigh (NC): North Carolina State College of Veterinary Medicine; 2004. p. 215.

[45] Tragauer V, Levine D, Millis DL. Percentage of normal weight bearing during partial immersion at various depths in dogs. In: Proceedings of the Second International Symposium on Physical Therapy and Rehabilitation in Veterinary Medicine. Knoxville (TN): University of Tennessee College of Veterinary Medicine; 2002. p. 189.

[46] Northrip JW, Logan GA, McKinney WC. Fluid mechanics. In: Introduction to biomechanic analysis of sport. 2nd edition. Dubuque (IA): Wm C Brown Company; 1979. p. 96–119.

[47] Marsolais GS, McLean S, Derrick T, et al. Kinematic analysis of the hind limb during swimming and walking in healthy dogs and dogs with surgically corrected cranial cruciate ligament rupture. J Am Vet Med Assoc 2003;222:739–43.

[48] Jackson AM, Stevens M, Barnett S. Joint kinematics during underwater treadmill activity. In: Proceedings of the Second International Symposium on Rehabilitation and Physical Therapy in Veterinary Medicine. Knoxville (TN): University of Tennessee College of Veterinary Medicine; 2002. p. 191.

Vet Clin Small Anim 35 (2005) 1287–1316

VETERINARY CLINICS
SMALL ANIMAL PRACTICE

Joint Mobilization

Deborah Gross Saunders, MSPT, CCRP[a],*,
J. Randy Walker, PT, PhD[b],
David Levine, PT, PhD, CCRP[b,c,d]

[a]Private practice, Middletown, CT, USA
[b]University of Tennessee at Chattanooga, Chattanooga, TN 37403–2598, USA
[c]Department of Small Animal Clinical Sciences, University of Tennessee College of Veterinary Medicine, 2407 River Drive, Knoxville, TN 37996, USA
[d]Department of Clinical Sciences, North Carolina State University College of Veterinary Medicine, 4700 Hillsborough Street, Raleigh, NC 27606, USA

Therapeutic touch has been used in human beings to soothe aches and pains. Most dogs also seem to enjoy being touched. Manual therapy techniques are skilled hand movements intended to improve tissue extensibility; increase range of motion (ROM); induce relaxation; mobilize or manipulate soft tissue and joints; modulate pain; and reduce soft tissue swelling, inflammation, or restriction [1]. The primary techniques included in manual therapy are mobilization and manipulation of joints and associated soft tissues. Mobilizations are passive movements that are oscillatory or sustained stretch performed in such a manner that the patient can prevent the motion if so desired. These motions are performed anywhere within the available ROM. The intent of this article is to provide an overview of the principles of manual therapy, followed by selected treatment techniques for the hip, stifle, elbow, shoulder, carpus, and thoracic and lumbar spine. The techniques of G.D. Maitland [2,3], an Australian physical therapist who developed a clinically based approach in the 1960s and 1970s, are emphasized. Maitland described four grades (I–IV) of mobilization (Fig. 1) and manipulation. Manipulation, a grade V mobilization, is a sudden passive movement that cannot be prevented by the patient and is typically performed near the end of available ROM.

There have been numerous randomized controlled trials (RCTs) in human beings that have demonstrated the efficacy of manual therapy for treating patients with a variety of disorders in the spine and peripheral joints. Many of these studies have compared "traditional treatments," such as exercise, pharmaceutic interventions, rest, and placebo, with manual therapy. Other RCTs

*Corresponding author. PO Box 287, Colchester, CT 06415, USA. E-mail address: wizofpaws@aol.com (D. Gross Saunders).

0195-5616/05/$ – see front matter
doi:10.1016/j.cvsm.2005.07.003

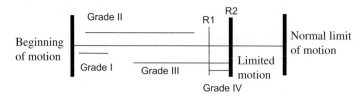

Fig. 1. Graphic description of grades of joint mobilization. R represents resistance. R1 represents the point in passive ROM at which the therapist senses resistance from a stretch on the noncontractile structures of a joint. R2 represents resistance felt at the end of available passive ROM.

have compared these traditional forms of therapy with groups receiving the traditional therapies plus manual therapy. Most of these studies have found that manual therapy is as effective as if not superior to traditional therapies [4–15]. Common outcome measures assessed have been pain, functional scales, disability levels, ROM, number of treatments needed, length of time in treatment, and cost-effectiveness of treatment. Despite the growing body of evidence for manual therapy, it is viewed as a complementary therapy in human medicine by many, even though its effectiveness seems well substantiated and the risks are low. The most likely reason for its slow acceptance is that the skill level required to apply these techniques properly is higher than with traditional therapies, such as exercise or modalities. Rationales for the reasons why manual therapies may work have been investigated and include reducing muscle inhibition [16], correcting joint displacement, adjusting joint subluxations, restoring bony alignment, reducing nuclear protrusion [17,18], and placebo effect [8]. More recent theories include evidence supporting the need for adequate stresses and normal movement as being critical to maintain the integrity of collagenous tissues, muscles, and bones [19]. Evidence of the effectiveness of manual therapy must be established in small animals. Although many anatomic similarities exist between human beings and small animals, we cannot assume that the techniques yield the same results.

INDICATIONS FOR MANUAL THERAPY
Manual therapy is indicated for pain and loss of motion that occurs secondary to neuromusculoskeletal dysfunction. The patient may have pain with motion or rest, pain in the midst of available ROM or at the end of available ROM, or pain or stiffness caused by postural changes. Specific examples include dogs with limited motion secondary to canine hip dysplasia, elbow dysplasia, intervertebral disk disease, and osteoarthritis. Manual therapy differs from stretching in that when a stretch is applied, a low load is placed on the tissues for a specified amount of time (usually 10–30 seconds) to help elongate them. In manual therapy, the force is applied in an oscillatory manner rather than in a sustained manner.

CONTRAINDICATIONS AND PRECAUTIONS FOR MANUAL THERAPY

The list of contraindications presented by Dutton [20] includes spinal instability, bacterial infection, malignancy, systemic localized infections, sutures over the area, recent fracture, cellulitis, febrile state, hematoma, acute circulatory condition, an open wound at the treatment site, osteomyelitis, advanced diabetes, hypersensitivity of the skin, inappropriate end feel (ie, spasm, empty, bony), constant severe pain, extensive radiation of pain, pain unrelieved by rest, any undiagnosed lesion, and severe irritability (pain that is easily provoked and does not go away within a few hours). Additional contraindications that are specific to dogs include contractures, such as fibrotic myopathy and quadriceps contracture, or other circumstances in which manual therapy is unlikely to effect any change and may be painful. An overly aggressive or fearful dog that may bite the therapist or a dog that does not relax to allow passive movement is also a contraindication. Total elbow replacements should be considered a contraindication for grades III through V accessory mobilizations until this procedure is further evaluated.

Precautions (proceed with caution) identified by Dutton [20] include joint effusion or inflammation, rheumatoid arthritis, presence of neurologic signs, osteoporosis, hypermobility, pregnancy (if the technique is to be applied to the spine), dizziness, and steroid or anticoagulation therapy.

BASIC PRINCIPLES OF MANUAL THERAPY

There a number of approaches to manual therapy, including those developed by physicians [21–23] and by physical therapists [2,3,24–26]. Regardless of the approach, there are several principles that should be considered as the patient is being examined and treated. Maitland [2] stresses the importance of communicating with the patient to "understand what the patient is enduring." Of course, in this case, the examiner must communicate with two constituents the dog and the owner.

Physiologic and Accessory Motion

Physiologic motion is the normal active motion that is available at any synovial joint. Another way to describe physiologic motion is the motion that occurs in the cardinal planes. Examples include flexion, abduction, and internal rotation. Accessory motions are movements that cannot be performed actively but can be performed passively. Examples are distraction, glides, spins, and rotations of a joint. Accessory motions must be present for full physiologic motion to be present.

Concave and Convex Relation of Joints

All synovial joints have a convex-concave relation. When the examiner is passively moving a joint, caution should be made to move the joint in a manner similar to how it moves when the joint is being actively moved by the dog. Osteokinematics is defined by how the bone is being moved through space (ie, flexion, abduction). Arthokinematics is defined by how the joint surfaces are moving as the bone is being moved (ie, rolling, sliding, spinning). When the joint surface is convex with respect to the other side of the joint, the articular surface moves in the opposite direction of the shaft of the bone. When the shoulder joint is being flexed (as in the swing phase of gait) by moving the humerus on the scapula, the convex surface of the proximal humerus is sliding and spinning on the concave glenoid of the scapula. When the joint surface is concave, the articular surface moves in the same direction of the shaft of the bone. When the distal radius is being moved on the stationary carpals (as in the stance portion of gait), the concave surface of the radius is rolling and sliding on the convex proximal row of carpal bones. Manual therapists strive to move joint surfaces physiologically to avoid injuries, such as joint subluxations and sprains.

Relation of Pain and Range of Motion

"During examination and assessment, pain should never be considered without relation to range nor range without relation to pain" [2]. Depending on the nature of the injury or disease, joints are affected by the presence of pain and stiffness. If pain is the primary problem, it may limit motion, as in hip dysplasia. When the pain diminishes, the ROM improves. If the primary problem is joint dysfunction or stiffness, pain is most evident at or near the end of available ROM. As the available ROM increases, pain becomes less of a factor. In those cases in which pain and loss of motion occur simultaneously, the examiner must decide which is the primary problem. These relations are the basis of deciding which grade of passive movement and other therapies should be used to treat the problem.

If pain occurs before resistance is felt by the examiner, the primary problem is pain; if the pain occurs when resistance is felt, the primary problem is limitation of motion with joint involvement. In addition, if active and passive motion is limited or painful in the same direction, the lesion is in the noncontractile tissues. For example, if the cranial joint capsule of the stifle is tight, flexion of the stifle is limited with active and passive flexion of the joint. Conversely, if active and passive motion is limited or painful in opposite directions, the lesion is in the contractile tissues   muscle and associated tendon. For example, if the biceps tendon is affected, active flexion of the elbow and passive extension of the elbow are painful, with a possible reduction in ROM. These presentations affect which grade and type of mobilization should be used to treat the problem.

The dog exhibits a capsular pattern if the entire capsule of the joint is inflamed or involved. Cyriax [21] described a capsular pattern as a joint-specific pattern of loss of motion with arthritis. This has not been described for dogs, but we know that limitations in movement accompany certain disorders. An example is that hip extension is typically the most limited motion in a dog with hip dysplasia.

End feel is the sensation imparted to the examiner when the end of passive ROM is encountered. The passive motion must be performed with a relatively quick movement, and the end of range is bumped briskly. Cyriax [21] described the quality of normal and abnormal end feels, which are defined in Table 1.

Assessment

The therapist participates in three activities while managing a patient problem: examination, treatment, and assessment. Although each is important to the provision of a complete and quality program, assessment is the keystone. Assessment involves "open-mindedness, mental agility and mental discipline, linked with a logical and methodical process of assessing cause and effect" [2]. The therapist is thinking and evaluating to make certain that the right task is being performed and that the task is being performed correctly. The therapist must continually assess the decision-making process during examination and treatment procedures. Assessment is implemented at three points of the patient interaction. The first assessment is implemented during the initial examination of the patient, making certain that all appropriate procedures are performed as signs are compared to reach the best diagnosis and formulate an appropriate plan of care. The second assessment occurs during the treatment session. The therapist assesses the appropriateness of the treatment techniques while the patient response is evaluated. The third assessment is an analytic process to consider the entire treatment program to determine whether the patient is progressing as a result of the treatment and to determine the prognosis for resolution of the current episode.

Table 1 End feels		
Name	Description	Example
Bony or hard	Bone approximates bone, resulting in an abrupt hard stop. Abnormal if occurs in joints other than stifle or elbow extension.	Bony overgrowth after a distal radial fracture
Soft tissue approximation	Motion is stopped by compression of soft tissues. Abnormal if occurs too early in the range because of edema.	Normal stifle flexion
Capsular or firm	A firm but slightly yielding stop, occurs because of tension in joint capsule or ligaments. Abnormal if occurs too early in the ROM.	Normal carpal extension
Springy block	A rebound is felt at the limit of motion; motion stops and then rebounds. Abnormal, may indicate joint effusion or a joint mouse.	Always abnormal
Empty	No end point is felt because the patient stops the motion because of pain; no resistance felt. Abnormal, indicates presence of sharp pain.	Always abnormal

CLINICAL ENVIRONMENT

What follows are concepts to make the clinical setting safe for the patient and the therapist so that the desired outcome of the examination and treatment session is more likely to be achieved. First, a quiet area that is free of distractions for the dog facilitates relaxation and cooperation. The area should also be safe for the dog and therapist. It may be necessary to muzzle the dog initially, especially with a fearful or apprehensive dog. Second, the therapist should make certain that he or she is using proper body mechanics to prevent undue stress on the spine and joints of the dog and the therapist. Third, approach the dog from a position where the dog can see you, and touch the dog with firm but not aggressive hands. Touch the dog at a place that is not painful and gradually move toward the involved area. Finally, the affected part should be cradled or held with a firm but gentle grip to encourage relaxation and trust by the dog.

Evaluation

The basic components of the initial examination for musculoskeletal dysfunction are observation, history of the present episode and relevant past history, active and passive ROM, functional tasks, strength assessment, and palpation. After the interview and examination are complete, all data should be evaluated to determine a diagnosis and a plan of care. The primary problem should be assessed to determine if it is primarily a painful (acute) or stiffness problem. Only after these decisions are made should joint mobilizations be considered as a part of the plan of care.

Treatment with Mobilization

The effectiveness of the manual therapy treatment program is affected by the environment and the skills of the therapist. Efforts must be made to facilitate relaxation of the dog to avoid excessive pain and stress to the animal. The therapist's grip should be firm enough to support the limb but not excessive. Good body mechanics and positioning by the therapist help to make the movements controlled and in the desired pattern.

Grades

Joint mobilization should be planned with a specific grade of mobilization in mind. Grades are assigned to the mobilizations depending on the range through which the mobilization is applied and the point in the range at which it is applied. A schematic is presented to describe a modification of Maitland's graded mobilization [2].

Grade I. Grade I mobilizations are small-amplitude movements that are performed with three to four oscillations per second. There should be no pain during the oscillations. The therapist should be working in the range opposite of the pain and avoid end range (R2). For example, if pain occurs during extension, do a grade I flexion.

Grade II. Grade II mobilizations are large-amplitude movements that are performed three to four oscillations per second. A grade II mobilization should not cause pain during the oscillations. The therapist should be in the range opposite of the pain and avoid either end range (R2).

Grade III. Grade III mobilizations are large-amplitude movements performed three to four oscillations per second at the end of range of the restricted motion (bump R2). This amplitude of motion may cause slight discomfort to the patient.

Grade IV. A grade IV mobilization is a small-amplitude movement that is performed three to four oscillations per second between R1 and R2. This amplitude of motion may cause slight discomfort for the patient.

How to choose the appropriate mobilization grade
When ROM is decreased because of pain:

- If the pain is treated, ROM increases.
- Grade I and II mobilizations should be performed.
- Grade I and II mobilizations should be performed in the pain-free range for 30 seconds. Function should be assessed after mobilization to determine whether any change has been achieved.

When ROM is decreased because of stiffness:

- Grade III and IV mobilizations should be used.
- Grade III and IV mobilizations should be performed in the direction of the stiffness for 60 seconds if possible. Function should be assessed after mobilization to determine whether any change has been achieved.

If pain and stiffness are present, the therapist must decide what the primary problem is. Does the pain limit ROM, or does the stiffness cause the pain? The sequence of pain and resistance can contribute to the treatment plan. For example:

- If pain occurs before resistance, use techniques to control the pain before progressing to more aggressive treatment.
- If pain occurs with resistance, mobilizations may be used with caution. It is customary to treat the pain and then the stiffness, however.
- If pain occurs after the resistance, vigorous mobilization may be used to treat the stiffness, followed by techniques for pain.

There are two types of mobilizations:

- Physiologic: mobilizations done in the same pattern of movement that is produced by voluntary muscle contraction.
- Accessory: mobilizations performed in a pattern of movement that must be done passively and cannot be produced by voluntary muscle contraction. These should be done in the midrange of the joint (open pack position), because this allows for more joint play or motion.

There are guidelines to help the therapist decide which type of mobilization to perform.

- If treating pain and physiologic mobilization grades I and II cause pain, accessory grades I and II should be performed.
- If 50% of physiologic active ROM is not available secondary to pain, use accessory grades I and II to treat the pain (50/50 rule).
- If treating stiffness (grades III and IV), the therapist should perform 60 seconds of an accessory mobilization, followed by 60 seconds of a physiologic mobilization and then assess the effect. During any mobilization treatment, an assessment should be made after each set of oscillations, whether for pain or stiffness, to determine the effect of the mobilization. This sequence should be performed three times.

Oscillation versus sustained stretch

Mobilization for joint restrictions should be oscillations. Mobilization for muscle, tendon, and skin restrictions should be sustained. Repetitive low-intensity stretches are beneficial to stimulate tissue elongation. Contracted tissues respond positively to sustained stretch [27].

Open versus closed kinetic chain

Dutton [20] defines open kinetic chain activities as when the "involved end segment of an extremity [is] moving freely through space, resulting in isolated movement of a joint." Examples of an open kinetic chain activity in a dog include when a paw is swinging forward in the gait cycle or when the dog is moving a forelimb while in lateral recumbency. Conversely, closed kinetic chain activity occurs when the distal segment of an extremity is in contact with a surface and the limb is weight bearing [28]. Examples of a closed kinetic chain activity include the stance phase of gait. It is of value to note whether a limb is being exercised in the open versus closed kinetic chain. Closed kinetic chain activities facilitate proprioception, muscles working in groups, and coordination of joint function. Conversely, it is easier to achieve isolated joint motion in the open kinetic chain.

Dogs perform a large array of movements to maintain function. The restoration of normal movement plays a significant role in the treatment of the dog. Joint mobilization offers one method of obtaining the motion required for the restoration of function through manual therapy skills.

Before beginning mobilization on the dog, it is essential that the therapist be completely familiar with the bony landmarks associated with the joint. The joints should be visible and easily palpated. The joint should be evaluated to be certain that pathologic joint luxation or subluxation is not present. Hair may need to be pulled out of the way or clipped to expose the joint. Active and passive ROM should be assessed and measured through function and goniometry before beginning the treatment. The assessment of passive and active ROM is an important aspect of the treatment process. The comparison of ROM before and after treatment demonstrates the effectiveness of the treatment.

Management of a dog's joint depends largely on the nature of the problem, particularly pain or stiffness. If the primary problem is pain, a relaxation technique, such as light massage, may be used to calm the dog and to gain trust. If the animal is not in pain but has lost ROM (has stiffness), the joint or joints to be mobilized should be prepared for treatment with a warming modality or light exercise. Moist heat, massage, or therapeutic ultrasound may be used before treatment. Active exercise, including aquatic therapy, may also be used. The joint mobilization treatment should then be followed with passive and active ROM accentuating the motion addressed. Therapeutic exercises prescribed should also address the motion. Ice may then be applied after the session to help prevent soreness from the mobilization and other activities.

Forelimb injuries are common in dogs. Elbow dysplasia and resultant osteoarthritis of the elbow occur quite frequently in dogs. In agility and jumping events, problems in the shoulder, elbow, and carpus are common secondary to the stresses placed on the forelimbs. Functional ROM at the carpus and elbow is essential to perform activities. For example, full elbow extension is required during normal ambulation. ROM demands in working and athletic dogs are greater than in pet dogs. For example, full shoulder extension is required for dogs participating in agility activities, such as jumping.

The hind limb is responsible for generating propulsion in the dog's body. Decreased ROM may result in a loss of power and function. The hind limb consists of the hip, stifle, and hock. Decreased joint motion in the hind limb is common with hip dysplasia, cruciate disease, muscle injuries, and osteoarthritis.

SHOULDER JOINT

The shoulder, or glenohumeral joint, is a ball and socket joint and follows the convex on concave rule of motion. The oval head of the humerus is twice the size of the glenoid cavity of the scapula [29]. Impairment in shoulder ROM may be seen after a fracture to the humerus, bicipital tenosynovitis, osteochondritis dissecans, infraspinatus contracture, scapular fracture, or other conditions. Compensations in the shoulder complex may also be seen as a result of hind limb or spinal problems, such as intervertebral disk disease, canine hip dysplasia, cruciate disease, or neurologic problems. It is believed that dogs increase the amount of weight placed on their forelimbs to compensate for a problem affecting their spine or hind limb. Over time, problems may develop in the forelimbs secondary to the increased weight placed on the joint. A brief overview of the mechanics of the shoulder joint is provided in Box 1.

Lateral Distraction of the Glenohumeral Joint

For lateral distraction of the glenohumeral joint (Fig. 2), the dog should be positioned in lateral recumbency with the shoulder to be treated facing the therapist. The therapist should be positioned ventral to the dog's shoulder, facing the shoulder to be mobilized.

The stabilizing hand is placed on the proximal scapula near the acromion. The web space, or the area of the hand between the thumb and index finger, of the mobilizing hand is placed under the axilla as close to the proximal humerus as possible.

> **Box 1: Brief overview of the mechanics of the shoulder joint**
>
> - As the glenohumeral joint extends, the humeral head moves in a caudal direction. Therefore, to increase extension, a caudal glide or mobilizing force should be applied.
> - As the glenohumeral joint flexes, the humeral head moves in a cranial direction. Therefore, to increase flexion, a cranial glide or mobilizing force should be applied.
> - As the glenohumeral joint abducts, the humeral head moves in a medial and ventral direction. Therefore, to increase abduction, a medial and ventral glide or mobilizing force should be applied.
> - As the glenohumeral joint adducts, the humeral head moves in a lateral and dorsal direction. Therefore, to increase adduction, a lateral and dorsal glide or mobilizing force should be applied.

Lateral distraction is applied with the mobilizing hand, while the stabilizing hand maintains the position of the scapula. The distraction is held for up to 5 seconds and then released. This may be repeated up to 10 times. This is a sustained mobilization. The objective is to stretch the capsule, relax the surrounding tissues, and prepare the joint for additional mobilizations.

This technique can be performed as a grade II mobilization to diminish pain in the shoulder joint. The mobilizing hand should be oscillated at a rate of two to three repetitions per second. The head of the humerus should be moved laterally only a minimal amount, making certain that no joint resistance is felt by the therapist and no pain is experienced by the dog. The oscillations are maintained for approximately 30 seconds; at that time, the dog should be assessed to determine whether there has been any change in function. The technique may be repeated up to three times if the dog's pain improves.

In addition to a lateral distraction, a grade III oscillation can be performed to improve a joint restriction. In this case, pain is not a major factor and should

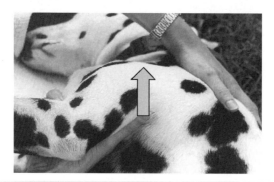

Fig. 2. Lateral distraction of the glenohumeral joint. Arrow indicates direction of mobilization.

only be present when the joint is moved to the point of limitation. To perform a grade III mobilization, the head of the humerus is oscillated to the point of end feel of the capsule, where the bone cannot be moved any further and the therapist feels a distinct stop in the available motion. These oscillations are maintained for up to 60 seconds, assuming the dog remains relaxed and allows this motion to occur. This mobilization can be followed with a physiologic motion to improve shoulder flexion, extension, or rotation. For example, the dog's shoulder should be passively moved through physiologic, or the normal range, of flexion. This may be followed with a movement of physiologic extension and then internal and external rotation.

Caudal Mobilization: Accessory Glide

For an accessory glide for caudal mobilization (Fig. 3), the dog should be positioned in lateral recumbency with the shoulder to be mobilized facing toward the therapist. The therapist should be positioned cranioventral to the dog's shoulder, facing the shoulder.

The stabilizing hand is placed over the scapula; the dog's arm may rest on the forearm of the stabilizing hand. The thenar eminence or the web space of the mobilizing hand is placed over the greater tubercle of the humerus.

A gentle lateral distraction should be performed before the caudal glide to facilitate movement. A caudal glide is applied to move the humerus in relation to the scapula. This glide should be sustained for 3 to 5 seconds. The objective is to increase shoulder extension.

A grade III accessory mobilization may be performed from the same grips by adding an oscillation of the mobilizing hand. The caudal oscillations are performed with the joint held in the loose packed position, and the oscillations should bump against the end of the available joint motion. The oscillations are performed at a rate of three to four repetitions per second and are continued for up to 60 seconds. The caudal glide is typically followed with a grade III

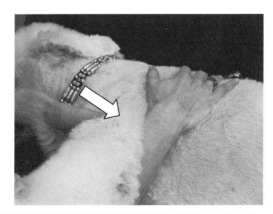

Fig. 3. Caudal mobilization of the humerus to increase shoulder extension. Arrow indicates direction of mobilization.

physiologic shoulder extension mobilization, oscillating for an additional 60 seconds.

To perform a grade III physiologic shoulder extension mobilization, the mobilizing hand and the stabilizing hand should exchange positions so that the therapist's mobilizing hand pushes the humerus rostrally into shoulder extension while the stabilizing hand is holding the scapula stable. The mobilizing hand should be gripped about the midshaft of the humerus.

With the scapula stabilized, the humerus is pushed into extension to the end of available ROM, bumping end feel of the joint. The humerus is moved back to near midposition of the joint. An oscillatory movement is performed by moving the humerus to end feel and back to midposition at a rate of three to four repetitions per second. The end feel should be sensed by the therapist with each oscillation. The mobilization is performed for up to 60 seconds.

The dog's shoulder extension should be assessed for improvement in ROM. If motion is improved, the grade III accessory mobilization and the grade III physiologic mobilization can be repeated up to three times in one treatment session.

Cranial Mobilization: Accessory Glide

For an accessory glide for cranial mobilization (Fig. 4), the dog should be positioned in lateral recumbency with the shoulder to be mobilized facing toward the therapist. The therapist should be positioned on the ventral side of the dog, caudal to the forelimb.

The stabilizing hand is placed over the scapula; the dog's forelimb may rest on the forearm of the stabilizing hand. The thenar eminence or web space of the mobilizing hand is placed on the caudal portion of the humerus as close to the joint as possible.

A cranial glide is applied to the humerus. The objective is to increase shoulder flexion.

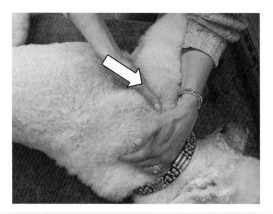

Fig. 4. Cranial mobilization of the humerus to increase shoulder extension. Arrow indicates direction of mobilization.

Further mobilizations for flexion include mobilizing the shoulder with an accessory cranial glide with a grade III or IV technique, followed by a physiologic mobilization to move the shoulder into the available shoulder flexion ROM.

Other motions about the shoulder joint in the dog, including rotation, abduction, and circumduction, are important, but less crucial to the overall function of the dog. Physiologic and accessory mobilizations to improve these motions can be performed but are not included in this article because of space limitations.

ELBOW JOINT

The elbow is a joint that is frequently problematic, with stiffness and pain secondary to degenerative joint disease. It is complex and consists of three joints: the humeroradial joint, the humeroulnar joint, and the radioulnar joint [29]. Clinically, stiffness in the elbow seems to respond well to a longitudinal distraction of the elbow joint. Pain and stiffness of the elbow may respond well to physiologic flexion and extension mobilizations. Full ROM of the elbow joint is necessary for proper function of the forelimb. Full elbow extension is necessary in the dog's normal gait cycle, and a significant amount of flexion is necessary to engage in functional activities, such as stair climbing and jumping [30,31].

The proximal portion of the radius is positioned laterally at the elbow, and the distal portion of the radius is positioned medially at the carpus. The articulation between the radius and ulna allows approximately 45° of rotational movement of the antebrachium. The articulation between the humerus and ulna provides the hinge motion responsible for elbow flexion and extension. The proximal ulna is positioned medially at the elbow. The trochlear notch is a deep half moon–shaped concavity that faces cranially and articulates with the convex trochlea of the humerus. Therefore, in an open kinetic chain, the concave ulna moves on the convex humerus.

Humeroulnar Longitudinal Distraction

For a humeroulnar longitudinal distraction (Fig. 5), the dog is positioned in lateral recumbency or in a sitting position with the elbow flexed to 90° and the radioulnar joint in slight supination. Approximately 45° of flexion allows the anconeal process to move more freely in relation to the humerus. The therapist is positioned on the ventral side of the dog, facing the elbow to be mobilized.

The stabilizing hand is located over the distal humerus. The mobilizing hand cradles the dog's forearm to maintain flexion and slight supination while grasping the proximal radius and ulna.

A longitudinal distraction is applied and maintained. In addition, the elbow may be moved into flexion as the distraction occurs. The objective is to decrease joint stiffness for elbow flexion or extension.

To perform a grade III physiologic elbow flexion mobilization, the therapist's mobilizing hand pulls the ulna ventrally and cranially with a scooping motion into elbow flexion while the stabilizing hand holds the distal humerus. With the humerus stabilized, the ulna is flexed to the end of available ROM, bumping

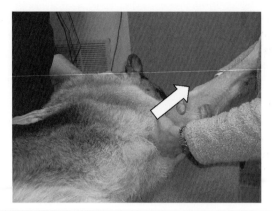

Fig. 5. Humeroulnar distraction for the elbow. Arrow indicates direction of mobilization.

end feel of the joint. The ulna is moved back to near midposition of the joint. An oscillatory movement is performed by moving the ulna to end feel and back to midposition at a rate of three to four repetitions per second. End feel should be sensed by the therapist with each oscillation. The mobilization is performed for up to 60 seconds.

The objective is to increase elbow flexion.

Elbow range of motion should be reassessed after the mobilization. If there is an improvement, three additional sets of the mobilization may be performed in a treatment session.

Physiologic Extension

For a physiologic extension, the dog should be positioned in lateral recumbency, although the mobilization may be performed while the dog is in a sitting position as well. The therapist is positioned ventrally, facing the cranial aspect of the elbow to be mobilized.

The stabilizing hand is wrapped around the distal portion of the humerus, placing the thenar and hypothenar eminences on the caudal aspect of the humerus and taking care to avoid the olecranon. The index and third fingers and the thumb of the mobilizing hand gently grasp the proximal radius and ulna.

To perform a grade III physiologic elbow extension mobilization, the therapist's mobilizing hand pushes the radius and ulna caudally into elbow extension while the stabilizing hand holds the distal humerus. With the humerus stabilized, the radius and ulna are pushed into extension to the end of available ROM, bumping end feel of the joint. The radius and ulna are moved back to near midposition of the joint. An oscillatory movement is performed by moving the radius and ulna to end feel and back to midposition at a rate of three to four repetitions per second. End feel should be sensed by the therapist with each oscillation. The mobilization is performed for up to 60 seconds. The objective is to increase elbow extension.

Elbow ROM should be reassessed after the mobilization. If there is an improvement, three additional sets of the mobilization may be performed in a treatment session.

Physiologic Flexion

For physiologic flexion, the dog should be positioned in lateral recumbency, although the mobilization may be performed while the dog is in a sitting position. The therapist should be positioned ventral to the elbow and facing the cranial aspect of the elbow to be mobilized.

The stabilizing hand is placed on the cranial aspect of the distal humerus. The web space of the mobilizing hand is placed over the proximal radius and ulna.

CARPUS

Despite its intricacy, the carpus functions primarily as a hinge joint, permitting flexion and extension [29]. The main movement occurs at the antebrachiocarpal joint, which consists of the distal radius and ulna, and at the radial and ulnar carpal bones. The distal radius and ulna offer a concave surface for the convex radial and ulnar carpal bones to move within. An overview of the kinematics of the antebrachiocarpal joint is provided in Box 2.

Caudal Glide of the Antebrachiocarpal Joint: Accessory Glide

For an accessory caudal glide of the antebrachiocarpal joint (Fig. 6), the dog should be positioned in lateral recumbency or in a sitting or sternal position. The therapist should be positioned ventrally, facing the carpus to be mobilized.

The stabilizing hand is placed over the caudal surface of the distal radius and ulna, just proximal to the joint. The mobilizing hand is placed on the dorsal portion of the radial and ulnar carpal bones.

A caudal mobilization is applied by directing the radial and ulnar carpal bones in a palmar direction while stabilizing the distal radius and ulna. This

---

Box 2: Overview of kinematics of the antebrachiocarpal joint

- As the antebrachiocarpal joint extends in an open kinetic chain, the convex articular surface of the radial and ulnar carpal bones moves in a caudal direction on the concave articular surface of the distal radius and ulna. Therefore, to increase carpal extension, a caudal glide of the radial and ulnar carpal bones on the distal radius and ulna should be applied.

- As the joint extends in a closed kinetic chain, the concave surface of the radius and ulna moves in a cranial direction on the proximal row of carpals.

- As the antebrachiocarpal joint flexes in an open kinetic chain, the convex articular surface of the radial and ulnar carpal bones moves in a cranial direction on the concave articular surface of the distal radius and ulna. Therefore, to increase carpal flexion, a cranial glide should be applied.

- As the joint flexes in a closed kinetic chain, the concave radius and ulna move in a caudal direction on the convex surface of the proximal row of carpals.

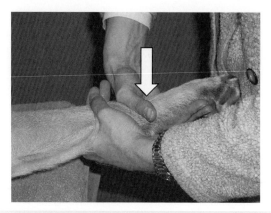

Fig. 6. Caudal accessory glide of the antebrachiocarpal joint. Arrow indicates direction of mobilization.

glide should be held for 3 to 5 seconds. The objective is to increase carpal extension.

A grade III accessory mobilization may be performed with the same hand position by adding an oscillation with the mobilizing hand. The caudal glide mobilizations are performed with the carpus held in a loose packed position or slight flexion, and the oscillations should bump against the end of the available motion. The oscillations are performed at a rate of three to four repetitions per second and are continued for up to 60 seconds. The accessory glide is typically followed by a grade III physiologic carpal extension glide for up to 60 seconds.

To perform a grade III physiologic carpal extension glide, the mobilizing hand is placed over the palmar portion of the radial and ulnar carpal bones and the stabilizing hand is placed on the cranial surface of the distal radius. The mobilizing hand pushes the distal radial and ulnar carpal bones dorsally into carpal extension. The distal radius and ulna are stabilized while the mobilizing hand moves the distal radial and ulnar carpal bones to the end of the available ROM and then back to the midposition of the joint. This oscillation between the available end range and the midrange should be performed at a rate of three to four oscillations per second for up to 60 seconds.

As always, the ROM should be assessed for an improvement. Further mobilizations may be repeated up to three times in one treatment session. Functional activities may then be prescribed for the dog to assist in maintaining the improved ROM, such as walking and stepping over obstacles to encourage carpal extension while in a weight-bearing position.

Cranial Glide of the Antebrachiocarpal Joint
For a cranial glide of the antebrachiocarpal joint (Fig. 7), the dog should be positioned in lateral recumbency or in a sitting or sternal position. The therapist should be positioned ventrally, facing the carpus to be mobilized.

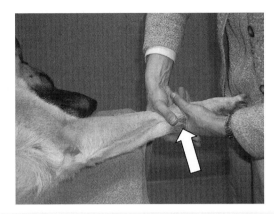

Fig. 7. Cranial antebrachiocarpal glide. Arrow indicates direction of mobilization.

The stabilizing hand is placed over the distal radius and ulna. The mobilizing hand is placed on the palmar portion of the radial and ulnar carpal bones, just distal to the accessory carpal pad.

A cranial mobilization is applied by directing the radial and carpal bones dorsally while stabilizing the distal radius and ulna. The objective is to increase carpal flexion.

A grade III accessory mobilization may be performed using the same hand positions by adding an oscillation of the mobilizing hand. The cranial glide mobilizations are performed with the joint held in a slight amount of flexion or the loose packed position. The oscillations should bump against of the available motion. The oscillations are performed at a rate of three to four repetitions per second and are continued for up to 60 seconds. The cranial glide is then typically followed with a grade III physiologic carpal flexion mobilization for an additional 60 seconds.

To perform a physiologic carpal flexion mobilization, the mobilizing hand is placed on the dorsal aspect of the radial and ulnar carpal bones and the stabilizing hand is placed on the palmar surface of the distal radius and ulna. With the distal radius and ulna stabilized, the mobilizing hand moves the radial and ulna carpal bones in a palmar direction into flexion. The radial and ulnar carpal bones are moved from the end feel of the joint back to the midposition of the joint at a rate of three to four repetitions per second for up to 60 seconds.

Carpal flexion should be assessed after the mobilization for an improvement. If the motion is improved, the grade III accessory and physiologic mobilizations may be repeated up to three times in one treatment session. Activities to be performed after mobilizations to maintain motion include high stepping over objects to encourage active flexion or walking in sand, snow, or tall grass.

HIP JOINT

A brief overview of the mechanics of the hip joint is provided in Box 3. The hip or the coxofemoral joint is a ball and socket joint. The convex on concave mobilization principles apply to this joint, similar to other joints. Hip compressions may be applied and seem to be beneficial in treating dogs afflicted with hip dysplasia and after femoral head and neck ostectomy.

Hip Compressions

For hip compressions, the dog should be positioned in lateral recumbency with the hip to be mobilized facing up. The hip should be held in slight abduction (25°–40° of abduction compared with a standing position) and slight flexion (25°–40° of flexion compared with a standing position). The therapist should be positioned on the ventral side of the dog, facing the hip to be mobilized.

The mobilizing hand is placed on the cranial lateral aspect of the proximal femur. The stabilizing hand may be placed on the ilium or sacral region.

The mobilizing hand applies the compressions in a rapid and rhythmic fashion at a rate of approximately 40 to 50 compressions per minute. The compression is aimed at the acetabulum (Fig. 8). Compressions should be repeated for 3 to 4 minutes if the dog relaxes. Normally, this is a relaxing technique for dogs. The objective is to increase firing of the mechanoreceptors; increase ligament tension, muscle stability, and proprioception; and enhance synovial fluid flow.

Caudal Glide: Accessory Glide

For an accessory caudal glide (Fig. 9), the dog should be positioned in lateral recumbency with the hip in slight abduction and slight flexion. The therapist should be positioned facing the hip to be mobilized on the ventral surface.

The stabilizing hand is placed over the sacrum. The forearm of the mobilizing hand may be placed under the hind limb to assist in guiding the limb. The web space of the mobilizing hand is placed at the cranial portion of the proximal femur, as close to the joint line as possible.

Box 3: Brief overview of the mechanics of the hip joint

- As the hip moves into flexion, the femoral head moves caudally with respect to the acetabulum. Therefore, to increase hip flexion, a caudal glide is applied to the femoral head.
- As the hip moves into extension, the femoral head moves cranially with respect to the acetabulum. Therefore, to increase hip extension, a cranial glide is applied to the femoral head.
- As the hip moves into abduction, the femoral head moves medially and dorsally in a rolling manner with respect to the acetabulum. Therefore, to increase hip abduction, a medial and dorsal glide is applied to the femoral head.
- As the hip moves into adduction, the femoral head moves laterally and ventrally in a rolling manner with respect to the acetabulum. Therefore, to increase adduction, a lateral and ventral glide is applied to the femoral head.

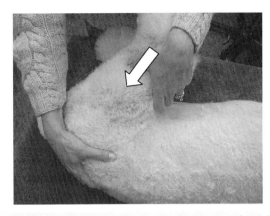

Fig. 8. Coxofemoral hip compressions. Arrow indicates direction of mobilization.

A caudal glide is applied with the mobilizing hand. The forearm may assist the hind limb into flexion as the guide is applied. The objective is to increase hip flexion.

A grade III accessory mobilization may be performed from the same described hand position by adding an oscillation of the mobilizing hand. The caudal glide oscillations are performed with the joint held in slight flexion and slight abduction or the loose packed position. The oscillations should bump against the end of the available motion at a rate of three to four repetitions per second and be continued for up to 60 seconds. The caudal glide is typically followed by a grade III physiologic hip flexion mobilization for an additional 60 seconds.

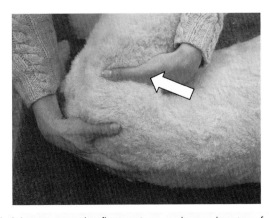

Fig. 9. Caudal glide to increase hip flexion. Arrow indicates direction of mobilization.

Physiologic Flexion

To perform a grade III physiologic hip flexion mobilization (Fig. 10), the mobilizing hand should be moved to the caudal portion of the proximal femur, just below the ischial tuberosity. The stabilizing hand should remain on the sacrum and cradle the distal portion of the hind limb if possible. With the pelvis stabilized, the femur is moved to the end of the available ROM and then back to near midposition of the joint. An oscillatory movement is performed by moving the femur to end feel and back to midposition at a rate of two to three repetitions per second for up to 60 seconds. It is important that the therapist move the limb with his or her body versus arm movements only with the physiologic mobilization, because this is a larger joint and requires proper body mechanics to avoid injury to the therapist.

Hip flexion should then be assessed after the mobilization to ascertain if there has been an improvement. If the motion is improved, the grade III accessory mobilization and the grade III physiologic mobilization may be repeated up to three times in one treatment session. Active movement after treatment includes high stepping to encourage active hip flexion.

Cranial Glide: Accessory Glide

For an accessory cranial glide (Fig. 11), the dog is positioned in lateral recumbency with the hip in slight abduction and slight flexion. The therapist is positioned caudal and ventral to the dog, facing the hip to be mobilized.

One hand may be placed at the distal femur to assist with control or placed at the sacroiliac region. Because this is a large joint to mobilize with a long lever arm, it is often easiest to place the hand not performing the mobilization at the

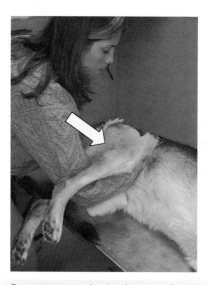

Fig. 10. Physiologic hip flexion. Arrow indicates direction of mobilization.

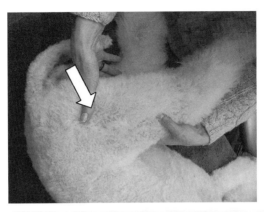

Fig. 11. Cranial mobilization to increase hip extension. Arrow indicates direction of mobilization.

distal femur. The pelvis is stabilized by the dog's weight in a lateral recumbent position. The forearm of the stabilizing hand may be used to assist the positioning of the hind limb. The web space of the mobilizing hand is placed under the ischial tuberosity, on the proximal and caudal aspect of the femur.

A cranial mobilization is applied by directing the proximal femur cranially, with a slight dorsal angulation. The objective is to increase hip extension.

A grade III accessory mobilization may be performed with the same hand positions as described previously. The cranial glide oscillation is performed with the hip in a loose packed position or in slight flexion and abduction. The oscillations should bump up against the end of the available motion. The oscillations are performed at a rate of three to four repetitions per second and are continued for up to 60 seconds. The cranial glide of the femur is typically followed by a grade III physiologic hip extension mobilization for an additional 60 seconds.

Physiologic Extension

To perform the physiologic mobilization for hip extension (Fig. 12), the mobilizing hand should be placed on the cranial and most proximal portion of the femur and the stabilizing hand should remain on the sacrum. The mobilizing hand applies a caudal force to the proximal femur to encourage hip extension. With the pelvis stabilized, the proximal femur is pushed into the available amount of extension, bumping the end feel of the joint. The femur is then moved back to the near midposition of the joint. Oscillatory movements are performed by moving the femur to the end feel and back to midposition at a rate of three to four repetitions per second for 60 seconds.

Hip extension should then be assessed after the mobilization for an improvement in ROM. If the motion is improved, the grade III accessory and physiologic mobilization should be repeated up to three times in one treatment

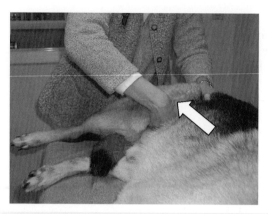

Fig. 12. Physiologic hip extension. Arrow indicates direction of mobilization.

session. Active hip extension should also be encouraged through resisted walking by having the dog pull against a leash or climbing stairs.

STIFLE JOINT

The femoral condyles are a convex surface sitting on the tibial plateau [29]. The stifle is a ginglymus joint, or a hinge joint, and flexion and extension are the primary motions at the joint. The concave tibia moves on the convex femur and is therefore following the convex on concave rule. Therefore, to increase stifle extension, the tibia glides cranially on the femur. To increase stifle flexion, the tibia glides caudally on the femur.

Restoration of stifle flexion and extension is essential in normal ambulation and function in the dog. The dog requires full stifle flexion to obtain a normal sitting posture and full stifle extension for proper ambulation. An overview of the kinematics of the stifle joint is provided in Box 4.

Box 4: Overview of kinematics of the stifle joint

- As the stifle joint flexes in the open kinetic chain, the concave plateau of the tibia moves in a caudal direction on the convex femoral condyles. Therefore, to increase stifle flexion, a cranial glide mobilization of the proximal tibia on the femur should be applied.

- As the stifle flexes in the closed kinetic chain, the convex femoral condyles roll caudally on the concave tibial plateaus.

- As the stifle joint extends in the open kinetic chain, the concave plateau of the tibia moves in a cranial direction on the convex femoral condyles. Therefore, to increase stifle extension, a caudal glide mobilization of the proximal tibia should be applied.

- As the stifle extends in the closed kinetic chain, the convex femoral condyles roll cranially and glide caudally on the concave tibial plateaus.

Femorotibial Cranial Glide

For a femorotibial cranial glide (Fig. 13), the dog is positioned in lateral recumbency with the stifle in a resting position. The therapist is positioned facing the ventral aspect of the dog and the stifle to be mobilized.

The stabilizing hand is on the cranial surface of the distal femur. The mobilizing hand is placed on the caudal surface of the proximal tibia.

A cranial glide is applied to the tibia while the distal femur is stabilized. The objective is to increase stifle joint flexion.

A grade III accessory mobilization may be performed from the same described hand position by adding an oscillation of the mobilizing hand. The cranial oscillations are performed with the joint held in slight flexion or the loose packed position. The oscillations should bump against the end of the available motion at a rate of three to four repetitions per second for up to 60 seconds. The cranial glide is typically followed by a grade III physiologic stifle flexion mobilization for an additional 60 seconds.

Physiologic Flexion

To perform a grade III physiologic stifle flexion mobilization (Fig. 14), the hand positions may remain the same or the mobilizing hand may be placed on the cranial aspect of the distal tibia while the stabilizing hand is placed on the cranial aspect of the distal femur. With the femur stabilized, the tibia is moved to the end of the available range of flexion and then back to near midposition of the joint. An oscillatory movement is performed by moving the tibia to end feel and back to midposition at a rate of three to four repetitions per second for up to 60 seconds.

Stifle flexion should then be assessed after the mobilization to ascertain if there has been an improvement. If the motion is improved, the grade III accessory mobilization and the grade III physiologic mobilization may be repeated up to three times in one treatment session. Active movement after treatment includes high stepping to encourage active stifle flexion.

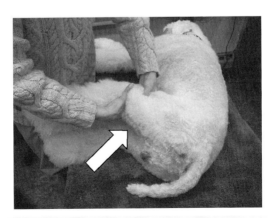

Fig. 13. Cranial glide to increase stifle flexion. Arrow indicates direction of mobilization.

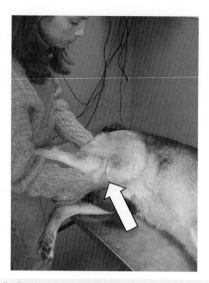

Fig. 14. Physiologic stifle flexion. Arrow indicates direction of mobilization.

Femorotibial Caudal Glide

For a femorotibial caudal glide (Fig. 15), the dogs should be positioned in lateral recumbency with the stifle in a resting position. The therapist is positioned facing the caudal aspect of the stifle to be mobilized.

The stabilizing hand is placed on the caudal aspect of the distal femur. The mobilizing hand is placed on the cranial aspect of the proximal tibia.

A caudal glide is performed by the mobilizing hand while the distal femur is stabilized. The objective is to increase stifle joint extension.

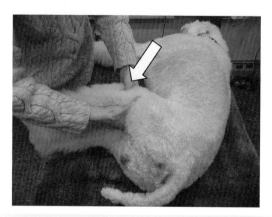

Fig. 15. Caudal glide to increase stifle extension. Arrow indicates direction of mobilization.

A grade III accessory mobilization may be performed from the same described hand position by adding an oscillation of the mobilizing hand. The caudal glide oscillations are performed with the joint held in slight flexion or the loose packed position. The oscillations should bump against the end of the available motion at a rate of three to four repetitions per second for up to 60 seconds. The caudal glide is typically followed by a grade III physiologic stifle extension mobilization for an additional 60 seconds.

Physiologic Extension

To perform a grade III physiologic stifle extension mobilization (Fig. 16), the hand positions may remain the same, or the mobilizing hand may be placed on the caudal aspect of the distal tibia while the stabilizing hand is placed on the cranial aspect of the distal femur. With the femur stabilized, the tibia is moved to the end of the available motion of extension and then back to near midposition of the joint. An oscillatory movement is performed by moving the tibia to end feel and back to midposition at a rate of three to four repetitions per second for up to 60 seconds.

Stifle extension should then be assessed after the mobilization to ascertain if there has been an improvement. If the motion is improved, the grade III accessory mobilization and the grade III physiologic mobilization may be repeated up to three times in one treatment session.

SPINE

The spinal region of the dog is complex in that it allows a significant amount of movement as it absorbs and distributes the forces from the four limbs. Each area of the spine (cervical, thoracic, lumbar, and coccygeal) possesses varying

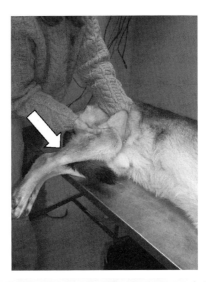

Fig. 16. Physiologic stifle extension. Arrow indicates direction of mobilization.

amounts of motion. The cervical region permits enough movement so that the dog may be able to touch any part of its body with its nose except between the scapulae. Observation of a running dog demonstrates the amount of thoracic and lumbar flexion and extension that may be present [29].

Movements of the spine include extension, flexion, side flexion, and rotation. The motions of each component of the spine contribute to the total movement of the entire spine.

The movement at the spinal level takes places between two vertebrae. Some regions of the spine demonstrate more mobility than other areas. For example, the lower thoracic region and the lumbosacral region are two of the most mobile areas of the spine. These are also the areas in which there are a significant number of injuries.

Mobilization techniques of the canine spine must be approached with extreme caution and knowledge of canine anatomy, medical conditions of the nervous system, and the anatomy of the individual breed of dog. For example, the angulation of the thoracic spine differs according to the breed of the dog and the topline [29,32]. A Labrador Retriever has a level topline. This differs from the arched topline of a Greyhound or a Whippet [29,33]. The differences in angulation of toplines alter the direction of the mobilization.

Because specialized training and clinical experience are necessary to perform spinal mobilizations safely, a limited number of basic mobilization techniques for the thoracic and lumbar regions are described. The cervical region is complex, and there are many contraindications associated with cervical mobilizations. It is essential that mobilization not be attempted without a clear comprehension of cervical anatomy, the nature of the dog's problem, and the contraindications of the region. Cervical ROM may become reduced secondary to arthritic conditions of the cervical spine, after surgery for a cervical disk, or secondary to conditions related to overuse of the forelimb muscles. It is common to see restrictions in the adjacent vertebrae after a ventral slot procedure. Changes in functional characteristics may result in decreased cervical extension while walking, lifting the head up from drinking or eating from a bowl off the floor, or flexing the head and neck as a dog ascends stairs. It is important to wait until after the surgical site has healed and is stable.

Thoracic Region

The dorsal spinous processes of the thoracic spine are narrow and long. Some dogs object to direct pressure over the spinous process. The lower thoracic region is one of the more common areas where problems secondary to increased mobility are present. Intervertebral disk disease, compensatory problems from canine hip dysplasia, and arthritic changes are common in this area. Dogs experiencing signs of hip dysplasia have decreased hip extension. Changes in the motion of the spinal column occur to compensate for the reduced extension.

There are 13 thoracic vertebrae in the dog. The eleventh vertebra is called the anticlinal vertebra [34]. It is a transition point along the thoracic vertebrae. The spinous processes cranial to T11 point caudally, and the spinous processes caudal to T11 point cranially. Therefore, when performing mobilizations to this area, it is essential to understand the topline of the dog as well as the inclination of the particular vertebral spinous process.

Thoracic Central Dorsal-to-Ventral Glides

For thoracic central dorsal-to-ventral glides (Fig. 17), the dog should be positioned standing or in a sitting position with the spine in a neutral position (no rotation or side flexion). The therapist should stand or kneel at the dog's side, with his or her shoulders directly over the dog. Kneeling may be necessary if the dog is on the floor or a mat.

The thumb of the mobilizing hand is placed over the spinous process of the vertebra to be mobilized. The remaining part of the mobilizing hand may be draped over the region. The stabilizing hand may be placed under the ventral position of the thoracic region. This hand helps to detect any changes in tension of the abdominal region in response to pain or discomfort as well as providing a light counterforce stabilization. The therapist's elbows should be slightly flexed to facilitate a smooth oscillation of the vertebra.

Depending on the angulation of the thoracic region of the dog, a dorsal-to-ventral glide is applied at an angle from approximately 90° to 75° degrees. Oscillations for a grade II mobilization should be performed gently so that the therapist senses only minimal resistance from joint structures and the dog does not experience any pain. Grade II mobilizations should be performed for up to 30 seconds. Oscillations for grade III mobilizations should be performed so that the therapist senses the end feel of the segment. This grade of mobilization should be performed for up to 60 seconds. After each mobilization, the dog should be assessed to determine whether there has been a functional change. Changes that may occur include an increase in functional mobility, such as with side flexion of the spine while the dog lies down or reaches for a treat near the base of the tail. Additional changes in thoracic mobility include the ability to ascend stairs with improved extension. Pain and muscle spasms should also be diminished.

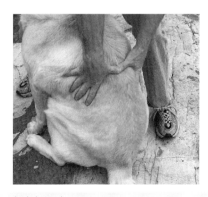

Fig. 17. Dorsal-to-ventral glide to thoracic spine.

Lumbar Region

The seven lumbar vertebrae possess blunt spinous processes, and the facet angles are positioned at an angle of approximate 90° to the floor when the dog is in a standing position. Therefore, mobilizations are mostly performed at an angle of 90° or perpendicular to the floor.

The areas of greatest mobility in the lumbar spine include the thoracolumbar region and the lumbosacral region [29,35]. This is also an area where intervertebral disk injuries are commonly seen [36].

Lumbar Dorsal-to-Ventral Glide

For a lumbar dorsal-to-ventral glide (Fig. 18), the dog is positioned standing with the spine in a neutral position. The therapist is positioned standing or kneeling directly over the area to be mobilized. The therapist's shoulders should be directly over the area to be mobilized.

The dominant thumb should be placed directly over the spinous process to be mobilized and then reinforced by the nondominant thumb. The remainder of the hand should be draped over the dog. If the therapist feels comfortable with performing the mobilization with one hand, the nondominant hand may be placed under the dog's abdomen to ascertain any signs of pain or discomfort. The shoulders should be directly over the area and the elbows and wrists slightly flexed to provide proper body mechanics.

A dorsal-to-ventral glide is applied at approximately 90° or perpendicular to the skin surface. Oscillations for a grade II mobilization should be performed gently so that the therapist senses only minimal resistance from joint structures and the dog does not experience any pain. Grade II mobilizations should be performed for up to 30 seconds. Oscillations for grade III mobilizations should be performed so that the therapist senses the end feel for the segment. This grade of mobilization should be performed for up to 60 seconds. After each mobilization, the dog should be assessed to determine whether there has been a functional change. If an increase in ROM and function has been made, the

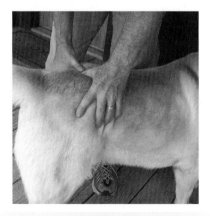

Fig. 18. Dorsal-to-ventral glide to lumbar spine.

mobilization may be repeated two more times. Functional improvements include an improved ability to ascend stairs, transition from a lying position to a sitting position, and possibly jumping. A decrease in pain and muscle spasms should be felt as well as increased comfort during palpation. Often, dogs contract their abdominal muscles when pressure is placed on a painful intervertebral segment.

Acknowledgments

The authors thank Shauna Miner and Brenda Walker for providing photographs. They also thank Ann and Champion Majessa Easy Rider "Tommy" Fischer, Latte Saunders, Cheryl and "Max" Brienza, and Fred for their photographs and the staff at Pieper-Olson Veterinary Clinic for their patience and understanding.

References

[1] Guide to physical therapist practice. 2nd edition. Alexandria, VA: American Physical Therapy Association; 2001. p. 118.

[2] Maitland GD. Peripheral manipulation. 3rd edition. London: Butterworth-Heinemann; 1991.

[3] Maitland GD. Vertebral manipulation. 5th edition. London: Butterworth-Heinemann; 1986.

[4] Blomberg S, Svardsudd K, Mildenberger F. A controlled, multicentre trial of manual therapy in low-back pain. Initial status, sick-leave and pain score during follow-up. Scand J Prim Health Care 1992;10(3):170–8.

[5] Koes BW, Bouter LM, van Mameren H, et al. A blinded randomized clinical trial of manual therapy and physiotherapy for chronic back and neck complaints: physical outcome measures. J Manipulative Physiol Ther 1992;15(1):16–23.

[6] Koes BW, Bouter LM, van Mameren H, et al. The effectiveness of manual therapy, physiotherapy, and treatment by the general practitioner for nonspecific back and neck complaints. A randomized clinical trial. Spine 1992;17(1):28–35.

[7] Blomberg S, Svardsudd K, Tibblin G. Manual therapy with steroid injections in low-back pain. Improvement of quality of life in a controlled trial with four months' follow-up. Scand J Prim Health Care 1993;11(2):83–90.

[8] Koes BW, Bouter LM, van Mameren H, et al. A randomized clinical trial of manual therapy and physiotherapy for persistent back and neck complaints: subgroup analysis and relationship between outcome measures. J Manipulative Physiol Ther 1993;16(4):211–9.

[9] Blomberg S, Hallin G, Grann K, et al. Manual therapy with steroid injections—a new approach to treatment of low back pain. A controlled multicenter trial with an evaluation by orthopedic surgeons. Spine 1994;19(5):569–77.

[10] Bang MD, Deyle GD. Comparison of supervised exercise with and without manual physical therapy for patients with shoulder impingement syndrome. J Orthop Sports Phys Ther 2000;30(3):126–37.

[11] Deyle GD, Henderson NE, Matekel RL, et al. Effectiveness of manual physical therapy and exercise in osteoarthritis of the knee. A randomized, controlled trial. Ann Intern Med 2000;132(3):173–81.

[12] Allison GT, Nagy BM, Hall T. A randomized clinical trial of manual therapy for cervicobrachial pain syndrome—a pilot study. Man Ther 2002;7(2):95–102.

[13] Aure OF, Nilsen JH, Vasseljen O. Manual therapy and exercise therapy in patients with chronic low back pain: a randomized, controlled trial with 1-year follow-up. Spine 2003; 28(6):525–31 [discussion: 531–2].

[14] Korthals-de Bos IB, Hoving JL, van Tulder MW, et al. Cost effectiveness of physiotherapy, manual therapy, and general practitioner care for neck pain: economic evaluation alongside a randomised controlled trial. BMJ 2003;326(7395):911.

[15] Hoeksma HL, Dekker J, Ronday HK, et al. Comparison of manual therapy and exercise therapy in osteoarthritis of the hip: a randomized clinical trial. Arthritis Rheum 2004;51(5): 722–9.

[16] Cleland J, Selleck B, Stowell T, et al. Short-term effects of thoracic manipulation on lower trapezius muscle strength. Journal of Manual and Manipulative Therapy 2004;12(2):82–90.

[17] Grieve G. The rationale of manipulation. Physiotherapy 1967;53(10):338–40.

[18] Mennell JM. Rationale of joint manipulation. Phys Ther 1970;50(2):181–6.

[19] Twomey LT. A rationale for the treatment of back pain and joint pain by manual therapy. Phys Ther 1992;72(12):885–92.

[20] Dutton M. Orthopaedic examination, evaluation, and intervention. New York: McGraw-Hill; 2004. p. 327.

[21] Cyriax J. Textbook of orthopaedic medicine, diagnosis of soft tissue lesions. 8th edition. London: Baillière Tindall; 1982.

[22] Mennell JM. Back pain. Diagnosis and treatment using manipulative techniques. Boston: Little Brown; 1960.

[23] Greenmann PE. Principles of manual medicine. 2nd edition. Baltimore: Williams & Wilkins; 1996.

[24] Kaltenborn FM. Manual mobilization of the extremity joints: basic examination and treatment techniques. 4th edition. Oslo: Olaf Norlis Bokhandel, Universitetsgaten; 1989.

[25] McKenzie R, May S. The lumbar spine, mechanical diagnosis and therapy, vols. 1 and 2. 2nd edition. Waikanae, NZ: Spinal Publications New Zealand Ltd; 2003.

[26] McKenzie R, May S. The human extremities, mechanical diagnosis and therapy. Waikanae, NZ: Spinal Publications New Zealand Ltd; 2000.

[27] Kubo K, Kanehisa H, Fukunaga T. Effects of transient muscle contractions and stretching on the tendon structures in vivo. Acta Physiol Scand 2002;175(2):157–64.

[28] Gray GW. Closed kinetic sense. Fitness Management 1992;31–3.

[29] Evans HE. Miller's anatomy of the dog. 3rd edition. Philadelphia: WB Saunders; 1983.

[30] Brown CM. Dog locomotion and gait analysis. Wheat Ridge, CO: Hoflin Publishing; 1986.

[31] Lyon M. The dog in action. New York: Howell Book House; 1988.

[32] Blythe LL, Gannon JR, Craig AM. Care of the racing greyhound. Corvallis (OR): American Greyhound Council; 1994.

[33] Gross DM. Canine physical therapy. East Lyme, CT; Wizard of Paws, 2002.

[34] Zink MC. Peak performance—coaching the canine athlete. 2nd edition. Lutherville, MD: Canine Sports Productions; 1997.

[35] Evans HE, deLaHunta A. Miller's guide to the dissection of the dog. 4th edition. Philadelphia: WB Saunders; 1996.

[36] Bloomberg MS, Dee JF, Taylor RA. Canine sports medicine and surgery. Philadelphia: WB Saunders; 1998.

ELSEVIER
SAUNDERS

Vet Clin Small Anim 35 (2005) 1317–1333

VETERINARY CLINICS
SMALL ANIMAL PRACTICE

Physical Agent Modalities

Janet E. Steiss, DVM, PhD, PT[a,*],
David Levine, PT, PhD, CCRP[b,c,d]

[a]Department of Anatomy, Physiology, and Pharmacology, College of Veterinary Medicine,
Auburn University, Auburn, AL 36849, USA
[b]Department of Physical Therapy, University of Tennessee at Chattanooga,
615 McCallie Avenue, Chattanooga, TN, USA
[c]Department of Small Animal Clinical Sciences, University of Tennessee College of Veterinary
Medicine, 2407 River Drive, Knoxville, TN, USA
[d]Department of Clinical Sciences, North Carolina State University College of Veterinary
Medicine, 4700 Hillsborough Street, Raleigh, NC 27606, USA

OVERVIEW

The purpose of this article is to review the use of cold, heat, therapeutic ultrasound (US), and electrical stimulation (ES) in small animal rehabilitation. The material in this article is a compilation from the veterinary and human literature [1–10]. Additional information is needed on how to adapt the techniques used in human beings to small animals and then to establish the efficacy of these techniques in animals [10].

COLD (CRYOTHERAPY)
Basic Properties

Cryotherapy refers to the application of cold as a method in rehabilitation and should not be confused with cryosurgery. The sensations reported by people after ice application are an initial sensation of cold followed by burning, aching, and eventual numbness. Cold penetrates deeper and lasts longer than heat because of the decreased circulation resulting from cold application.

Local application of cold decreases [1,2,5] the following:

1. Blood flow because of vasoconstriction
2. Edema formation
3. Hemorrhage
4. Histamine release
5. Local metabolism
6. Muscle spindle activity
7. Nerve conduction velocity (NCV)
8. Pain
9. Spasticity
10. Response to acute inflammation or injury

*Corresponding author. E-mail address: steisje@vetmed.auburn.edu (J.E. Steiss).

0195-5616/05/$ – see front matter
doi:10.1016/j.cvsm.2005.08.001

Local application of cold increases [1,5] the following:

1. Connective tissue stiffness (with decreased tensile strength)
2. Temporary muscle viscosity (with decreased ability to perform rapid movements)

Generalized application of cold over the whole body or large portions of it causes [1,5] the following:

1. Decreased respiratory and heart rates
2. Generalized vasoconstriction in response to cooling of the hypothalamus
3. Increased muscle spindle bias, which can increase spasticity (opposite to the effect of localized cold application)
4. Increased muscle tone, which may be accompanied by shivering

Indications

Cold is indicated in small animal rehabilitation for the management of several conditions:

1. Acute injury or inflammation: "RICE" stands for rest (to halt further injury), ice (to minimize cell death), compression (to decrease edema), and elevation (to decrease edema). In animals with acute injury, rest and ice can be readily used. Compression bandages may be applied to certain sites, such as the stifle joint. Elevation is seldom possible, although keeping the edematous side up when in lateral recumbency is advocated. Application of cold to minimize postsurgical swelling is also recommended.
2. To increase range of motion (ROM) which is limited by pain and inflammation
3. To provide emergency care for burns
4. To stimulate muscle function using a brief application of cold
5. To decrease spasticity attributable to upper motor neuron disorders (using local application of cold while keeping the rest of the body warm). Spasticity associated with spinal cord disorders in small animals can be difficult to treat, and this use of cold application deserves further study.

Contraindications and Precautions

The primary precaution is avoidance of frostbite. It is difficult to check skin color on dogs because of pigmentation and hair coat. The guideline in human beings is that treatment should be stopped if the skin is cyanotic. To be safe and avoid prolonged application, use a timer and inspect the skin every few minutes. Downer [2] recommended never applying ice directly on the animal because of possible discomfort and tissue damage; she recommended covering ice packs with at least one layer of moist towel. The insulating effect of the hair coat in dogs may be a factor to consider, although one study indicated that the extent of caudal thigh muscle cooling was similar with clipped and unclipped hair coats when cold packs (two parts ice to one part isopropyl alcohol) were applied [11]. Research is needed in dogs to document the amount and duration of tissue cooling with various forms of cold application. Other precautions and contraindications include the presence of cardiac or respiratory disease, uncovered open wounds, and ischemic areas.

Treatment Guidelines

1. In the absence of specific clinical research in companion animals, many of the recommendations for cryotherapy in dogs are extrapolated from human rehabilitation until additional data are available.
2. A general rule for deciding when to apply cold versus heat is that cryotherapy should be used for the first 24 to 72 hours after acute injury when the acute signs of inflammation are present (swelling, redness, heat, and pain). If in doubt, use cold.
3. If ROM is decreased because of pain, apply cold. If ROM is decreased because of stiffness, apply heat.
4. Cover ice packs with a single layer of wet towel (moisture enhances heat exchange) or nothing between the skin and the ice pack. Otherwise, therapeutic temperatures may not be reached.
5. Apply ice packs for up to 10 to 20 minutes. The duration may vary for different types of commercial ice packs. Until studies are performed on dogs to determine specific tissue temperatures achieved with ice packs and cold packs, the recommendation is to avoid prolonged cold because of the risk of tissue damage.
6. The recommendations on how often to apply ice vary. Therapists treating people often follow the rule of "15 minutes on, 15 minutes off." Other recommendations include spacing cold treatments at least 2 hours apart.
7. It is recommended not to apply cold to open wounds after 48 to 72 hours because of the vasoconstriction that occurs with cryotherapy.
8. Ice packs made with crushed ice in a plastic bag are inexpensive, convenient, and indicated when a cold source is desired. The pack can be applied directly to the skin (Fig. 1A) or wrapped in a moist towel, covered with bandaging tape, and left in place for 10 to 20 minutes. Vannatta and colleagues [11] studied the effects of cold packs on skin and muscle temperature in dogs and intramuscular muscle blood flow in the caudal thigh muscles during cryotherapy and subsequent rewarming. Temperature was measured at the skin surface and at depths of 1 and 3 cm below the skin using needle thermistor probes inserted beneath the site of cold pack application. Blood flow was measured using laser Doppler flowmetry. Treatment consisted of a standard cold pack applied for 20 minutes. Tissue cooling with the hair coat intact and clipped was evaluated. Temperature and blood flow measurements were recorded every minute for 100 consecutive minutes (5 minutes for baseline data, 20 minutes for cold pack treatment, and 75 minutes after treatment). There was a significant reduction in cutaneous temperature with rapid rewarming of the skin after cold pack removal. At depths of 1 and 3 cm, tissue cooling was less profound but still significant. Temperatures at depths of 1 and 3 cm continued to decrease after cold pack removal until they reached a plateau and began to ascend back toward baseline. The maximum temperature reductions were 14.2°C, 2.3°C, and 1.6°C at the skin surface and at depths of 1 and 3 cm, respectively. Although blood flow was reduced in the tissues during the cold pack application, blood flow in deeper tissues actually increased above baseline level after removal of the cold pack, possibly as a result of vasodilation to bring more blood to the superficial cooled region for rewarming.

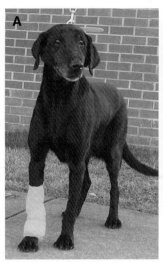
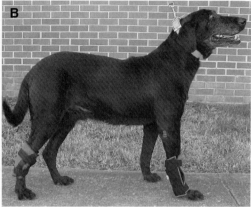

Fig. 1. Cryotherapy is indicated in the treatment of acute carpal sprain. (A) A 15-year-old Labrador Retriever's carpus is wrapped with crushed ice in a plastic bag and secured with elastic bandage (Vetrap bandaging tape; 3M Animal Care Products, St. Paul, MN). Alternatively, commercially available custom-fitted wraps with cold pack inserts can be applied. (B) Dog is fitted with carpal and hock wraps (Canine Icers; Canine Icer, LLC, Charlottesville, VA) with Cryopak flexible inserts (Cryopak Industries, Delta, British Columbia, Canada).

9. Commercial reusable cold packs are made of silica gel in plastic or canvas covers. Custom-fitted neoprene wraps with pockets for reusable cold packs are now commercially available for dogs (see Fig. 1B). The packs maintain a low temperature for a considerable time, but most do not lower skin temperature as much as ice. For horses, Kaneps [12] stated that commercial cold packs are convenient to use and may be applied for more than 30 minutes but result in smaller changes in tissue temperature than ice. In people, commercial cold packs are sometimes applied for up to several hours for the acute treatment of burns [5]. Temperature changes were recorded in dogs during application of cold gel packs over the thigh for up to 30 minutes in one study [13]. The authors found that the superficial tissues, such as skin and subcutaneous tissues, had the most rapid and profound cooling, whereas deeper tissues, such as bone and muscle, exhibited smaller and more gradual declines in temperature. The time for the intramuscular layers to return to baseline ranged from 60 minutes for 10 minutes of cold application up to 145 minutes for 30 minutes of cold application.
10. Iced towels are towels soaked in ice-water slush. In people, iced towels are used to treat spasticity or painful muscle guarding when relatively large areas are involved. Two iced towels should be alternated because towels warm up quickly and should be exchanged to prevent unwanted rewarming.
11. Ice wrap bandages are marketed for use in horses and people and can be used on dogs. They may be stored in the refrigerator or at room temperature. Some wraps are made from a gel material, which can be messy if applied directly to the skin.

12. Ice gels are commercially available for other species. Penetration through canine skin has not been studied to the authors' knowledge.

13. Ice massage is appropriate for treating small areas. Water frozen in paper cups, with a popsicle stick or tongue depressor as a handle, is inexpensive and convenient. The frozen water may be removed from the cup just before use, and the ice is gently rubbed over the area to provide a massage while cooling tissues.

14. Cold and compression systems have the advantage of providing compression during cold application. Some commercially available ice boots can be adapted to small animals. A commercial compression splint with circulating coolant was applied to the limbs of standing horses [14]. After 1 hour, the average core temperature of the superficial digital flexor tendon was reduced by 22°C (with a mean minimum temperature of 10°C), with no loss in cell viability.

15. Cold baths involve immersing the affected body part in cool or icy water. This method is frequently used for treating extremities in horses. For people, the temperature ranges of the cold bath are graded as cool (19°C–27°C, 67°F–80°F), cold (13°C–19°C, 55°F–67°F), or very cold (0°C–13°C, 32°F–55°F) [5].

16. Vapocoolant sprays (eg, fluoromethane, ethyl chloride) are highly volatile liquids that cause evaporative cooling when sprayed on the skin. Although the technique of "cool and stretch" seems to be beneficial for treating trigger points in people, the technique is more difficult in small animals because of the hair coat and the difficulty of having awake animals sufficiently relaxed to stretch, particularly if they are in pain.

17. Contrast baths consist of alternately immersing the body part in warm and cold water. The goal is to produce alternating vasodilation and vasoconstriction. Contrast baths are used as a "vascular exercise" to stimulate blood flow and healing.

HEAT

Heating agents are classified as superficial or deep heating. Superficial heating agents penetrate to tissue depths up to approximately 2 cm, whereas deep heating agents elevate tissue temperatures at depths of 3 cm or more. Heat sources are classified as radiant, conductive, or convective heat. An infrared lamp is an example of a radiant superficial heating device, a hot pack is an example of a conductive superficial heating device, and a whirlpool is an example of moist heat delivered by conduction and convection.

Superficial Heat

Superficial heating agents include hot packs, heat wraps, hosing with warm water, whirlpools, paraffin baths, circulating warm water blankets, electric heating pads, and infrared lamps. The last two are considered to have a higher risk of burn in animals.

Basic properties

The effects of heat are opposite to those of cold, except that heat and cold both relieve pain and muscle spasm [6]. Heat is carried away by the circulation; thus, tissues do not hold heat after treatment for the same length of time that they retain cold.

Local application of heat decreases [6] the following:

1. Blood pressure (if heat is applied for a prolonged time or over a large surface area)
2. Muscle spasm
3. Pain

Local application of heat increases [6] the following:

1. Body temperature, respiratory rate, and heart rate if heat is applied for a prolonged time
2. Capillary pressure and permeability (which can promote edema)
3. Leukocyte migration into the heated area
4. Local circulation (promoting healing in subacute and chronic inflammation)
5. Local metabolism
6. Muscle relaxation
7. Tissue elasticity

Indications

1. Subacute and chronic traumatic and inflammatory conditions
2. Decreased ROM attributable to stiffness and/or contracture (basis for the principle of "heat and stretch")
3. Pain relief, because heat may render sensory nerve endings less excitable

Precautions

1. There is risk of overheating in dogs immersed in a heated whirlpool. They should be observed and their rectal temperature measured if in doubt.
2. Use caution in treating sedated animals or areas of decreased sensation.
3. The skin response can be difficult to monitor because of the hair coat and skin pigmentation.
4. The weight of a hot pack could be deleterious if it aggravates tenderness or risks injury from the weight of the pack itself. In some instances, the pack can be placed under the area to be treated.
5. Open or infected wounds should be treated with caution.

Contraindications

1. Electric heating pads and infrared lamps have a higher risk of burns. Electric heating pads should never be placed under an anesthetized animal or an animal with decreased superficial sensation. In general, animals should never be left unattended during treatment, and the skin should be monitored frequently.
2. Active bleeding
3. Acute inflammation
4. Cardiac insufficiency
5. Decreased impaired circulation in the area to be treated (to avoid overheating)
6. Fever
7. Malignancy
8. Poor body heat regulation

Treatment guidelines
   1. Heat is generally applied for 15 to 30 minutes.
   2. The guideline in people is that if white areas (attributable to rebound vasocon-striction) or red mottled areas appear on the skin, treatment should be stopped.
   3. Hot packs are relatively safe because they cool during treatment, minimizing the risk of burn. Padding is applied around the pack. Hot packs may be made from canvas filled with silica gel and maintained in a hydrocollator (self-contained moist heating storage unit) with the water temperature near 75°C (167°F). The pack retains heat for approximately 30 minutes. The heat is absorbed mostly by the skin and subcutaneous fat. The reader is referred to another source [6] for specific instructions on wrapping hot packs before application. Studies need to be conducted in dogs to allow specific recommendations for hot pack applications.
   4. Heat wraps are marketed for people. Some products provide up to 8 hours of continuous low level heat and could be fitted to small animals.
   5. Whirlpools have the advantage of also providing increased hydrostatic pressure to submerged body parts. Increased hydrostatic pressure helps to increase lymphatic and venous flow from a distal-to-proximal orientation. Agitation within a whirlpool decreases the thermal gradient so that the temperature of the water in the tank is consistent throughout. The temperature of a whirlpool is based on the needs of the individual animal. For example, patients with chronic conditions may be treated with warmer water than patients with more acute disorders. For human patients, the recommendation is that the whirlpool temperature for full body immersion should not be higher than 38°C (100°F) [15]. For dogs, it is probably safe to extrapolate temperature recommendations from underwater treadmills, where the temperature ranges from approximately 80°F to 95°F (27°C to 35°C), depending on how vigorously the dog is exercising.
   6. Hosing with warm water is frequently used for horses. Kaneps [12] reported that water as warm as a human being could comfortably tolerate yielded surface temperatures in horses of 39.5°C to 41°C, with subcutaneous and deeper tissues stabilizing at 39°C to 40°C approximately 9 minutes after starting treatment.

Deep Heat: Therapeutic Ultrasound

The conventional terms *superficial* and *deep* heat are relative terms. In some anatomic sites in small animals, superficial heat, such as hot packs, may be providing heat to the deepest portions of the body part. For example, superficial heat that penetrates 1 to 2 cm may heat sufficiently deeply around the stifle joint, especially in small-breed dogs.

Deep heating agents include therapeutic US and shortwave diathermy. Diathermy units produce heat by electromagnetic energy. Diathermy in dogs has been discussed in previous articles [2,3,16]. To the authors' knowledge, however, diathermy is rarely used in veterinary practice; the patient would need to be quite still, because frequent movement could alter the amount of heating. Diathermy could offer the advantage of heating larger areas compared with US. Penetration of diathermy through canine skin and hair coat remains to be studied.

Basic properties

US refers to high-frequency acoustic waves above range of human hearing (approximately 20 KHz). Sound waves are produced within a transducer head (also termed *sound head*). The advantages of US are that it produces localized heating in deeper tissues and the duration of therapy is short, approximately 10 minutes. A disadvantage is that the dosage is difficult to monitor.

Energy within a sound beam decreases as it travels through tissue because of scatter and absorption. Absorption is high in tissues with a high proportion of protein and minimal in adipose tissue. Only 1% of US energy is absorbed by the skin and subcutaneous tissues.

The hair coat presents a problem when treating animals that is not encountered with human patients. Because US energy is absorbed by tissues with high protein content and deflection of the US beam occurs at tissue interfaces, US penetration through a dog's hair coat into underlying tissues is poor [17]. In addition, US waves do not penetrate through air, and a large amount of air is trapped within the hair coat, even with wetting. It is recommended to clip the hair to ensure optimal tissue heating.

In human medicine, debate persists over the effectiveness of US [18–21]. Draper [22] has argued that many clinical trials evaluating US did not use correct technique to achieve sufficient heating.

Therapeutic US has thermal and nonthermal (mechanical and biomechanical) effects on tissues. Continuous mode emission at intensities of 1.0 W/cm^2 or higher and a duration of approximately 10 minutes heat tissues, whereas continuous mode at low intensity or pulsed mode is selected for nonthermal effects.

Thermal effects. Similar to the effects listed previously for superficial heat, deep heating produced by US can yield increases in collagen extensibility, blood flow, pain threshold, macrophage activity, nerve conduction velocity, and enzyme activity, and it also decreases muscle spasm. To achieve the thermal effects, the tissue temperature should be raised 1°C to 4°C, depending on the desired outcome. In a study in healthy people [23], thermistors were placed in muscle at depths of 2.5 and 5.0 cm for 1-MHz treatment and at depths of 0.8 and 1.6 cm for 3-MHz treatment. The rate of temperature increase per minute at the two depths for 1-MHz exposure ranged from 0.04°C at an intensity of 0.5 W/cm^2 up to 0.38°C at an intensity of 2.0 W/cm^2; corresponding values for treatment with 3 MHz ranged from 0.3°C at an intensity of 0.5 W/cm^2 up to 1.4°C at 2.0 W/cm^2. The 3-MHz frequency heated faster at all intensities.

Nonthermal effects. Nonthermal effects result from sound waves causing molecules to vibrate, resulting in compression and rarefaction. The term *acoustic streaming* has been used to describe this phenomenon. Nonthermal effects include alterations in cell membrane permeability to ions like calcium, phagocytosis, and histamine release as well as stimulation of collagen deposition, angiogenesis, and fibroblast proliferation because of increased release of growth factors.

Indications

- Tendonitis and bursitis: For chronic tendonitis, one therapeutic approach is heating with US followed by cross-frictional massage. In human beings, lateral epicondylitis ("tennis elbow"), subacromial bursitis, and bicipital tendonitis are typical indications. Experimental animal studies indicate that there also may be a role for US in the early stages of tendon repair. The stage of healing at which US is administered and the intensity of the US seem to be important factors [24]. One experimental study using dogs reported that pulsed US at 0.5 W/cm^2 enhanced healing of the Achilles tendon [25]. In that study, US was started the third day after surgically severing the tendon and was performed daily for 10 days.
- Joint contracture: To treat limited ROM associated with joint contracture, patients may receive US in conjunction with stretching. A study performed in dogs demonstrated increased hock flexion after an US and stretching treatment compared with the control group, which received stretching alone [26].
- Wound healing: US has been shown in multiple studies to have an effect on soft tissue healing. More research is needed to establish the mechanism of action at different stages of healing and the optimal treatment parameters. The results seem to depend on the intensity and duration of treatment and time after injury. For additional information, the reader is referred to articles by Dyson and coworkers [27] and Enwemeka and colleagues [24].
- Bone healing: Warden [28] recently reviewed research evidence of the beneficial effect of low-intensity pulsed US on bone fractures. He stated that for fresh fractures, US reduced healing times by 30% or more; for nonunions, US treatment yielded unions in 86% of cases. A report on dogs with experimentally created ostectomies of the radius with an intact ulna indicated no effect of low-intensity US using parameters typically employed in human beings, however [29].
- Other conditions: Pain and muscle spasm are additional indications for US therapy. With chronic injury, US can be administered before exercise to assist in the warm-up and provide some pain relief. Additionally, US may enhance calcium resorption. A clinical trial of people with calcific tendonitis of the shoulder indicated that the rate of calcium resorption was enhanced by US [30].

Contraindications and precautions

Tissue burns can occur if the intensity is too high or the transducer is held stationary, thereby concentrating energy in a small area. These factors put the patient at risk for cavitation, a phenomenon whereby bubbles of dissolved gas form in the tissues and grow during each rarefaction phase. When they burst, they release energy, which may cause damage to tissues.

Contraindications. Avoid direct exposure to cardiac pacemakers, the carotid sinus, cervical ganglia, eyes, ears, the heart, lumbar and abdominal areas in pregnant animals, near a malignant growth, the spinal cord if exposed by laminectomy, the testes, and contaminated wounds. As a safety measure, avoid the physes in immature animals.

Precautions. Exert precaution in areas with bony prominences, decreased blood circulation, acute injuries that should not receive heat, and areas of decreased sensation attributable to denervation or application of cold. When applying US over the paraspinal muscles, the transducer may be moved across the dorsal midline to change sides but the transducer should not dwell over the spine. The effects of US on bone cement are unknown. Precaution should be used over incision sites for the first 14 days to minimize the risk of dehiscence.

Equipment maintenance and safety

US equipment falls under the rules and regulations of the radiation safety performance standards of the US Food and Drug Administration (FDA). Verification of output accuracy and timer accuracy as well as verification of safety relating to the electrical components is advised on an annual basis or more often if the unit is used frequently (multiple times per day).

Treatment guidelines

The US beam is not conducted by air and is reflected at air-tissue interfaces. Consequently, a coupling medium must be placed between the sound head and the skin. Direct coupling is preferred. Water-soluble gel is spread on the skin, and the sound head is placed in contact with the gel. Commercial US gels are most practical. Coupling agents that are not recommended include substances that may irritate or penetrate through the skin, electroconductive gels, lanolin-based compounds, and petroleum gel. Mineral oil transmits US waves effectively (97% transmission) but is not as convenient as water-soluble gel to clean. If there are bony prominences or the surface to be treated is small, smaller transducers (1–2-cm diameter) are available.

The immersion method was popular before smaller transducer heads were available. Immersion can be considered when the surface to be treated is so uneven that direct contact is not possible. The limb is immersed in a pail of degassed water (tap water that has been allowed to sit for 4–24 hours), and the sound head is held in the water approximately 1 to 2 cm from the skin. Immersion does not heat as effectively as direct coupling; thus, the intensity is increased approximately 0.5 W/cm^2.

A commercially available coupling cushion, comparable to the stand-off pad used in diagnostic US, can be used when the surface of the area to be treated is not congruent with the surface of the sound head or when the additional distance through the pad allows the therapist to treat at the desired level. Surgical gloves filled with water do not transmit as well as commercial coupling pads [31].

Frequency. Frequency determines the depth of penetration. One megahertz heats at a depth of 2 to 5 cm and 3 MHz heats at a depth of 0.5 to 2 cm. Therapeutic levels of soft tissue heating have been documented in dogs for frequencies of 1 MHz [17] and 3 MHz [32]. Long wave (low-frequency) US refers to frequencies in the kilohertz range (eg, 0.75 MHz). That equipment has been used primarily in the United Kingdom [33]. Long-wave US is less attenuated and could offer advantages of penetrating deeper and passing through bone.

Intensity. Intensity is the rate of energy per unit area. Intensity on commercially available equipment typically ranges from 0.25 to 3.0 W/cm^2. The higher the intensity, the larger and faster the tissue temperature increases. Generally, intensities required to increase tissue temperature to a range of 40°C to 45°C are in the range of 1.0 to 2.0 W/cm^2 continuous wave heating for 5 to 10 minutes. If using US for acute injuries or open wounds, low intensity with the pulsed mode is recommended (eg, <0.3 W/cm^2 of 20% pulsed US) [28]. Most therapists use intensities that produce no sensation in human patients. Some dogs may indicate discomfort (mild vocalizing or avoidance movements) 5 to 10 minutes after commencing US. Any distress that dogs show should be assumed to be attributable to pain and verified by reducing the intensity or stopping.

Duty cycle. Duty cycle is the fraction of time that the sound is emitted during one pulse period. In continuous mode, energy is emitted continuously from the sound head. In pulsed mode, energy is delivered in an on/off manner. Typical duty cycles range from 0.05 (5%) to 0.5 (50%).

Duration of treatment. Duration of treatment is typically 4 minutes for an area the size of the sound head, with a recommended maximum area of four times the area of the sound head.

Treatment area. An area two to four times the size of the effective radiating area of the transducer head is recommended [23]. Increasing total area decreases the dosage. The speed at which the transducer is moved is recommended to be 4 cm/s. Moving the transducer too quickly may encourage the therapist to cover too large an area, resulting in insufficient heating. The transducer should be constantly moving to avoid overheating or tissue damage (cavitation) because of standing waves. Without motion, some tissues could receive an excessive amount of energy, because the US beam is nonuniform (hot spots).

Treatment schedule. A general guideline is that treatment may be administered daily initially and then less frequently as the condition improves. Bromiley [34] recommended that treatment be administered daily for up to 10 days but should not exceed two 10-day courses without a 3-week rest; however, this has not been validated.

ELECTRICAL STIMULATION
Basic Properties
Electrotherapy, or ES, has been used in human medicine for a variety of purposes, including improving ROM [35], increasing muscle strength [36], enhancing function [37], pain control [38], accelerating wound healing [39], edema reduction [40], and enhancing transdermal administration of medication (iontophoresis) [41]. This article focuses on two uses of ES: neuromuscular dysfunction and pain management. When using ES for neuromuscular dysfunction, such as weakness or deceased endurance, the goal is to depolarize a motor nerve and cause a muscle contraction. When using ES for pain management, the goal is to depolarize sensory nerves to suppress the pain.

Terminology relating to ES was ambiguous and has been standardized [42] to avoid confusion. The use of ES to stimulate a motor nerve and cause a muscle contraction is termed *neuromuscular electrical stimulation* (NMES). This is the most commonly used type of ES and includes all applications of ES for strengthening, except in cases of denervated muscle. The use of ES to excite denervated muscle directly, such as in patients with spinal cord injuries, is called electrical muscle stimulation (EMS). The term *transcutaneous electrical nerve stimulation* (TENS) is the use of an electrical stimulator for pain control.

Types of Stimulators

There are several hundred ES units on the market. Many claims of superiority of one machine over another seem to be unfounded. There are stimulators that are better suited for a particular use (ie, strengthening, pain reduction, edema reduction). Adequate knowledge of the devices and their capabilities is needed to make an informed decision about the purchase of an ES unit. Veterinary-specific devices (Fig. 2) have been developed and have canine and equine protocols.

Electrodes

There are many types of surface electrodes on the market. The main criteria in choosing electrodes are that they (1) should be flexible enough to conform to

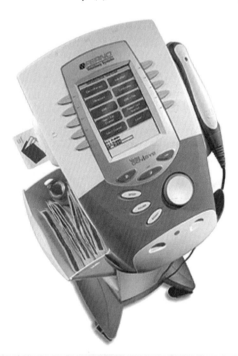

Fig. 2. Veterinary-specific therapeutic US electrical stimulator (Courtesy of Ferno Veterinary Systems, Wilmington, OH; with permission).

the tissue, (2) may be trimmed to a specific size, (3) have a low resistance, (4) are highly conductive, (5) may be used repeatedly, and 6) are inexpensive. There are many types of electrodes on the market; some are good for only a few uses, and some may be used more than 100 times (carbon-impregnated silicon rubber electrodes). Conductive performance of any electrode decreases over time. Electrodes require a medium to transmit current. Commonly used media include gels (disposable electrodes typically have gel pads already applied), sponges, or paper towels. Sponges and paper towels tend to dry out, and rewetting is necessary every 30 minutes. Electrodes should be of the appropriate size to stimulate the desired muscle without stimulating unwanted muscles in close proximity. The smaller the electrode, the higher is the current density and the more painful the stimulus may be.

Typical Parameters Available in Electrical Stimulation Devices
- Frequency: the rate of oscillation in cycles per second, expressed as pulses per seconds (pps) or hertz. Frequency may also be labeled as in terms of pulse rate or pulses per second or as frequency on stimulators.
- Phase or pulse duration (Fig. 3): the duration of a phase or a pulse, usually measured in microseconds
- Amplitude (see Fig. 3): the current value in a monophasic pulse or for any single phase of a biphasic pulse
- Waveform: the shape of the visual representation of pulsed current on a current-time plot or voltage-time plot. Wavforms can be symmetric, asymmetric, balanced, unbalanced, biphasic, monophasic, or polyphasic, for example.
- On/off time: the amount of time the stimulator is delivering current compared with the rest period between contractions, usually measured in seconds
- Polarity: when using direct current (DC), the electrode may be the anode (positive electrode) or cathode (negative electrode) type.

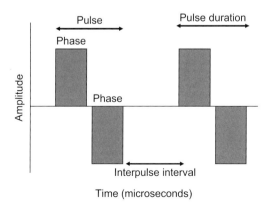

Fig. 3. Amplitude, phase, pulse, pulse duration, and interpulse interval for a biphasic pulsed current.

- Ramp: the time elapsed between the current being first applied to the patient and the current reaching its peak, usually measured in seconds

Recruitment

ES recruits muscle fibers in a different order than in a volitional contraction. ES tends to recruit more fast-twitch fibers with a submaximal contraction than with a volitional contraction [43]. An increase in pulse duration increases recruitment of smaller diameter motor units at the same depth. Increasing the amplitude or the pulse duration affects the strength of contraction because of recruitment of additional fibers. Increasing the frequency results in the existing motor units firing at a faster rate and increases the strength of contraction but also causes more rapid fatigue. Using the optimal frequency gives the optimal physiologic response while minimizing fatigue. This is commonly between 35 and 50 Hz. In a healthy individual, a maximal voluntary muscle contraction always produces greater torque, or strength of muscle contraction, than in an electrically induced contraction. In disease conditions or in patients recovering from surgery, however, an electrically induced muscle contraction may produce a stronger contraction than a volitional contraction [36].

Treatment Guidelines

NMES is used to minimize muscle atrophy in patients when weight-bearing exercises are contraindicated or not possible. For example, NMES may be used in patients recovering from the surgical stabilization of a cranial cruciate ligament injury or may be used in patients with prolonged limb disuse resulting from a femoral head and neck ostectomy.

Current Parameters for Strengthening

Optimal parameters have not been adequately studied; however, in one trial using the following parameters in dogs with postoperative extracapsular repairs for cruciate tears, atrophy was minimized compared with the control group [44]:

- Frequency generally between 25 and 50 Hz (this range has been shown to produce strong tetanic contractions while minimizing fatigue)
- Waveforms: many shapes are available with limited evidence of one being optimal. Many prefer a symmetric biphasic pulse, because some people report that this is more comfortable than other waveforms.
- Pulse duration between 100 and 400 microseconds
- Ramp up or down 2 to 4 seconds up to increase comfort and 1 to 3 seconds down
- On/off time at a ratio of 1:3 to 1:5; an example would be 10 seconds on and 40 seconds off.
- Frequency of treatment between three and seven times per week

Current Parameters for Pain Control

Optimal parameters have not been adequately studied; however, in one trial using the following parameters in dogs with chronic stifle osteoarthritis, peak vertical forces as measured by force plate were significantly improved 30, 60, 120, 150, and 180 minutes after treatment compared with pretreatment values [45]:

- Frequency generally between 50 and 150 Hz for acute pain and between 1 and 10 Hz for chronic pain; we used 50 to 150 Hz for chronic pain.
- Waveforms: there are many types on the market; commonly used waveforms include interferential, premodulated interferential, and various other pulsed alternating current (AC) and DC waveforms.
- Pulse or phase duration between 2 and 50 microseconds for acute pain and 100 and 400 microseconds for chronic pain
- On/off time: continuously on for 20 to 30 minutes for acute pain and 30 minutes for chronic pain
- Treatment may be performed daily.

Animal Reaction and Safety

Precautions should be taken to avoid injury to the handler and animal. A muzzle should be applied and the animal placed in lateral recumbency during the initial treatment. In some cases, sedation may be necessary if the animal is anxious. Treatment should only be administered under the supervision of trained personnel.

Preparation and Electrode Placement

The hair over the area to which ES is to be applied should be clipped to lower impedance. If the dog is short haired, this may not be necessary if the proper electrodes and coupling media are used. The skin should also be cleaned with alcohol before treatment to remove oils from the skin surface. When performing ES for muscle contraction, the electrodes are placed on the muscle to be stimulated. When performing ES for pain control, the electrodes are most commonly positioned around the painful area. An indelible marking pen may be used to draw a circle around the electrode for future placement.

Precautions and Contraindications

Avoid direct exposure to cardiac pacemakers, the carotid sinus, cervical ganglia, eyes, ears, the heart, lumbar and abdominal areas in pregnant animals, near a malignant growth, areas of decreased sensation, animals with seizure disorders, over areas of thrombosis or thrombophlebitis, and any time active motion is contraindicated [46].

Equipment Maintenance and Safety

Verification of output accuracy and timer accuracy as well as safety relating to the electrical components is advised on an annual basis.

References

[1] Heinrichs K. Superficial thermal modalities. In: Millis DL, Levine D, Taylor RA, editors. Canine rehabilitation and physical therapy. St. Louis, MO: WB Saunders; 2004. p. 277–88.
[2] Downer A. Physical therapy for animals. Springfield, IL: Charles C. Thomas; 1978.
[3] Blythe LL, Gannon JR, Craig AM. Physical therapy of training and racing injuries. In: Care of the racing greyhound. Portland, OR: Graphic Arts Center; 1994. p. 165–73.

[4] Steiss JE, McCauley L. Therapeutic ultrasound. In: Millis DL, Levine D, Taylor RA, editors. Canine rehabilitation and physical therapy. St. Louis, MO: WB Saunders; 2004. p. 324–36.

[5] Hayes K. Cryotherapy. In: Physical agents. 4th edition. Norwalk, CT: Appleton & Lange; 1993. p. 49–59.

[6] Hayes K. Conductive heat. In: Physical agents. 4th edition. Norwalk, CT: Appleton & Lange; 1993. p. 9–15.

[7] Oestmann RE, Downer AH. Downer's physical therapy procedures: therapeutic modalities. 6th edition. Springfield, IL: Charles C. Thomas; 2004.

[8] Prentice WE. Therapeutic modalities in sports medicine. St. Louis, MO: Mosby–Year Book; 1995.

[9] Michlovitz S. Thermal agents in rehabilitation. 2nd edition. Philadelphia: FA Davis Co; 1990.

[10] Belanger AY. Evidence-based guide to therapeutic physical agents. Baltimore (MD): Lippincott Williams & Wilkins; 2002.

[11] Vannatta ML, Millis DL, Adair S, et al. Effects of cryotherapy on temperature change in caudal thigh muscles of dogs. In: Marcellin DJ, editor. Proceedings of the Third International Symposium on Rehabilitation and Physical Therapy in Veterinary Medicine [abstract]. Raleigh (NC): Department of Continuing Education, North Carolina State College of Veterinary Medicine; 2004. p. 205.

[12] Kaneps AJ. Superficial cold and heat. In: Levine D, Millis DL, editors. Proceedings of the Second International Symposium on Rehabilitation and Physical Therapy in Veterinary Medicine. Knoxville (TN): University of Tennessee, University Outreach and Continuing Education; 2002. p. 41–7.

[13] Akgun K, Korpinar MA, Kalkan MT, et al. Temperature changes in superficial and deep tissue layers with respect to time of cold gel pack application in dogs. Yonsei Med J 2004;45: 711–8.

[14] Petrov R, MacDonald MH, Tesch AM, et al. Influence of topically applied cold treatment on core temperature and cell viability in equine superficial digital flexor tendons. Am J Vet Res 2003;64:835–44.

[15] Hayes K. Hydrotherapy. In: Physical agents. 4th edition. Norwalk (CT): Appleton & Lange; 1993. p. 17–25.

[16] Christie RV, Binger CAL. An experimental study of diathermy: IV. Evidence for the penetration of high frequency currents through the living body. J Exp Med 1927;46:715–34.

[17] Steiss J, Adams C. Rate of temperature increase in canine muscle during 1 MHz ultrasound therapy: deleterious effect of hair coat. Am J Vet Res 1999;60:76–80.

[18] Robertson VJ, Baker KG. A review of therapeutic ultrasound: effectiveness studies. Phys Ther 2001;81:1339–50.

[19] Ebenbichler G. Critical evaluation of ultrasound therapy. Wien Med Wochenschr 1994;144:51–3.

[20] Gam A, Johannsen F. Ultrasound therapy in musculoskeletal disorders: a meta-analysis. Pain 1995;63:85–91.

[21] Feine J, Lund J. An assessment of the efficacy of physical therapy and physical modalities for the control of chronic musculoskeletal pain. Pain 1997;71:15–23.

[22] Draper DO. Letter to the editor. Phys Ther 2002;82:190.

[23] Draper DO, Castel JC, Castel D. Rate of temperature increase in human muscle during 1 MHz and 3 MHz continuous ultrasound. J Orthop Sports Phys Ther 1995;22:142–50.

[24] Enwemeka CS, Rodriguez O, Mendosa S. The biomechanical effects of low-intensity ultrasound on healing tendons. Ultrasound Med Biol 1990;16(8):801–7.

[25] Saini NS, Roy KS, Bansal PS, et al. A preliminary study on the effect of ultrasound therapy on the healing of surgically severed Achilles tendons in five dogs. J Vet Med A Physiol Pathol Clin Med 2002;49:321–8.

[26] Loonam JE, Millis DL. The effect of therapeutic ultrasound on tendon heating and extensibility. In: Proceedings of the 30th Annual Conference of the Veterinary Orthopedic Society. Newmarket (NH): Veterinary Orthopedic Society; 2002. p. 69.

[27] Dyson M, Pond JB, Joseph J, et al. The stimulation of tissue regeneration by means of ultrasound. Clin Sci 1968;35:273–85.

[28] Warden SJ. A new direction for ultrasound therapy in sports medicine. Sports Med 2003;33:95–107.

[29] Lidbetter D, Millis DL. Effect of ultrasound stimulation on bone healing in dogs [abstract]. Vet Comp Orthop Traumatol 2002;15(2).

[30] Ebenbichler GR, Erdogmus CB, Resch KL, et al. Ultrasound therapy for calcific tendinitis of the shoulder. N Engl J Med 1999;340:1533–8.

[31] Klucinec B, Scheidler M, Denegen C, et al. Transmissivity of coupling agents used to deliver ultrasound through indirect methods. J Orthop Sports Phys Ther 2000;30:263–9.

[32] Levine D, Millis DL, Mynatt T. Effects of 3.3 MHz ultrasound on caudal thigh muscle temperature in dogs. Vet Surg 2001;30:170–4.

[33] Bradnock B, Law HT, Roscor K. A quantitative comparative assessment of the immediate response to high frequency ultrasound and low frequency ultrasound (longwave therapy) in the treatment of acute ankle sprains. Physiotherapy 1996;82:78–84.

[34] Bromiley M. Physiotherapy in veterinary medicine. Oxford, UK: Blackwell Scientific Publications; 1991.

[35] de Kroon JR, Ijzerman MJ, Lankhorst GJ, et al. Electrical stimulation of the upper limb in stroke: stimulation of the extensors of the hand vs. alternate stimulation of flexors and extensors. Am J Phys Med Rehabil 2004;83:592–600.

[36] Fitzgerald GK, Piva SR, Irrgang JJ. A modified neuromuscular electrical stimulation protocol for quadriceps strength training following anterior cruciate ligament reconstruction. J Orthop Sports Phys Ther 2003;33:492–501.

[37] Popovic MB, Popovic DB, Sinkjaer T, et al. Clinical evaluation of functional electrical therapy in acute hemiplegic subjects. J Rehabil Res Dev 2003;40:443–53.

[38] Rakel B, Frantz R. Effectiveness of transcutaneous electrical nerve stimulation on postoperative pain with movement. J Pain 2003;4:455–64.

[39] Houghton PE, Kincaid CB, Lovell M, et al. Effect of electrical stimulation on chronic leg ulcer size and appearance. Phys Ther 2003;83:17–28.

[40] Faghri PD, Van Meerdervort HF, Glaser RM, et al. Electrical stimulation-induced contraction to reduce blood stasis during arthroplasty. IEEE Trans Rehabil Eng 1997;5:62–9.

[41] Nirschl RP, Rodin DM, Ochiai DH, et al. Iontophoretic administration of dexamethasone sodium phosphate for acute epicondylitis. A randomized, double-blinded, placebo-controlled study. Am J Sports Med 2003;31:189–95.

[42] American Physical Therapy Association, Section on Clinical Electrophysiology. Electrotherapeutic terminology in physical therapy. Alexandria, VA: American Physical Therapy Association; 2000. p. 36–9.

[43] Knaflitz M, Merletti R, De Luca CJ. Inference of motor unit recruitment order in voluntary and electrically elicited contractions. J Appl Physiol 1990;68(4):1657–67.

[44] Millis DL, Levine D, Weigel JP. A preliminary study of early physical therapy following surgery for cranial cruciate ligament rupture in dogs [abstract]. Vet Surg 1997;26:434.

[45] Levine D, Johnston KD, Price MN, et al. The effect of TENS on osteoarthritic pain in the stifle of dogs. In: Levine D, Millis DL, editors. Proceedings of the Second International Symposium on Rehabilitation and Physical Therapy in Veterinary Medicine. Knoxville (TN): University of Tennessee, University Outreach and Continuing Education; 2002. p. 199.

[46] Johnson J, Levine D. Electrical stimulation. In: Millis DL, Levine D, Taylor RA, editors. Canine rehabilitation and physical therapy. St. Louis, MO: WB Saunders; 2004. p. 289–302.

Vet Clin Small Anim 35 (2005) 1335–1355

VETERINARY CLINICS
SMALL ANIMAL PRACTICE

ELSEVIER
SAUNDERS

Emerging Modalities in Veterinary Rehabilitation

Darryl L. Millis, MS, DVM, CCRP[a],*,
David Francis, MS, DVM[b],
Caroline Adamson, MSPT, CCRP[c]

[a]Department of Small Animal Clinical Sciences, College of Veterinary Medicine, University of Tennessee, 2407 River Drive, Knoxville, TN 37996, USA
[b]Vancouver, Canada
[c]Alameda East Veterinary Hospital, 9770 East Alameda Avenue, Denver, CO 80247, USA

Many new modalities have been introduced in human and veterinary physical rehabilitation. In many instances, there is sound theory of how they may impact the physiology of various cells, tissues, or organs. Nevertheless, the impact of these modalities in diseased or injured tissues, or in the entire body, is not known in some cases; therefore, it is inappropriate to make the assumption that the modalities may have similar effects on diseased and healthy tissues. Studies of the clinical effects of various modalities are often lacking, and sometimes, existing studies are flawed in terms of study design and the conclusions drawn. This article reviews some of the modalities that have been introduced recently in human and veterinary rehabilitation. Low-level laser, phototherapy, and extracorporeal shock wave treatment, in particular, are discussed.

LOW-LEVEL LASER THERAPY

The concept of using light for therapeutic purposes, called phototherapy, originates from the belief that the sun and other sources of light, such as infrared and ultraviolet light, have therapeutic benefit. Low-power laser devices, a form of artificial light, were first used as a form of therapy more than 30 years ago. The term *laser* is an acronym for Light Amplification by Stimulated Emission of Radiation. Many different types of lasers are available for medical and industrial purposes. The types of lasers used for rehabilitation purposes, commonly known as low-level laser therapy (LLLT), are also called cold lasers. Surgical lasers are high power and capable of thermal destruction of cells and tissues,

*Corresponding author. E-mail address: dmillis@utk.edu (D.L. Millis).

0195-5616/05/$ – see front matter
doi:10.1016/j.cvsm.2005.08.007

whereas those used in rehabilitation are low power and help to modulate cellular processes, known as photobiomodulation.

Properties of Lasers

Basic light sources emit electromagnetic radiation that is visible to the normal eye. Natural light sources, such as sunlight, are forms of electromagnetic radiation. Lasers are fabricated sources that emit radiation in the form of a flow of photons. The process of light emission begins with the activation of electrons in the laser component, generally helium-neon or gallium, aluminum, and arsenide, to an excited state [1]. When the electrons drop from their excited state to their ground state, photons are emitted. Although some photons are absorbed by the laser chamber wall, others stimulate the emission of other photons, and, together, they travel in a chamber, amplifying the stimulated emission and leading to a chain reaction. Some of these photons are released through a semireflective mirror to form a beam of light.

The major difference between laser light and the light generated by normal sources is that laser light is monochromatic, coherent, and collimated. Monochromatic means that all light produced by the laser is of one wavelength and a single color. The coherent properties of light mean that the photons travel in the same phase and direction. Laser light is also collimated, which means that there is minimal divergence in the laser beam over a distance. These properties allow low-level laser light to penetrate the surface of the skin with no heating effect, no damage to the skin, and few or no side effects.

Using a monochromatic light source allows the absorption of the light to be targeted to specific wavelength-dependent chromophores [1]. The properties of coherence and collimation allow the light to be focused precisely on small areas of the body.

Lasers are classified according to the power that is produced. Class 1 lasers are mild and include supermarket scanners and post office readers. Class 2 lasers are always visible and include items such as laser pointers and, occasionally, therapy lasers. Class 3A lasers are therapy lasers that produce visible light, whereas class 3B lasers are therapy lasers and survey lasers that produce nonvisible light. Class 4 lasers are surgical lasers and industrial cutting lasers.

Most lasers used in physical rehabilitation are class 3A lasers that normally would not produce injury if viewed momentarily with the unaided eye. An example is the helium-neon (HeNe) laser that has a radiant power above 1 mW but not exceeding 5 mW. Class 3B lasers can cause severe eye injuries if the beams are viewed directly, or if the reflection of the laser light is viewed, and include visible HeNe lasers above 5 mW but not exceeding 500 mW of radiant power.

LLLT devices are low power, typically less than 100 mW, and do not heat tissues. In comparison, surgical lasers have energy ranging from 3000 to 10,000 mW. LLLT devices typically have small treatment beam diameters up to 1 cm. They are most effective for surface level conditions. They do not penetrate deep tissues or large joint capsules. Light that is not absorbed by water, hemoglobin, or melanin is gradually attenuated as it passes through tissues. The level of scattering and absorption is such that HeNe (632.8 nm) laser light loses about one-third of its intensity during the first 0.5 to 1 mm of tissue depth [2]. The depth (in centimeters) at which the energy of a laser beam is 36% of its original value is termed the *first depth of penetration* [3]. This attenuation of energy is derived by dividing the original value by a constant, 2.78. Subsequent depths of penetration can be determined by dividing by 2.78 again; therefore, the level of energy at the second depth of penetration is 13%. Because biologic effects may be noted with relatively low energy (0.01 J/cm^2), lasers that typically deliver 1 to 4 J/cm^2 may penetrate up to 0.5 to 2 cm before the energy level is so low that they have no effect. Because animal skin is different from human skin, and most areas have hair that may prevent penetration of the laser light, additional research is needed in small animal practice to determine the depth of penetration.

In addition to the direct effects of lasers at a particular depth of tissue, indirect effects may be seen. These cellular and tissue effects are decreased in the deeper tissues and are catalyzed by the energy absorption in the more superficial tissues.

The basic types of lasers used for LLLT are gaseous HeNe and gallium-arsenide (GaAs) or gallium-aluminum-arsenide (GaAlAs) semiconductor or diode lasers. HeNe lasers emit a visible red light with a wavelength of 632.8 nm, whereas GaAs and GaAlAs emit invisible light near the infrared band with a wavelength of 820 to 904 nm. The wavelengths of photons determine their effect. Longer wavelengths are more resistant to scattering than are shorter ones; therefore, GaAs and GaAlAs lasers penetrate more effectively (direct effect at up to 2 cm, indirect effect to 5 cm) than HeNe lasers (direct effect up to 0.5 cm, indirect effect up to 1 cm) because there is less absorption or scattering in the epidermis and dermis. Light waves in the near-infrared ranges penetrate the deepest of all light waves in the visible spectrum (Box 1). Although this spectrum of light is not visible, commercial lasers have a light-emitting diode that allows the therapist to see where the laser light is aimed. Most lasers have a finite lifespan that generally varies from 5000 to 20,000 hours.

Box 1: Wavelengths of various components of the electromagnetic spectrum

AM radio: 10, 000 cm

Television and FM radio: 100 cm

Microwave: 10 cm

Infrared light: 700 nm

Ultraviolet light: 10 nm

X-rays: 1 nm

Biologic Effects of Low-Level Lasers

Most studies of laser use in rehabilitation have focused on wound healing and pain management; however, information regarding their efficacy in reducing pain or promoting tissue repair is incomplete [4]. Recently, interest has been generated in the United States regarding their use in treating humans, and a natural extension has been an interest in treating animals. In evaluating the potential usefulness of LLLT in rehabilitation, the reader is encouraged to be critical of studies that have been performed and should evaluate these studies in light of recent advances in laser technology and the application of new information. Until recently, low-energy lasers were not approved for medical treatment in the United States. As more evidence becomes available, they will most likely be used increasingly.

Most of the potential responses of cells and tissues to laser energy have been studied in in vitro models. Photons delivered to the cells and tissues trigger biologic changes within the body. Photons are absorbed by chromophores and respiratory chain enzymes (cytochromes) within the mitochondria and at the cell membrane, resulting in oxygen production and the formation of proton gradients across the cell and mitochondrial membranes. The enzyme flavomononucleotide is activated and initiates the production of ATP. DNA production is also stimulated. Changes in cell membrane permeability occur. Photons also seem to affect tissues by activating enzymes that trigger biochemical reactions in the body. Because cellular metabolism and growth are stimulated, lasers have the potential to accelerate tissue repair and cell growth of structures such as tendons, ligaments, and muscles. Although low doses of laser energy appear to stimulate tissues, higher doses may actually inhibit responses such as tissue healing.

Wound Healing

Laser light stimulates fibroblast development and may affect collagen production to repair tissues. Laser light may also accelerate angiogenesis and increase the formation of new capillaries in damaged tissues, possibly improving the rate of wound healing; therefore, laser therapy may aid healing of open wounds and burns. There is an increased growth factor response within cells and tissues, which may be related to increased ATP and protein synthesis. Laser light therapy causes vasodilation and may also improve lymphatic drainage. This effect may result in decreased edema and swelling caused by bruising or inflammation.

One study reported the results in 100 clinical cases in which healing wounds were treated with LLLT [5]. There was a marked increase in collagen formation, increased vasodilation, and accelerated DNA synthesis. These researchers recommended 1 J/cm^2 of laser treatment. A statistical meta-analysis was performed to determine the overall treatment effects of laser phototherapy on tissue repair [4]. After a literature search was performed, the effectiveness of laser treatment was calculated from each study using standard procedures. Thirty-four peer-reviewed articles met the inclusion criteria for tissue repair. There was a positive effect of laser phototherapy on tissue repair. Collagen formation, the rate of healing, tensile strength, the time needed for wound closure, tensile stress, the number and rate of degranulation of mast cells, and flap survival were improved with laser therapy. Laser treatment with a wavelength of 632.8 nm had the greatest effect, whereas 780 nm had the least effect. This review article concluded that LLLT was an effective treatment for tissue repair.

LLLT may also be beneficial for difficult wounds in metabolically compromised patients. Laser photostimulation accelerated wound healing in diabetic rats in one study [6]. Diabetes was induced in male rats by streptozotocin injection, and two 6-mm diameter circular wounds were created on either side of the spine. The left wound of each animal was treated with a 632.8-nm HeNe laser at a dose of 1.0 J/cm^2 5 days per week until the wounds closed (3 weeks). There was a marginal increase of biomechanical properties in the laser-treated wounds, including an increase in maximum load (16%), stress (16%), strain (27%), energy absorption (47%), and toughness (84%) in a comparison with control wounds. The amount of total collagen was significantly increased in laser-treated wounds. It was concluded that laser photostimulation promoted tissue repair by accelerating collagen production and promoting overall connective tissue stability in healing wounds of diabetic rats.

Another study reviewed the literature regarding the in vitro and in vivo effects of LLLT on the wound-healing process, especially in diabetic patients [7]. Although many of the in vivo studies lacked specific information on dosimetric data and appropriate controls, the data from appropriately designed studies indicated that LLLT should be considered as an adjuvant therapy for refractory wound-healing disorders, including in diabetic patients.

LLLT may also be useful for other forms of soft-tissue injury, such as ligament healing. In one study, 24 rats underwent surgical transection of the right medial collateral ligament, whereas eight underwent a sham operation [8]. After surgery, 16 received a single dose of the GaAlAs laser to the transected ligament for 7.5 minutes or 15 minutes, and eight served as controls with treatment from a placebo laser. The sham group did not receive any treatment. The ligaments were biomechanically tested 3 or 6 weeks postoperation. The ultimate tensile strength and stiffness in the laser and sham groups were larger than in controls. The laser and sham groups had improved stiffness from 3 to 6 weeks. It was concluded that a single dose of LLLT improved the biomechanical properties of healing in the repair of medial collateral ligaments 3 and 6 weeks after injury.

The results from other controlled and blinded studies have been less clear regarding the efficacy of LLLT for the treatment of wounds [2]. Studies in laboratory animals have suggested that LLLT may improve healing during the early stages of wound healing, but the effect may not result in improved total healing time [9,10]. Another large review article did not find unequivocal evidence that LLLT was beneficial for the treatment of wound healing [11]. A randomized clinical trial of LLLT for the treatment of ankle sprains in humans found that laser treatment was not effective [12].

Bone and Cartilage Effects

Bone and cartilage may be affected by laser treatment. In one study of bone healing, rats received a defect to a femur [13]. The rats were then treated for 12 sessions (4.8 J/cm^2 per session, 28 day follow-up) or three sessions (4.8 J/cm^2 per session, 7 day follow-up) with 40 mW 830 nm laser light. Treatments were applied three times per week, and two other groups served as untreated controls. The rats were sacrificed on day 7 or 28 after surgery. Although there were significant differences between the treated and control animals regarding the area of mineralized bone at 7 days, there were no differences at 28 days. It was suggested that LLLT may have some effect on early bone repair.

Another study evaluated osteochondral lesions of the knee treated intraoperatively with LLLT in rabbits [14]. Bilateral osteochondral lesions were created in the femoral medial condyles. All of the left lesions underwent immediate stimulation using a GaAlAs laser (780 nm), whereas the right knees were untreated and served as a control group. After 24 weeks, the condyles were examined histomorphometrically. The condyle treated with the laser had better cell morphology and repair of osteocartilaginous tissue. A more complete review of the effects of LLLT for bone repair has been published [15]. Most of the research regarding bone healing has been performed in cell culture or rodent models. More study on the laser properties, wavelength, and energy dosage is needed, alone with improved study design.

The effect of LLLT on cartilage has been investigated. One study evaluated whether intraoperative laser biostimulation could enhance healing of cartilaginous lesions of the knee in rabbits [16]. Bilateral chondral lesions were created in the medial femoral condyles. The lesion in the left knee of each animal was treated intraoperatively using the diode GaAlAs 780-nm laser (300 J/cm^2, 1 W, 300 Hz, 10 minutes), whereas the right knee was untreated. Cartilage was then examined at 2, 6, or 12 weeks after surgery. The rabbits receiving LLLT had progressive filling with fibrous tissue of the cartilaginous lesion, whereas no changes were apparent in the untreated group.

LLLT may also help maintain the health of cartilage during periods of disuse and immobilization. The influence of LLLT (632.8 nm, He-Ne, 13 J/cm^2, three times a week) on the articular cartilage of rabbit stifles immobilized for 13 weeks was examined in one study [17]. The number of chondrocytes and the depth of articular cartilage in the treated rabbits were significantly higher than in the sham-treated group. The cartilage surface of the sham-treated group was rough and fibrillated, whereas the surface of the experimental group was intermediate between that of a nonimmobilized control group and the sham-treated group. It was concluded that low-power He-Ne laser irradiation reduced the adverse effects on the articular cartilage of rabbits immobilized for 13 weeks. Another study evaluated the use of 810 nm LLLT on bone and cartilage during joint immobilization of rat knees [18]. Three groups of rats received 3.9 W/cm^2, 5.8 W/cm^2, or sham treatment. After six treatments over a 2-week period, tissues were harvested for testing. The results indicated that cartilage stiffness, assessed by indentation testing, was preserved in both LLLT groups.

Analgesia and Pain Management

The results of studies of pain management with use of the laser have been controversial. Nevertheless, the studies performed have resulted in approval of 635 nm low-level lasers for the management of chronic minor pain, such as osteoarthritis and muscle spasms, by the US Food and Drug Administration (FDA). Laser therapy may have some analgesic effects by blocking pain transmission to the brain. Some studies have shown a change in the conduction latencies of the radial and median nerve after LLLT [19,20], whereas others have shown no effect [21]. Laser treatment may also increase the release of endorphins and enkephalins, which may further provide analgesic benefits. Laser therapy has been used to stimulate muscle trigger points and acupuncture points, which may provide pain relief.

Although the precise mechanism by which LLLT may provide analgesia is unknown, several studies have investigated possible mechanisms. One study evaluated the effects of diode laser irradiation of peripheral nerves [22]. The response was evaluated by monitoring neuronal discharges from the L5 dorsal nerve roots elicited by application of various stimuli to the hind-paws of rats, including brush, pinch, cold, heat stimulation, and chemical stimulation by injection of turpentine. Diode laser irradiation (830 nm, 40 mW, 3 minutes, continuous wave) of the saphenous nerve significantly inhibited neuronal discharges elicited by pinch, cold, heat, and chemical stimulation, but not discharges induced by brush stimulation. These data suggest that laser irradiation may selectively inhibit nociceptive neuronal activities.

Another study evaluated the effect of LLLT on the head of rats [23]. Rats received various combinations of laser energy (0, 6.4, and 12 J/cm^2) and naloxone (0, 5, and 10 mg/kg) before a hot plate test. LLLT (820 nm, pulsing) was applied to the rats' skulls. Hind-paw lick latencies (in seconds) in response to the hot plate test were recorded immediately, 30 minutes, and 24 hours after the administration of treatment. When the animals were tested immediately following laser irradiation at 12 J/cm^2, significant analgesia resulted. Treatment with naloxone at either dose antagonized this effect, but naloxone produced no significant hyperalgesia when given alone. The findings suggest that opioid peptide mechanisms may mediate the analgesic action of LLLT on the cranium.

A meta-analysis was performed to evaluate the effect of LLLT on pain relief [4]. Nine articles met the inclusion criteria for pain control. The overall treatment effect for pain control was positive. Another review of LLLT with location-specific doses for pain from chronic joint disorders suggested that some benefit might be derived from the use of lasers [24]. A literature search identified 88 randomized controlled trials, of which 20 included patients with chronic joint disease. LLLT was applied within the suggested dose range to the knee or temporomandibular joint capsule to reduce pain in chronic joint disorders. The results showed a mean difference in change of pain using a visual analogue scale by 45.6% in favor of LLLT. Global status was also improved for 33.4% more patients in the LLLT group. Although LLLT appeared to reduce pain in patients with chronic joint diseases, the heterogeneity in the patient samples, treatment procedures, and trial design calls for cautious interpretation of the results.

A randomized, double-blind study of 100 patients with neck and shoulder pain indicated that 90% of the patients in the treatment group had at least a 30% improvement in the degree of pain relief compared with 14% of the patients in the placebo group [25]. Most patients had a reduction of their pain immediately after treatment, and the improvement was typically maintained for 24 hours. A follow-up study of another 100 patients indicated that 65% of the treated patients had an improvement of their pain, whereas 12% of untreated patients improved.

Treatment of Osteoarthritis with Low-Level Laser Therapy

LLLT has been used for the treatment of osteoarthritis in humans. The effect of laser therapy on osteoarthritis of the knee was investigated in a double-blind study [26]. One group received infrared laser (GaAlAs) treatment, and the other received HeNe laser treatment. Patients were treated for 15 minutes twice daily for 10 days. The total dose for each session was 10.3 J for the HeNe group and 11.1 J for the GaAlAs group. The laser-treated groups were significantly less painful when compared with the placebo groups, but there was no difference between the HeNe and GaAlAs groups. The Disability Index Questionnaire also revealed an improvement in the laser groups. Patients receiving laser treatment had less pain for 2 months to 1 year after treatment.

Laser treatment was also performed on 20 human patients with osteoarthritis of the knee, ranging from 42 to 60 years of age [27]. All of the patients had previously received conservative treatment with poor results. The laser device used for this treatment was a pulsed infrared diode laser with an 810-nm wavelength. The device was used once per day for 5 consecutive days followed by a 2-day rest interval. The total number of applications was 12 sessions. Laser treatment was performed on five periarticular tender points for 2 minutes each. Pain relief and functional ability were assessed using a numerical rating scale, self-assessment by the patient, an index of severity for osteoarthritis of the knee, and analgesic requirements for comfort. There was significant improvement in pain relief and quality of life in 70% of patients when compared with their previous status, but there was no significant change in range of motion of the knee. Although the investigators indicated that laser treatment was beneficial, there was no untreated control group; therefore, the results should be interpreted with caution.

A double-blind randomized study was conducted on 90 patients with osteoarthritis of the knee to evaluate a GaAs laser in combination with 30 minutes of exercise [28]. One group received 5 minutes of LLLT, with 3 J delivered. Another group was treated for 3 minutes and received 2 J, whereas a third group received placebo laser therapy and exercise. Patients received a total of 10 treatments and were studied for 14 weeks. Patients receiving laser treatment had significantly improved pain, function, and quality of life measures after treatment and improved scores when compared with the placebo laser group.

A similar randomized, placebo-controlled study of 60 patients with osteoarthritis of the knee indicated no significant improvement using 50 mW, 830 nm, GaAlAs LLLT at 3 weeks or 6 months [29]. In that study, patients received 3 or 1.5 J per painful joint or placebo laser treatment five times per week, with 10 total treatments.

Low-Level Laser Therapy and the Spinal Cord

Spinal cord injuries can be devastating to patients of all species. Recently, the effects of LLLT on nerve tissue have been investigated [30]. In an initial study, laminectomy and transection of the spinal cord at T12-L1 were performed in 17 dogs. An autograft of the sciatic nerve was implanted in the injured area. Ten dogs received LLLT for 20 days, and the others did not. The seven that did not receive LLLT were paralyzed, whereas the 10 treated dogs stood up between 7 to 9 weeks and walked between 9 to 12 weeks. The treated dogs did not have prominent scar tissue, and there were new axons and blood vessels originating in the spinal tissue and extending into the graft.

Subsequent studies in rat sciatic nerve injuries indicated that there was increased functional activity, decreased scar tissue formation, decreased degeneration of motor neurons, and increased axonal growth and myelinization with LLLT applied to the spinal cord immediately after wounding and for 30 minutes daily for 21 days using the 16-mW, 632-nm, HeNe laser [31]. The study suggested that LLLT applied directly to the spinal cord might improve the recovery from corresponding peripheral nerve injuries. A study of patients with incomplete peripheral nerve or brachial plexus injuries present for 6 months to several years indicated that LLLT resulted in progressive improvement of peripheral nerve function [30].

Application of Low-Level Laser Therapy

Before applying LLLT to a patient, two fundamental attributes must be established. First, the type of laser must be known as well as the wavelength. The output power must also be known. Based on these attributes and the problem to be treated, the dose must be calculated. Unfortunately, the optimal wavelengths, intensities, and dosages have not been studied adequately in animals, and information obtained in humans is difficult to interpret because of different conditions and treatment regimens. Power is measured in watts and is often expressed as milliwatts. Power density is the power delivered under the area of the probe. One watt is equivalent to one joule per second. The energy density is the amount of energy, or dose, per square centimeter of tissue. The difference between the power density and the energy density is the time, with power density expressed as W/cm^2 and energy density expressed as J/cm^2. The greater the power density and higher the wavelength, the deeper the penetration through tissues. More laser dosage is not better, and overdosing may retard the desired effect.

The three variables for lasers used for LLLT are (1) the wavelength (typically in the infrared or near-infrared range of 600–1000 nm), (2) the number of watts or milliwatts (usually between 5 and 600 mW), and (3) the number of seconds to deliver joules of energy (1 to 8 J of energy are typically applied to treat various conditions). With these factors known, the length of time needed to hold the laser on a point to deliver the appropriate joules of energy must be calculated. For example, if a 904-nm laser with a maximum output power of 250 mW is used, it will take 4 seconds to deliver 1 J as follows:

$$0.250\,W = 1\,J/x \text{ seconds}$$
$$(0.250\,W)(x \text{ seconds}) = 1\,J$$
$$x \text{ seconds} = 1\,J/0.250\,W$$
$$x = 4 \text{ seconds}$$

With this particular laser, it will be necessary to hold the laser on one point for 4 seconds to deliver 1 J of energy.

LLLT is generally administered with a handheld probe, with a small beam area that is useful to treat small surfaces (Fig. 1). Laser energy may be applied with the laser probe in contact with the skin, which eliminates reflection and minimizes beam divergence, or with the probe not held in contact. With the noncontact method, it is necessary to hold the probe perpendicular to the treatment area to minimize wave reflection and beam divergence. The appropriate dosage may be applied to larger areas by administering the calculated dose to each individual site in a grid fashion, or by slowly moving the probe over the entire surface, being certain to distribute the energy evenly to each site.

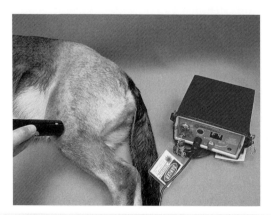

Fig. 1. Application of LLLT.

Regardless, the probe should be held perpendicular to the skin. A coupling medium is not necessary, as in ultrasound, because the laser beam is not attenuated by air.

To maximize laser application, the hair should be clipped, because 50% to 99% of the light may be absorbed by hair. Little is known about the transmission of laser light to deeper tissues in darker dogs, but HeNe laser energy is likely to be absorbed because of the pigment. Any iodine or povidone iodine should be washed off the area. Any topical medications, especially corticosteroids, should be removed. The therapist should wear protective ear wear, because damage may occur to the retina if the laser shines into the eyes.

LLLT has been used for the treatment of osteoarthritis, muscle, ligament, and tendon injuries, ulcerations and open wounds, and postsurgical and soft-tissue trauma. Contraindications and precautions to LLLT include pregnancy, treatment over open fontanels or growth plates of immature animals, treatment over malignancies, treatment directly into the cornea, and treatment over photosensitive areas of the skin [1].

Summary

Low-level lasers may be a potentially useful tool in veterinary rehabilitation. Although their use remains controversial, several studies have demonstrated a benefit using LLLT. Especially promising for their use in veterinary rehabilitation are studies showing preservation of cartilage properties with treatment, improvement in peripheral nerve injuries, and efficacy as a possible adjunct to managing pain, such as in patients with osteoarthritis. LLLT also appears to have some benefit in early wound healing. Regardless of whether the use of LLLT for this indication is cost effective, LLLT is noninvasive, and there are no reported side effects when it is used properly.

EXTRACORPOREAL SHOCK WAVE THERAPY

Extracorporeal shock wave therapy (ESWT) has been used for the treatment of renal calculi in humans since 1980 [32,33]. Investigators noted changes in the pelvis as a result of shock waves striking the pelvis [32]. Since that time, orthopedic applications for which shock wave therapy has been found to be useful in humans include delayed or nonunion fractures, plantar fasciitis, lateral epicondylitis, Achilles and patellar tendonitis, and, with limited experience, osteoarthritis. Focal ESWT is currently approved by the FDA for use in chronic heel pain (plantar fasciitis) and tennis elbow (lateral epicondylitis). Other potential applications include the use of ESWT to provide analgesia for persons with avascular necrosis of the femoral head, to treat calcified tendonitis of the shoulder, and to stabilize loose press-fit total hip replacements [34–46]. Patients with humeral epicondylitis or plantar fasciitis tend to respond better to ESWT if the condition is chronic (>35 months) in nature rather than acute (3 to 12 months) [47]. Similar findings may be identified in dogs with osteoarthritis.

In veterinary medicine, ESWT has been used in horses for the treatment of suspensory ligament desmitis, tendinopathies, navicular disease, back pain, osteoarthritis, and stress fractures [48,49]. Although the treatment of dogs with shock wave therapy is relatively new, tendonitis, desmitis, spondylosis, non-union fractures, and osteoarthritis have all been treated.

Shock Wave Characteristics

Extracorporeal shock waves are acoustic waves initiated outside the body. Shock waves are high-energy, high-amplitude acoustic pressure waves (20–100 megapascals [MPa]) (Fig. 2). Shock waves are characterized by an extremely short build-up time of approximately 5 to 10 nanoseconds with an exponential decay to baseline with a negative deflection of approximately 10 MPa. The entire wave cycle time is approximately 300 nanoseconds [32,48,49].

There are three primary methods of generating shock waves: electrohydraulic, electromagnetic, and piezoelectric [50]. All of these techniques produce shock waves in a fluid medium by converting electrical energy to mechanical energy. Shock waves behave like sound waves in tissue in that the waves travel through soft tissue and fluid and release their energy into the tissues when a change in tissue density is encountered, such as the interface between bone and ligament. When a shock wave travels through the target area, very high pressures build up for a short period, energy is released, and the pressure returns to normal. The larger the change in impedance, the greater the energy released. This energy release is thought to stimulate healing. Shock waves should not be focused on gas-filled cavities or organs because of the potential damage to surrounding tissues that may occur as a result of the release of significant energy [40].

In addition to the methods of producing extracorporeal shock waves, there are two primary methods to deliver the energy. Focused shock waves have the ability to focus the energy to different tissue depths. The shock waves are focused by means of a parabola so that they may be delivered to a relatively focused depth up to 110 mm. With this form of shock wave, the energy may be

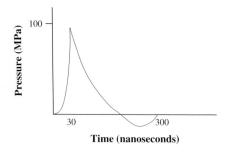

Fig. 2. Profile of an extracorporeal shock wave. Note the rapid rise in energy and the relatively short duration of the acoustic wave. There is negative tissue pressure as the energy is released in the tissues.

focused in an intense manner to a relatively small area. Radial shock waves are delivered to the surface of the body. From there, they rapidly disperse through the tissues, releasing their energy rapidly to a wide area. Because of the energy dissipation, it is relatively difficult to deliver energy to deeper tissues.

Biologic Effects of Extracorporeal Shock Waves

The clinical effects of shock wave treatment include reduced inflammation and swelling, short-term analgesia, improved vascularity and neovascularization (which may stimulate soft-tissue healing), increased bone formation, realignment of tendon fibers, and enhanced wound healing. It may also provide analgesia [33,40,51,52]. The precise mechanisms of action that underlie the clinical effects are not clearly understood, but current research has focused on the effect of pressure waves on cells and their responses, including the production and release of growth factors.

Studies have indicated that there is induction of cytokines and growth factors, such as transforming growth factor β1, substance P, vascular endothelial growth factor, proliferating cell nuclear antigen, and osteocalcin [51]. In addition, there is induction of endothelial nitric oxide synthase, which influences bone healing osteoblastic activity. Bone morphogenetic proteins (BMPs) have been implicated as having an important role in bone development and fracture healing. Research has shown that ESWT promotes fracture healing and is linked to an increase in the expression of BMPs at the fracture site [52]. There may also be stimulation of nociceptors, which, in turn, appears to inhibit afferent pain signals.

When performing ESWT, surrounding tissues may be affected. Numerous studies have used animal models to investigate the effect of shock waves on skin, tendons, neurovascular bundles, bone, and cartilage [34,42,51,53–61]. Various energy levels were used in these studies. Significant negative side effects were produced only when high-energy shock waves were administered. Although it appears that at lower energy levels vital structures are spared, it is recommended that one be familiar with anatomic landmarks and structures in the treatment field.

Shock wave treatment to immature rats caused focal tibial growth plate dysplasia [61]. Although there was little soft-tissue coverage and the bones were relatively small, the researchers cautioned against using ESWT near or over open growth plates in animals. When compared with other soft tissues, joint cartilage seems less susceptible to the negative side effects of shock waves. Even with the use of high-energy ESWT, no changes were reported for up to 24 weeks after treatment in one study [59]. Cartilage resistance to damage from shock waves may be explained by the lack of vascularization, because free fluid is necessary for the formation of cavitation bubbles, which are damaging to tissue [53].

Shock waves have direct and indirect effects on target tissues. Direct effects include compression and tension generated as the shock wave travels through the tissue. An indirect effect is that the tension and shear forces caused by the shock wave may result in the development of cavitation bubbles in tissues and fluid. These cavitation bubbles collapse or expand with subsequent shock waves [32,33,49]. The transient cavitation is responsible for the disruption of uroliths with lithotripsy. It is also likely responsible for microscopic damage to tissues within the shock wave treatment field, which may ultimately lead to beneficial changes. There is an apparent dose-response effect with ESWT. As is true for most treatments, there are most likely levels that are too low that have a subtherapeutic effect. There is likely a range of energy that results in a positive effect, and a high level that may produce toxic or injurious effects on the cells and tissues [32,48,50].

Use of Extracorporeal Shock Wave Treatment in Dogs

Although it is relatively new, there are several reports of the use of ESWT in dogs [62–64]. These reports describe the use of ESWT to treat shoulder tendonopathies with calcifications in the tissues [62,63] and chronic osteoarthritis of the elbow or hip joint [64]. Clinical improvement was noted for the tendonopathies, but the two dogs treated for osteoarthritis were not improved when evaluated 4 and 12 weeks after treatment. Only subjective evaluation was used in these reports.

A blinded prospective study evaluated the effect of ESWT on hip and elbow osteoarthritis in dogs [65]. Animals with moderate-to-severe radiographic and clinical signs of hip or elbow osteoarthritis were evaluated. Objective parameters included measuring ground reaction forces with a force platform and determining comfortable joint range of motion (CROM) with a goniometer. Dogs were randomly assigned to 4 weeks of ESWT or sham treatment. ESWT of the hips and elbows involved 500 shocks at 0.14 mJ/mm^2 and 0.13 mJ/mm^2, respectively. Two treatments 2 weeks apart were directed to joint capsule insertion points. Dogs in the sham group were crossed over to the ESWT group after 4 weeks of sham treatment. The mean improvements in peak vertical force and CROM were 3.7% and 20%, respectively, at 28 days in the treated dogs, with no change in the sham-treated dogs (Fig. 3). The dogs that initially received the sham treatment and then ESWT showed improvement following ESWT, but there were no changes during the period of sham treatment. The improvements in weight bearing and CROM were similar to what is typically expected with the use of nonsteroidal anti-inflammatory drugs (NSAIDs). It was concluded that ESWT may be beneficial as part of the treatment program for osteoarthritis in dogs. Further studies involving larger sample groups are required to evaluate the effects of age, weight, the joint treated, the duration and severity of disease, and the concurrent use of other therapies on the outcome.

Application of Extracorporeal Shock Wave Therapy

ESWT may be beneficial in patients that cannot tolerate NSAIDs or other forms of treatment owing to gastrointestinal upset or liver or kidney disease, or may be useful as a nonpharmacologic form of adjunctive treatment along

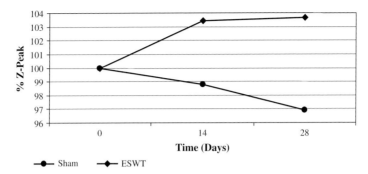

Fig. 3. Change in peak vertical force, as measured with a force plate, in patients with osteoarthritis of the hip or elbow treated with ESWT or sham treatment.

with medical management to obtain additional improvement. It is critical to be certain that the diagnosis is correct before instituting shock wave treatment because ESWT is not indicated for some conditions.

Heavy sedation or anesthesia is required for most forms of ESWT. Because many patients requiring treatment are geriatric, adequate health screening should be performed before treatment, including a complete physical examination and appropriate ancillary tests, such as radiographs, a complete blood count, serum chemistry profile, and urinalysis.

Shock wave treatment is a local treatment and not systemic; therefore, a complete understanding of the anatomy of the treatment area and of the spatial relationships of various anatomic landmarks is critical. Careful palpation and use of skeletal models and anatomy textbooks may be necessary to locate specific areas for appropriate treatment.

Because shock waves may cause petechiation and bruising, aspirin and other non–cyclooxygenase-selective drugs should be discontinued before treatment, because these drugs inhibit platelet function and may worsen the bruising.

The treatment area should be clipped, and the skin should be cleansed with alcohol if it is excessively oily. Ultrasound gel is liberally applied to the area. One should not use other lotions or creams because they contain too much air, which attenuates the sound waves.

Currently, the optimal energy level and the number of shocks for various conditions are not known. The energy level and number of shocks to be delivered are selected based on the manufacturer's directions and the areas to be treated. In general, treatments should not be repeated more frequently than 2 weeks. Most conditions are treated two or three times.

When treating joints, one should direct the probe at the insertion sites of the joint capsule and not the articular cartilage (Fig. 4). When treating the supraspinatus or biceps tendons, the probe should be directed over these areas from proximal to distal. The probe should not be directed over the thorax or lungs when treating conditions of the forelimbs. Patients may be a bit sedate for the

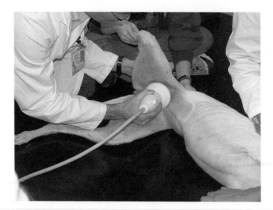

Fig. 4. Application of ESWT to the ventral aspect of a coxofemoral joint.

rest of the day after treatment and may develop some bruising, petechiation, or a hematoma over the treatment site. Some patients may be sore for several days after treatment and then have relative relief from pain. During this time, one can consider the use of NSAIDs or other medications to provide analgesia. Continued improvement may be seen for up to several weeks after treatment. Some conditions seem to be more responsive to shock wave treatment than others are. The hips and back may respond more favorably than other areas, whereas stifles may not respond to the same extent. Anecdotally, initial response rates of up to 80% may be seen, and the effects may last as long as 1 year.

Precautions When Using Extracorporeal Shock Wave Therapy

Shock waves can have adverse effects if they are applied at excessively high energy levels, if a large number of shocks are used, or if they are focused on structures sensitive to their effects. Negative side effects associated with ESWT include tissue damage by thermal and mechanical mechanisms. As tissues absorb the energy generated by ESWT, heat is generated. If the energy is too high, there is the potential for thermal damage to the tissues [66]. Excessive and violent cavitation can lead to the production of free radicals, which can cause chemical damage to cells and tissues [66].

Local hematomas, petechial hemorrhages, and local swelling have been documented with the use of high-energy flux densities. Even though these effects are not caused when lower-energy flux densities are used, the concurrent use of NSAIDs that affect platelet function is not recommended before ESWT.

ESWT should not be administered for the treatment of infectious arthritis, immune-mediated joint disease, neoplastic disease, diskospondylitis, acute unstable fractures, or neurologic deficits. In addition, shock waves should not be delivered over the lung field, brain, heart, major blood vessels, nerves, neoplasms, or a gravid uterus.

STATIC MAGNET FIELD THERAPY

The use of static magnets for medical purposes is relatively common in humans and is becoming more popular in animals. Owners can purchase magnets that are embedded in wraps, collars, or pet beds. Static magnets provide a continuous magnetic field that is thought to alter physiologic processes. Proposed therapeutic mechanisms involve an increase in local blood flow, possible release of endorphins, and anti-inflammatory effects. Despite much research, there is little evidence to confirm these theories [2].

The strength of static magnets is measured in gauss. Therapeutic magnets range from 2500 to 6000 G, whereas the earth's magnetic field is 0.5 G. MRI units produce magnetic fields that are two to four times greater than therapeutic magnetic pads. In contrast, common refrigerator magnets are about 50 to 200 G. In general, the amount of gauss delivered to the skin is less than that directly in contact with the magnet because the magnetic field decreases rapidly with distance. In fact, the amount delivered to the skin may be only one-third of the amount of the magnet.

Studies of Static Magnets

The original theory that static magnets influence blood flow may have come from an experiment in which exposure of a concentrated saline solution (five times as much as normal blood) in a glass capillary tube to a static magnetic field increased the flow of the solution in the tube. Extrapolation of these results to suggest that magnetic fields may increase blood flow is highly questionable. One study of horses used nuclear scintigraphy to assess blood flow to the cannon bone with a magnet placed over the limb [67]. Vascular, soft-tissue, and bone phases were evaluated following magnet placement. Although radionuclide uptake was significantly increased in all three phases, concern was expressed about the experimental design, especially the method of nuclear scintigraphy.

Another study involved the placement of two magnetic wraps over the third metacarpal region of six horses [68]. The magnet from one wrap was removed to serve as a control. Treatments were applied for 48 hours. Red blood cells were labeled in vivo with ^{99m}Tc-PYP, and quantitative scintigraphic determinations were made pre- and postwrapping to evaluate blood flow to the metacarpal region. Regions of interest with mean pixel counts were used to assess blood flow. No significant differences were noted in perfusion of the region. In addition, the peak magnet strength of 450 G declined to 200 G at a distance of 1 to 2 mm and to 1 G at 1 cm. Other studies of blood flow have also failed to show any effect, including the use of dental magnets applied to the human cheek [69], magnetic foil applied to human forearms [70], and magnets over equine tendon [71].

The possible anti-inflammatory effects of magnets were investigated using an experimental inflammatory synovitis model in rats [72]. Eight of ten rats treated with a 3800-G magnet had decreased inflammation. Inflammation in the test group was half as much as in the control group.

Use of Static Magnets

Static magnets are relatively cheap and easy to apply. There are no known side effects, and there may be some biologic effects in some individuals. Nevertheless, there is little evidence that they have clinical effects, and there are few well-designed, blinded, placebo-controlled studies to evaluate them properly.

Static magnets may be combined with other treatments, which is a benefit. They must be placed directly over affected joints because of the rapid decrease in magnetic field over short distances. It may be somewhat difficult to maintain them over the affected areas, and they should not be used with a pacemaker. Static magnets should be considered as a complement to osteoarthritis treatment and not as a sole or alternative treatment. In fact, the biggest potential danger of static magnets is that they may delay conventional treatment and result in progression of disease or undue discomfort.

SUMMARY

Low-energy lasers, ESWT, and magnets are some of the more commonly used modalities that are emerging in veterinary rehabilitation. Unfortunately, despite some evidence that there are biologic effects in tissue culture or laboratory experiments, there are few published well-designed clinical studies in veterinary medicine to make firm recommendations for their use. In particular, questions regarding adequate energy or power, the length of treatment, and the most effective treatment protocols for specific conditions are lacking. Users should demand proper studies of products before purchasing them, and veterinary funding agencies should provide adequate resources for investigators to test such devices independently.

References

[1] Bélanger A-Y. Laser. In: Bélanger A-Y, editor. Evidence-based guide to therapeutic physical agents. Philadelphia: Lippincott, Williams & Wilkens; 2002. p. 191–221.

[2] Ramey DW, Rollin BE. Scientific aspects of CAVM. In: Ramey DW, Rollin BE, editors. Complementary and alternative veterinary medicine considered. Ames (IA): Iowa State Press; 2004. p. 117–63.

[3] Baxter GD, Walsh DM, Allen JM, et al. Effects of low-intensity infrared laser irradiation upon conduction in the human median nerve in vivo. Exp Physiol 1994;79:227–34.

[4] Enwemeka CS, Parker JC, Dowdy DS, et al. The efficacy of low-power lasers in tissue repair and pain control: a meta-analysis study. Photomed Laser Surg 2004;22(4):323–9.

[5] Mester E, Spiry T, Szende B, et al. Effect of laser rays on wound healing. Am J Surg 1971;122:532–8.

[6] Reddy GK, Stehno-Bittel L, Enwemeka CS. Laser photostimulation accelerates wound healing in diabetic rats. Wound Repair Regen 2001;9(3):248–55.

[7] Schindl A, Schindl M, Pernerstorfer-Schoen H, et al. Low intensity laser therapy in wound healing: a review with special respect to diabetic angiopathies. Acta Chir Aust 2001;33(3):132–7.

[8] Fung DT, Ng GY, Leung MC, et al. Therapeutic low energy laser improves the mechanical strength of repairing medial collateral ligament. Lasers Surg Med 2002;31:91–6.

[9] Surinchak JS, Alago ML, Mellamy RF, et al. Effects of low-level energy lasers on the healing of full-thickness skin defects. Lasers Surg Med 1983;2(3):267–74.

[10] Braverman B, McCarthy RJ, Ivankovich AD, et al. Effect of helium-neon and infrared laser irradiation on wound healing in rabbits. Lasers Surg Med 1989;9(1):50–8.

[11] Lucas C, Criens-Poublon LJ, Cockrell CT, et al. Wound healing in cell studies and animal model experiments by low level laser therapy: were clinical studies justified? A systematic review. Lasers Med Sci 2002;17(2):110–34.

[12] De Bie RA, de Vet HC, Lenssen TF, et al. Low-level laser therapy in ankle sprains: a randomized clinical trial. Arch Phys Med Rehabil 1998;79(11):1415–20.

[13] Pinheiro ALB, Oliveira MG, Martins PPM, et al. Biomodulatory effects of LLLT on bone regeneration. Laser Ther 2001;13:73–9.

[14] Guzzardella GA, Tigani D, Torricelli P, et al. Low-power diode laser stimulation of surgical osteochondral defects: results after 24 weeks. Artif Cells Blood Substit Immobil Biotechnol 2001;29(3):235–44.

[15] Barber A, Luger JE, Karpf A, et al. Advances in laser therapy for bone repair. Laser Ther 2001;13:80–5.

[16] Guzzardella GA, Morrone G, Torricelli P, et al. Assessment of low-power laser biostimulation on chondral lesions: an "in vivo" experimental study. Artif Cells Blood Substit Immobil Biotechnol 2000;28(5):441–9.

[17] Bayat M, Ansari A, Hekmat H. Effect of low-power helium-neon laser irradiation on 13-week immobilized articular cartilage of rabbits. Indian J Exp Biol 2004;42(9):866–70.

[18] Akai M, Usuba M, Maeshima T, et al. Laser's effect on bone and cartilage change induced by joint immobilization: an experiment with animal model. Laser Surg Med 1997;21(5):480–4.

[19] Snyder-Mackler L, Bork CE. Effect of helium-neon laser irradiation on peripheral sensory nerve latency. Phys Ther 1988;68:223–5.

[20] Lowe AS, Baster GD, Walsh DM, et al. The effect of low-intensity laser (830 nm) irradiation upon skin temperature and antidromic conduction latencies in the human median nerve: relevance of radiant exposure. Lasers Surg Med 1994;14:40–6.

[21] Basford JR, Daube JR, Hallman HO, et al. Does low-intensity helium-neon laser irradiation alter sensory nerve action potentials or distal latencies? Lasers Surg Med 1990;10:35–9.

[22] Tsuchiya K, Kawatani M, Takeshige C, et al. Laser irradiation abates neuronal responses to nociceptive stimulation of rat-paw skin. Brain Res Bull 1994;34(4):369–74.

[23] Wedlock PM, Shephard RA. Cranial irradiation with GaAlAs laser leads to naloxone reversible analgesia in rats. Psychol Rep 1996;78(3):727–31.

[24] Bjordal JM, Couppè C, Chow R, et al. A systematic review of low level laser therapy with location-specific doses for pain from chronic joint disorders. Aust J Physiother 2003;49:107–16.

[25] Kleinkort JA. Low-level laser therapy: new possibilities in pain management and rehab. Orthopaedic Prac 2005;17(1):48–51.

[26] Stelian J, Gil I, Habot B, et al. Laser therapy is effective for degenerative osteoarthritis: improvement of pain and disability in elderly patients with degenerative osteoarthritis of the knee treated with narrow-band light therapy. J Am Geriatr Soc 1992;40:23–6.

[27] Djavid GE, Mortazavi SMJ, Basirnia A, et al. Low level laser therapy in musculoskeletal pain syndromes: pain relief and disability reduction. Lasers Surg Med 2003;152(Suppl 15):43.

[28] Gur A, Cosut A, Sarac AJ, et al. Efficacy of different therapy regimes of low-power laser in painful osteoarthritis of the knee: a double-blind and randomized-controlled trial. Lasers Surg Med 2003;33:330–8.

[29] Tascioglu F, Armagan O, Tabak Y, et al. Low power laser treatment in patients with knee osteoarthritis. Swiss Med Wkly 2004;134(17–18):254–8.

[30] Rochkind S. The role of laser phototherapy in nerve tissue regeneration and repair: research development with perspective for clinical application. In: Proceedings of the World Association of Laser Therapy, Sao Paulo, Brazil. 2004. p. 94–5.

[31] Rochkind S, Nissan M, Alon M, et al. Effects of laser irradiation on the spinal cord for the regeneration of crushed peripheral nerve in rats. Lasers Surg Med 2001;28(3):216–9.

[32] Ogden JA, Toth-Kischkat A, Schultheiss R. Principles of shock wave therapy. Clin Orthop 2001;387:8–17.
[33] Thiel M. Application of shock waves in medicine. Clin Orthop 2001;387:18–21.
[34] Haupt G. Use of extracorporeal shock waves in the treatment of pseudarthrosis, tendinopathy and other orthopedic diseases. J Urol 1997;158(1):4–11.
[35] Haupt G, Haupt A, Ekkernkamp A, et al. Influence of shock waves on fracture healing. Urology 1992;39(6):529–32.
[36] Johannes EJ, Kaulesar Sukul DM, Matura E. High-energy shock waves for the treatment of nonunions: an experiment on dogs. J Surg Res 1994;57(2):246–52.
[37] Lee GP, Ogden JA, Cross GL. Effect of extracorporeal shock waves on calcaneal bone spurs. Foot Ankle Int 2003;24(12):927–30.
[38] Ludwig J, Lauber S, Lauber HJ, et al. High-energy shock wave treatment of femoral head necrosis in adults. Clin Orthop 2001;387:119–26.
[39] Maier M, Steinborn M, Schmitz C, et al. Extracorporeal shock-wave therapy for chronic lateral tennis elbow—prediction of outcome by imaging. Arch Orthop Trauma Surg 2001;121(7):379–84.
[40] Ogden JA, Alvarez RG, Levitt R, et al. Shock wave therapy (Orthotripsy) in musculoskeletal disorders. Clin Orthop 2001;387:22–40.
[41] Rompe JD, Hope C, Kullmer K, et al. Analgesic effect of extracorporeal shock-wave therapy on chronic tennis elbow. J Bone Joint Surg Br 1996;78(2):233–7.
[42] Schaden W, Fischer A, Sailler A. Extracorporeal shock wave therapy of nonunion or delayed osseous union. Clin Orthop 2001;387:90–4.
[43] Wang CJ, Chen HS, Chen CE, et al. Treatment of nonunions of long bone fractures with shock waves. Clin Orthop 2001;387:95–101.
[44] Wang CJ, Chen HS, Chen WS, et al. Treatment of painful heels using extracorporeal shock wave. J Formos Med Assoc 2000;99(7):580–3.
[45] Wang CJ, Huang HY, Chen HH, et al. Effect of shock wave therapy on acute fractures of the tibia: a study in a dog model. Clin Orthop 2001;387:112–8.
[46] Weinstein JN, Oster DM, Park JB, et al. The effect of the extracorporeal shock wave lithotriptor on the bone-cement interface in dogs. Clin Orthop 2004;235:261–7.
[47] Helbig K, Herbert C, Schostok T, et al. Correlations between the duration of pain and the success of shock wave therapy. Clin Orthop 2001;387:68–71.
[48] McClure SR, Merritt DK. Extracorporeal shock-wave therapy for equine musculoskeletal disorders. Compend Contin Educ Pract Vet 2003;25(1):68–75.
[49] McClure SR, Van Sickle D, White MR. Effects of extracorporeal shock wave therapy on bone. Vet Surg 2004;33(1):40–8.
[50] Wild C, Khene M, Wanke S. Extracorporeal shock wave therapy in orthopedics: assessment of an emerging health technology. Int J Technol Assess Health Care 2000;16(1):199–209.
[51] Wang CJ, Wang FS, Yang KD, et al. Shock wave therapy induces neovascularization at the tendon-bone junction: a study in rabbits. J Orthop Res 2003;21(6):984–9.
[52] Wang FS, Yang KD, Kuo YR, et al. Temporal and spatial expression of bone morphogenetic proteins in extracorporeal shock wave–promoted healing of segmental defect. Bone 2003;32(4):387–96.
[53] Delius M, Draenert K, Al Diek Y, et al. Biological effects of shock waves: in vivo effect of high energy pulses on rabbit bone. Ultrasound Med Biol 1995;21(9):1219–25.
[54] Haupt G, Chvapil M. Effect of shock waves on the healing of partial-thickness wounds in piglets. J Surg Res 1990;49(1):45–8.
[55] Rompe JD, Bohl J, Riehle HM, et al. Evaluating the risk of sciatic nerve damage in the rabbit by administration of low and intermediate energy extracorporeal shock waves. Z Orthop Ihre Grenzgeb 1998;136(5):407–11.
[56] Rompe JD, Kirkpatrick CJ, Kullmer K, et al. Dose-related effects of shock waves on rabbit tendon Achilles: a sonographic and histological study. J Bone Joint Surg Br 1998;80(3): 546–52.

[57] Schelling G, Delius M, Gschwender M, et al. Extracorporeal shock waves stimulate frog sciatic nerves indirectly via a cavitation-mediated mechanism. Biophys J 1994;66(1): 133–40.

[58] Steinbach P, Hofstaedter F, Nicolai H, et al. Determination of the energy-dependent extent of vascular damage caused by high-energy shock waves in an umbilical cord model. Urol Res 1993;21(4):279–82.

[59] Vaterlein N, Lussenhop S, Hahn M, et al. The effect of extracorporeal shock waves on joint cartilage: an in vivo study in rabbits. Arch Orthop Trauma Surg 2000;120(7–8):403–6.

[60] Wang CJ, Huang HY, Yang K, et al. Pathomechanism of shock wave injuries on femoral artery, vein and nerve: an experimental study in dogs. Injury 2002;33(5):439–46.

[61] Yeaman LD, Jerome CP, McCullough DL. Effects of shock waves on the structure and growth of the immature rat epiphysis. J Urol 1989;141(3):670–4.

[62] Danova NA, Muir P. Extracorporeal shock wave therapy for supraspinatus calcifying tendinopathy in two dogs. Vet Rec 2003;152:208–9.

[63] Venzin C, Ohlerth S, Koch D, et al. Extracorporeal shockwave therapy in a dog with chronic bicipital tenosynovitis. Schweir Archiv fur Tierheilkunde 2004;146(3):136–41.

[64] Laverty PH, McClure SR. Initial experience with extracorporeal shock wave therapy in six dogs. Part 1. Vet Comp Orthop Traumatol 2002;15:177–83.

[65] Francis DA, Millis DL, Evans M, et al. Clinical evaluation of extracorporeal shockwave therapy for the management of canine osteoarthritis of the elbow and hip joints. In: Proceedings of the 31st Veterinary Orthopedic Society. Okemos (MI): Veterinary Orthopedic Society; 2004.

[66] Bushberg J, Seibert J, Leidholdt E Jr, et al. The essential physics of medical imaging. 2nd edition. Philadelphia: Lippincott Williams & Wilkins; 2002.

[67] Kobluk CN, Johnston GR, Lauper L. A scintigraphic investigation of magnetic field therapy on the equine third metacarpus. J Comp Orthop Traumatol 1994;7:9–13.

[68] Steyn PF, Ramey DW, Kirschvink J, et al. Effect of a static magnetic filed on blood flow to the metacarpus in horses. J Am Vet Med Assoc 2000;217(6):874–7.

[69] Saygili G, Avdinlik E, Ercan MT, et al. Investigation of the effect of magnetic retention systems used in prosthodontics on buccal mucosal blood flow. Int J Prosthodont 1992;5(4): 326–32.

[70] Barker A, Cain M. The claimed vasodilatory effect of a commercial permanent magnet foil: results of a double blind trial. Clin Phys Physiol Meas 1985;6(3):261–3.

[71] Turner T, Wolfsdorf K, Jourdenais J. Effects of heat, cold, biomagnets and ultrasound on skin circulation in the horse. In: Proceedings of the 37th Annual Meeting of the American Association of Equine Practitioners. Lexington (KY): American Association of Equine Practitioners; 1991. p. 249–57.

[72] Weinberger A, Nyska A, Giler S. Treatment of experimental inflammatory synovitis with continuous magnetic field. Isr J Med Sci 1996;32(12):1197–201.

Vet Clin Small Anim 35 (2005) 1357–1388

ELSEVIER
SAUNDERS

VETERINARY CLINICS
SMALL ANIMAL PRACTICE

Rehabilitation for the Orthopedic Patient

Jacqueline R. Davidson, DVM, MS, CCRP, CVA[a],*,
Sharon C. Kerwin, DVM, MS[b],
Darryl L. Millis, MS, DVM, CCRP[c]

[a]Veterinary Clinical Sciences, School of Veterinary Medicine, Louisiana State University,
Skip Bertman Drive, Baton Rouge, LA 70803, USA
[b]Small Animal Clinical Sciences, College of Veterinary Medicine, Texas A&M University,
College Station, TX 77843, USA
[c]Small Animal Clinical Sciences, College of Veterinary Medicine, University of Tennessee,
2407 River Drive, Knoxville, TN 37996, USA

Rehabilitation of orthopedic conditions is one of the most important areas of canine rehabilitation. An understanding of these conditions and their medical and surgical treatment is important to help the therapist develop a treatment plan that will help the patient return to function quickly with minimal complications. The therapist must constantly assess the patient for improvement or complications and adjust the therapy plan accordingly. Knowledge of the stages of tissue healing and the strength of tissues is critical to avoid placing too much stress on the surgical site, yet some challenge to tissues must be provided to optimize the return to function.

FRACTURES

Rehabilitation is an important part of the overall management of fracture. Although, traditionally, the focus of the surgeon has been on repair of the fracture, attention more recently has moved toward concurrent management of soft-tissue injury and maintaining full range of motion of involved or adjacent joints. As veterinary surgeons have advanced from external coaptation to internal fixation and an earlier return to weight bearing, a balance has been sought between protecting the repair and encouraging limb use. Many veterinary surgeons are reluctant to add rehabilitation exercises as part of their postoperative protocol, fearing implant failure. Nevertheless, with a thorough understanding of the fracture and implant biomechanics and the various rehabilitation modalities available, an appropriate and safe rehabilitation plan can be made for every patient, with increased patient comfort, faster return to function, and increased client satisfaction.

*Corresponding author. E-mail address: jdavidson@vetmed.lsu.edu (J.R. Davidson).

Rehabilitation of the patient with a fracture actually begins preoperatively, beginning at the time of presentation. Cryotherapy (cold-packing) is an essential and simple modality that can be applied in any practice setting. Cryotherapy generally consists of commercial or homemade ice packs that are directly applied over the closed fracture before temporary stabilization (cast, Robert Jones bandage, or splint) for 10 to 20 minutes. These applications are repeated every 2 to 4 hours if practical. Cryotherapy reduces blood flow, resulting in decreased edema, hemorrhage, and inflammation in the soft tissues surrounding the fracture site. It also reduces cellular metabolism, decreases nerve conduction velocity, is analgesic, and may decrease muscle spasm [1]. In the authors' practice, ice packs are applied during triage of the fracture patient, assuming that body temperature is above 98°F. The combination of appropriate cryotherapy plus supportive bandaging can dramatically decrease soft-tissue damage and swelling, facilitating surgical repair and decreasing muscle fibrosis postoperatively. As soon as the patient is stable, analgesics should be administered on a humane basis and to facilitate postoperative rehabilitation by preventing hyperesthesia associated with the "wind-up" phenomenon caused by untreated preoperative and intraoperative pain [2].

Before surgery, the rehabilitation plan should be based on several factors, including the location of the fracture (articular, physeal, long bone), the stability of the repair, whether more than one limb or bone is involved, pre-existing patient disease (obesity, osteoarthritis), the degree of soft-tissue injury (low-energy versus high-energy fracture), and the presence or absence of open wounds. If the practice employs a veterinarian, physical therapist, certified veterinary rehabilitation technician, or a technician who is primarily responsible for the postoperative rehabilitation of the patient, that person should be involved in discussions with the surgeon and in examination of the patient preoperatively.

Articular Fractures

Articular fractures are unique in that they demand rigid fixation and anatomic reduction to maintain an even stable cartilage surface. Because of the necessity for anatomic reduction, the surgical approach may be extensive, particularly in acetabular or humeral condylar fractures, which may include tendon incisions or osteotomies. The surgeon must carefully balance the degree of soft-tissue manipulation with the need for exposure of the fracture to facilitate reduction. Extensive dissection will increase postoperative pain and swelling and may increase the degree of muscle scarring and periarticular fibrosis after surgery. In the authors' experience, excessive postoperative scarring and fibrosis leading to decreased range of motion is particularly likely after articular fractures involving the distal humerus or distal femur in the dog and cat. The use of more minimally invasive techniques, such as closed reduction and fixation via the use of fluoroscopy, as well as arthroscopic-assisted fracture reduction, should be considered [3]. Wherever possible, osteotomies rather than tenotomies should be performed to gain access to the fracture, because osteotomies heal by reforming normal bone, whereas tenotomies heal via scar tissue. When osteotomies are repaired, the surgeon must pay particular attention to pin and wire placement. Inadvertent wire placement into the joint (Fig. 1) will cause mechanical loss of range of motion and pain for the patient, rendering even the most sophisticated rehabilitation strategy useless.

In addition to the demand for anatomic reduction, rigid fixation in articular fractures may rely on implants placed across a small epiphyseal segment, resulting in a somewhat tenuous repair. In distal humeral fractures, particularly Salter-Harris type IV fractures in young dogs, the surgeon may be tempted to splint the limb or place a carpal flexion bandage to prevent weight bearing. Although these strategies may effectively prevent mechanical overload of the repair during the healing process, they may have the unintended effect of promoting muscle scarring around the operative site as well as cartilage atrophy [4]. Although a carpal flexion bandage will allow some range of motion exercises, contracture of muscles around the carpus may lead to long-standing pain, loss of range of motion, and poor limb use despite good fracture healing.

Physeal Fractures

Fractures involving the growth plate are a common presentation in veterinary practice and are usually described based on severity using the Salter-Harris classification as follows:

> A Salter-Harris I fracture traverses only the growth plate (ie, femoral capital physeal separations).

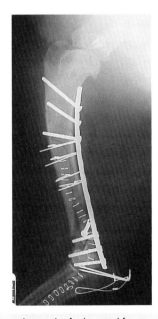

Fig. 1. Lateral postoperative radiograph of a humeral fracture accessed via an olecranon osteotomy. Note that the K-wires of the pin and tension band apparatus penetrate the joint. Rehabilitation will not be effective until the fixation is revised.

A Salter-Harris II fracture partially traverses the growth plate and involves the metaphysis (ie, distal femoral fracture).

A Salter-Harris III fracture traverses the growth plate and extends into the articular surface.

A Salter-Harris IV fracture starts at the articular surface, crosses the growth plate, and exits through the metaphysis (ie, lateral humeral condylar fracture).

A Salter-Harris type V fracture involves a crushing of the growth plate (ie, distal ulnar fracture).

Generally, articular fractures are considered more severe than nonarticular fractures, with the exception of a crushing injury that usually causes premature physeal closure, and may result in angular limb deformity and joint incongruity.

Because, by definition, physeal fractures occur in animals with open growth plates, the potential for rapid healing is high. Nevertheless, young animals present a challenge because of their high activity level and, in some cases, low tolerance for potentially painful procedures such as range of motion exercises. As is true for articular fractures, fixation devices often engage a relatively small epiphyseal fragment, resulting in a less than sturdy repair. In addition, the bone in young dogs and cats tends to be soft, and care must be taken not to cause fragmentation of fracture segments during reduction and fixation. Placement of Kirschner wires must be precise so that they do not impinge on major muscle groups, causing pain during rehabilitation (Fig. 2). The three most

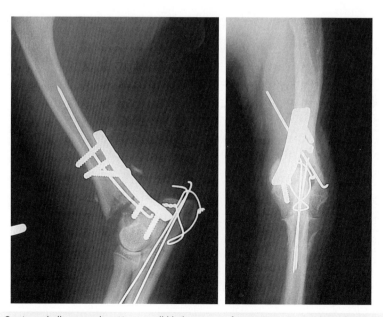

Fig. 2. A medially protruding K-wire will likely cause soft-tissue irritation and interfere with rehabilitation postoperatively.

commonly seen physeal fractures in veterinary practice are the Salter-Harris type II fracture involving the distal femur, the type I femoral capital physeal separation, and the Salter-Harris IV fracture of the lateral aspect of the humeral condyle. Each type can present unique challenges for postoperative rehabilitation.

Distal femoral physeal fractures

Although many different repair techniques are described, the most commonly used repair is cross-pinning. Repaired distal physeal fractures can be difficult to reduce, particularly if they are more than 48 hours old. In addition, distal femoral physeal fractures are predisposed to a devastating postoperative complication characterized by quadriceps contracture (Fig. 3). In a frequent scenario, surgical repair is performed, the patient seems to have good range of motion of the stifle joint immediately postoperatively, but, by the time of suture removal, excessive extension and severe loss of range of motion occur have occurred.

Quadriceps contracture is characterized by scarring of the quadriceps muscle group with adhesions to the distal femur and fracture callus. The likelihood of quadriceps contracture is greatly increased when the limb is maintained in extension, that is, with a cast or splint. Once fibrosis has occurred, attempts to break down the scar tissue by performing range of motion exercises, even under anesthesia, will often lead to refracture of the femur. Surgical release will result in reformation of scar tissue within a few weeks, although this complication has been managed successfully with a combination of surgical release, dynamic stifle flexion apparatus, and passive range of motion exercises (PROM)

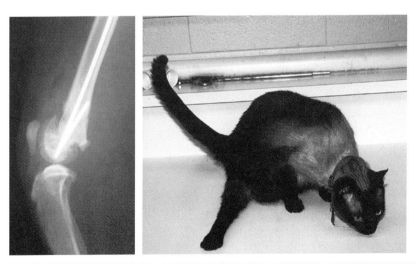

Fig. 3. Insufficient fracture reduction and inadequate postoperative management of a Salter-Harris type II fracture of the distal femoral epiphysis led to quadriceps muscle group contracture in this cat.

[5]. Generally, the prognosis is poor, and many patients end up with an amputation after what initially appeared to be a successful fracture repair.

Prevention of quadriceps contracture depends on several factors. First, the fracture should be repaired as soon as possible, preferably within 24 hours. Gentle tissue dissection and the use of surgical techniques that minimize tissue trauma, such as fluoroscopic guidance of pins, should be employed. Although cross-pins may be bent over distally to prevent migration, excess pin protruding into the soft tissues may inhibit rehabilitation exercises. Some surgeons prefer to countersink these pins rather than bend them, resulting in less interference with range of motion. The fracture must be reduced anatomically. Postoperatively, it is critical that the quadriceps muscle group be kept in flexion rather than extension to prevent shortening. To accomplish this, many surgeons place a 90-90 muscle sling to maintain the stifle in flexion for 72 hours postoperatively, which has been shown to decrease greatly the risk of contracture [6]. In some cases, if the range of motion of the stifle is good after repair and there is no obvious tendency for the stifle joint to be in extension, a more physiologic rehabilitation program may be employed. Cryotherapy is used immediately postoperatively, and gentle PROM exercises are done after cryotherapy before recovery from anesthesia. Aggressive treatment of pain, often achieved using a combination of nonsteroidal anti-inflammatory drugs (NSAIDs) and narcotics, is mandatory to successful rehabilitation efforts and should begin before recovery from anesthesia. The authors often administer an injectable nonsteroidal agent immediately postoperatively (eg, carprofen or meloxicam) while continuing a narcotic for at least 24 hours (eg, hydromorphone or buprenorphine). Caution should be used with NSAIDs, taking into consideration the history of preoperative NSAID use, corticosteroid use, renal disease, the risk of gastrointestinal ulceration, and hypotension that may have occurred during surgery.

Once the patient has recovered, cryotherapy and range of motion exercises are continued three to six times daily. Immediately after cryotherapy, gentle massage is used starting from the distal aspect of the limb and working proximally for 2 to 3 minutes. Although the stifle is the primary area of interest, it is important to treat the whole limb; therefore, gentle flexion and extension range of motion of the digits with some stretching is done first, moving up the hock, stifle, and hip, using 15 to 20 repetitions per joint. For the stifle, it may be helpful to use gentle stretching (holding the joint at maximal flexion or extension for 15 seconds). The process must not be painful for the patient, and vigorous manipulations that may tear tissue should be avoided [7]. The authors generally continue cryotherapy for 72 hours. For patients that do not tolerate NSAIDs or that remain painful on appropriate NSAIDs, additional analgesics may be used. Oral sustained release morphine given once to twice daily may be a good choice and can safely be combined with a NSAID.

Once the patient has completely recovered from anesthesia, it should be observed while walking. Many patients will begin to bear some weight on the limb at this time. If the patient resents range of motion or tends to hold the limb in extension, a 90-90 flexion bandage should be applied after sedation. If the patient allows range of motion and is beginning to use the limb, early active exercises may be performed, primarily with slow leash walks and balancing exercises that encourage the patient to bear weight on the limb. If the patient is released to its' owners, a recheck should be performed within a few days to ensure that range of motion is not being lost in the stifle joint. If range of motion is preserved and limb function is improving, the patient should be rechecked weekly until the time of radiographic healing, usually by 4 weeks. After about 3 days, cryotherapy may be replaced with heat therapy before rehabilitation exercises.

Heat therapy can be used after the acute inflammatory phase of wound healing is over. Heat causes vasodilation of the cutaneous blood vessels, improves muscle and connective tissue extensibility, increases the pain threshold, and can be useful before stretching, range of motion, and exercise sessions. Some therapists recommend using heat before exercise and cryotherapy afterward.

If a 90-90 flexion bandage has been applied, cryotherapy is continued over the bandage while it is in place, along with analgesic therapy. As soon as the bandage comes off, massage and range of motion exercises should be initiated as described previously. Assuming a stable repair and compliant owners, a good prognosis is associated with distal femoral physeal fractures in the dog and cat.

Femoral capital physeal separations

These fractures are typically repaired with lag screws or divergent K-wires. As is true for distal femoral fractures, early repair and minimal soft-tissue dissection will result in fewer complications. Although, in general, these fractures are not associated with the muscle contracture noted with distal femoral fractures, because of the small epiphyseal segment and possible tenuous repair, surgeons may occasionally elect to place these limbs in an Ehmer or 90-90 sling for up to 3 weeks after surgery. Ideally, such slings should be removed as early as possible, and cryotherapy, PROM, and early weight-bearing active range of motion should begin within a few days. Collapse of the fracture around the pins can occur. If crepitus, loss of range of motion, or an increase in pain occurs during rehabilitation exercises postoperatively, the surgeon should be contacted immediately or radiographs obtained to assess for loss of reduction or implant penetration into the articular space.

Lateral humeral condylar fractures

As described in the section on articular fractures, the surgeon must balance stability versus postoperative fibrosis and loss of range of motion of the elbow, which is a common complication after repair of these fractures. Cryotherapy, analgesia, massage, and PROM as described for distal femoral fractures may also be used for lateral humeral condylar fractures. In difficult to handle small breed dogs, the use of a therapy ball may be helpful to encourage limb use and flexion of the elbow without direct manipulation of the limb. Exercises should be continued until the fracture is radiographically healed and may be continued after this time if flexion of the elbow has been lost in an attempt to regain some range of motion. The use of heat therapy may be helpful before exercise in improving extensibility of fibrous tissue to allow increased stretching and range of motion of the affected joint over time.

Long Bone Fractures

Diaphyseal and metaphyseal fractures of the long bones occur in a large number and variety in veterinary practice. The rehabilitation plan must be made by a team including the rehabilitation technician, surgeon, and client. The surgeon's opinion regarding the risk of implant failure should be communicated to the team. Implant failure can result from single catastrophic overload or from fatigue, implying a greater number of normal weight-bearing cycles than the implant can bear before fracture healing. In general, plates, interlocking nails, and some external fixators tend to be more biomechanically stable than intramedullary pin and cerclage wire constructs. Cryotherapy and PROM of the limb are always indicated. Judgment and experience come into play when using active modalities, including exercises such as dancing, sit-to-stand, negotiating Cavaletti rails, walking on a land treadmill and water treadmill, and other types of active rehabilitation exercises. In addition, external fixation devices such as linear and circular fixators present some special considerations. Patients most in need of aggressive rehabilitation are those with multiple limb fractures. The risk of implant failure is much higher in these patients when compared with animals with single limb injuries because the patient is unable to protect the injured limb.

External fixators

Rehabilitation is important in patients with external fixators. During surgical planning, the surgeon should place pins through safe corridors without crossing large muscle masses and neurovascular bundles or entering joints [8,9]. A pin inadvertently placed through a large muscle mass (as can occur with femur fractures) or major tendon (eg, Achilles tendon perforation with a ring fixator applied to the tibia) will cause enough pain or mechanical difficulty that the patient will not tolerate range of motion exercises or weight bearing on the limb. Because, by necessity, some muscle masses must be entered, analgesia and careful attention to pin tract maintenance are important. The frame can present a problem in that it may be difficult to apply cryotherapy or other modalities. Some clinicians use ice packs applied to the frame for a short time to allow cold to travel down the pins to the limb. In addition, if an open wound is present, cold or heat therapy should generally not be applied directly to the wound. Massage, PROM exercises of the joints, and stretching can be applied to fractures repaired with external linear or ring fixators.

Patients with external fixators may be reluctant to flex and extend the limbs fully in the early postoperative period. Active exercises that improve proprioception and that encourage limb flexion may be useful, including using a therapy ball, walking over Cavaletti rails or other objects that the patient can step over (many therapists use pool noodles), or walking on a land or water treadmill. Although patients with open wounds are generally not treated with water treadmill therapy or swimming, external fixator patients may be placed in the water treadmill or pool after their incisions have healed, as is true for any fracture patient.

Multiple Limb and Bilateral Pelvic Fractures

Patients with multiple limb fractures are often nonambulatory immediately after surgical repair. Aggressive rehabilitation, keeping in mind the biomechanical limitations of the fracture repair, should be started immediately postoperatively with analgesia, cryotherapy, and PROM exercises. The following day if the patient is stable, sling therapy should begin. Short 5-minute sessions initially once or twice daily can be started. Advantages of sling therapy include psychologic benefits of the patient being in a more normal stand up position, the ability to begin assisted active motion and early limited weight bearing, and improved access for the technician to perform massage and range of motion exercises. Rear limb slings can be homemade or commercial. Whole body slings can be used for patients with forelimb and rear limb trauma. Once the incisions are sealed and the patient no longer has intravenous catheters or other invasive lines, water treadmill or swimming therapy should be considered.

Water treadmill therapy for polytrauma patients is useful because it allows the therapist to tailor the amount of weight bearing (a water level up to the level of the greater trochanter allows the dog to walk with only 38% of normal weight bearing on its limbs) [10]. The temperature, hydrostatic pressure, and buoyancy of the water can also help improve blood flow, decrease edema, and decrease stress on the joints. Many dogs seem to enjoy being in the underwater treadmill. Because it can be very demanding for the dog to walk for any length of time after trauma, the cardiovascular status of the dog should be monitored, and short (3–5 minute) sessions should be used for the first few treatments.

Summary

Rehabilitation of fracture patients is a process that should begin at presentation before surgery, with aggressive pain management and control of further soft-tissue injury and swelling being the starting point. The surgeon should strive for a stable repair with minimal soft-tissue dissection. Although concerns about the effects of rehabilitation exercises on the biomechanical stability of the fracture repair should be considered, in the authors' experience, rehabilitation using the techniques described herein improves the early return to weight bearing, which, in turn, stimulates bone to heal. Communication among the surgeon, therapist, and client when making the rehabilitation plan will maximize the outcome, resulting in not only a healed fracture but also a functional limb.

JOINTS

The joints can be affected by a variety of congenital, developmental, and acquired conditions. Surgery has role in the treatment of many joint conditions. Although there may be specific considerations for individual joints, some general guidelines can be applied to rehabilitation of any joint.

General Guidelines for Surgery

Immediately after joint surgery while the patient is recovering from anesthesia, cryotherapy can be helpful to reduce the inflammatory reaction and pain caused by the surgical procedure. The skin should be monitored carefully to avoid damage if the patient is not conscious enough to react to stimuli. PROM is beneficial in most cases, providing it does not place too much stress on the surgical repair. PROM helps maintain the normal range of joint motion, improves blood and lymphatic circulation, and stimulates sensory awareness. After 15 to 30 minutes of cryotherapy, a pressure bandage may be applied to the limb to limit swelling and edema. The bandage is usually removed within 12 to 24 hours to begin a rehabilitation program. Massage can be performed intermittently to reduce edema formation. Appropriate analgesic medication is also important to allow pain-free rehabilitation to begin. NSAIDs may be used before each rehabilitation session. Transcutaneous electrical stimulation (TENS) may help control pain in the early postoperative period. Therapeutic exercise is often begun within a few days of surgery to encourage muscle strengthening and re-education. Weight-bearing exercise is needed to prevent atrophy of bone and cartilage and to maintain the strength of ligaments and other soft tissues. The initial exercises are controlled, low-impact activities such as leash walking. If the patient is not using the limb, this may be encouraged by weight-shifting activities. Aquatic therapy may improve range of motion, particularly if increased flexion is desired [11,12]. Aquatic therapy also reduces the load on the joint, which is desirable in some cases; however, the increased resistance provided by water promotes muscle strengthening. Underwater treadmill walking may begin when the incision line is sealed and free of drainage. Swimming may be too strenuous in the early postoperative period. Neuromuscular electrical stimulation (NMES) once daily or every other day may be used for muscle strengthening if the patient is painful or unable to bear weight on the limb. Cryotherapy may be used after an exercise session to reduce pain and inflammation. After the acute inflammation has resolved (about 4 or 5 days), hot packs or therapeutic ultrasound may be used before range of motion or therapeutic exercises to warm the tissues, increase tissue elasticity, improve comfort, and relax the muscles. Table 1 summarizes the goals of joint rehabilitation after surgery.

The rate of progression of the rehabilitation program is based on the patient's response. Useful parameters to measure include the limb circumference to assess muscle mass and goniometry to assess the range of motion. Gait analysis is useful to assess function and pain. If the patient appears to have increased stiffness, lameness, or pain after a therapy session, the activity level

Table 1	
Joint rehabilitation after surgery	
Goals	Treatment
Control inflammation and edema	Cryotherapy
	Pressure bandage
	Massage
	NSAIDs
Maintain or improve range of motion	PROM or stretching
	Therapeutic ultrasound after inflammation resolves
Control pain	Analgesics
	TENS
	Heat
	Cryotherapy
Strengthen muscle	NMES if nonambulatory or painful
	Weight shifting to encourage weight bearing
	Therapeutic exercise—slow leash walking
	Aquatic therapy after incision has sealed

may need to be decreased. The rehabilitation program should proceed with the patient being as pain free as possible.

Excision arthroplasty

Excision arthroplasty involves the surgical removal of part of the joint, allowing a pseudoarthrosis (false joint) to from fibrous tissue. It can be performed in various joints but is most commonly performed by excision of the femoral head and neck. Excision arthroplasty is performed as a treatment for severe osteoarthritis, irreparable fractures involving the joint, severe or recurrent joint luxation, or congenital joint deformities. Elimination of the joint and the bony contact relieves the joint pain. The goal is for fibrous tissue to create a pseudoarthrosis with no bony contact, which will provide pain-free function. Normal function and gait are not expected owing to the biomechanical changes. After excision arthroplasty, early active use of the limb is encouraged to prevent excessive fibrosis and loss of motion. Adequate analgesia throughout the rehabilitation program is a key factor for a successful outcome. Opiods may need to be combined with NSAIDs for optimum pain control. Cryotherapy can also help reduce pain and early inflammation. PROM exercises are begun the second day postoperatively and are continued until the patient is using the limb well. Once the acute inflammation has subsided, hot packs or therapeutic ultrasound can be used to promote PROM and stretching. Massage may also be helpful before passive or active exercises. Active weight-bearing activities are begun and are progressed to higher levels as tolerated by the patient to improve limb use and muscle strength.

Femoral head and neck ostectomy is the most common excision arthroplasty. After this procedure, the femur tends to be located more dorsally than normal; therefore, there is a functional shortening of the limb, which can cause gait abnormalities. In addition, the hindquarters may appear to be asymmetrical.

Rehabilitation after femoral head and neck ostectomy follows the same guidelines as for any excision arthroplasty, but there is an emphasis on regaining hip extension range of motion. Sit-to-stand exercises may be used soon after surgery to build gluteal muscles without requiring the pain associated with full hip extension. Walking up hills or steps will build the gluteal muscles and encourage active hip extension. Dancing exercises encourage muscle strengthening with maximal hip extension. Although swimming is a good conditioning exercise, it does not promote hip extension. Cryotherapy may be used at the end of each session to reduce inflammation. Patients can usually toe touch in 1 to 2 weeks, partially weight bear in 3 weeks, and actively use the leg by 4 weeks. The patient should regain near-normal walking and trotting gaits but will rarely achieve full range of motion, with hip extension being the most limited. The prognosis is generally good but varies with the surgical technique and the chronicity of the pre-existing lameness [13]. Adherence to a rehabilitation program may also affect the outcome; therefore, it is important to manage pain during the rehabilitation period to facilitate patient compliance.

Arthrodesis

Arthrodesis is the surgical fusion of a joint performed to salvage limb function when there is severe joint damage or in certain cases of nerve damage to a distal limb. To create bony fusion, the joint must be immobilized rigidly after destroying the articular cartilage and placing a bone graft. The joint is usually fused in a functional standing angle and is most commonly stabilized with a bone plate. Alternatively, pins, screws, or an external fixator may be used. Because of the massive inflammation and edema that can result from the surgical procedure, a pressure bandage is maintained during the immediate postoperative period. Cryotherapy and NSAIDs are also used to minimize the inflammatory reaction. The repair is supported by external coaptation (cast or splint) if internal fixation is used. This rigid support is usually applied in 3 to 5 days after the edema and swelling have resolved. The external coaptation is usually maintained for 6 to 8 weeks or until there are radiographic signs of fusion. During this time, PROM is performed on adjacent joints. Muscle-strengthening exercises may be instituted. Although other joints in the limb can compensate to some degree, the gait will never be normal. As the bone heals, gait training should be performed to restore the gait to the most normal pattern possible. Arthrodesis of joints that are located more distally on the limb is associated with better limb function and prognosis than is arthrodesis of more proximal joints. Arthrodesis is performed more commonly on the carpus and tarsus than on other joints.

Amputation

Limb amputation may be performed as a treatment for neoplasia, or for severe soft-tissue, orthopedic, or neurologic disorders. The patient should be encouraged to stand on the first postoperative day but may need assistance. Therapeutic exercise may begin with standing and walking and progresses to more challenging activities that help the animal adapt to the new center of gravity.

Uneven terrain or balance boards can be used to improve limb strength and proprioception. Most patients do well after amputation, whether it is a forelimb or hindlimb [14]. Patients that are overweight or that have impaired function of other limbs may have more difficulty adapting to an amputation.

Joint Disruption

Shoulder, elbow, and hip luxation

Joint luxations are generally a result of trauma. Hip dysplasia or congenital shoulder or elbow malformations may cause joints to be more unstable and predisposed to luxation. The diagnosis of a luxation can often be made by palpation of bony displacement, but radiographs are helpful to evaluate for the presence of concomitant fractures. In addition, the shoulder and elbow should be evaluated for congenital malformations, and the hip should be evaluated for hip dysplasia. These abnormalities may affect the treatment choice and prognosis.

If the diagnosis is made within a few days of an injury and there are no congenital malformations, closed reduction and immobilization in a sling or splint for 1 to 3 weeks may be successful. Medial shoulder luxations are immobilized with the limb flexed in a Velpeau sling. Lateral shoulder luxations and elbow luxations are immobilized with the limb extended in a spica splint. Hip luxations are immobilized with the femur abducted and internally rotated in an Ehmer sling. Open reduction and surgical stabilization are indicated if closed reduction is not successful, the joint is unstable after reduction, or luxation recurs while the leg is immobilized. Surgical treatment often involves repair of periarticular soft tissues such as ligaments or joint capsule. In some cases, the joint may be stabilized with heavy suture material. After surgery, joint healing is often protected by immobilization in the sling or splint for 1 to 3 weeks, depending on the degree of tissue damage and the type of repair.

Regardless of whether the treatment is by closed or open reduction, rehabilitation is begun after the sling or splint is removed. Range of motion must be restored without causing the joint to reluxate. In all joint luxations, cryotherapy and NSAIDs are used to minimize inflammation in the early postoperative period. During the first 3 weeks of shoulder rehabilitation, PROM is limited to the sagittal plane to avoid stress on the medial or lateral joint capsule, and weight-bearing exercises are limited. After elbow luxation, passive and active range of motion exercises should be limited to the sagittal plane, and varus or valgus stresses should be minimized. Muscle strengthening and re-education after hip luxation begins with walking on a level surface or a downhill grade. External rotation and adduction of the hind limb should be avoided during the healing phase of a craniodorsal hip luxation. In all cases, activity is gradually increased, but aggressive activities such as jogging, swimming, or uncontrolled play are limited until the joint has healed, which may take 1 to 3 months depending on the degree of tissue damage.

Joint reduction may not be recommended if there are irreparable fractures involving the joint, severe congenital malformations, hip dysplasia, or significant damage to the articular cartilage. In these cases, a joint salvage procedure may be a better choice. Common salvage procedures include excision arthroplasty, arthrodesis, or limb amputation.

The prognosis for traumatic joint luxations is generally good, although osteoarthritis is a common sequela. If damage to the articular cartilage is noted at the time of surgery, long-term problems with osteoarthritis may be expected. If the osteoarthritis becomes severe, a salvage procedure may be indicated.

Carpal hyperextension

Carpal hyperextension injuries occur after jumping or falling from a height, damaging the palmar fibrocartilage and carpal ligaments. Damage may occur to antebrachiocarpal, middle carpal, carpometacarpal, or any combination of these joints. Carpal hyperextension may also be caused by immune-mediated joint disease. Affected animals are lame and walk with the carpus hyperextended. In severe cases, the carpus may touch the ground. Healing of a sprain (ligament injury) may take months and occurs by the formation of fibrous connective tissue to replace the torn ligament, rather than by primary healing of the ligament. Conservative management of carpal hyperextension injuries is generally unsuccessful [15]. The recommended treatment is panarthrodesis (surgical fusion of all three joint levels) or partial arthrodesis (fusion of only the middle and distal joints), depending on the level of the injuries. Rehabilitation is performed as for any arthrodesis, with an emphasis on gait training after the initial healing period. The prognosis for limb function is good after carpal arthrodesis. The prognosis is guarded if instability is due to rheumatoid arthritis, because multiple joints are typically affected.

Stifle luxation

Total derangement of the stifle with rupture of one or both cruciate ligaments and one or both collateral ligaments occurs as a result of severe trauma. The meniscus is often damaged as well. Surgical repair is recommended and may involve suturing stretched or torn ligaments, or the use of prosthetic material (eg, suture and screws or bone anchors) to replace the torn ligaments. If the damage is severe or if injury to other limbs will result in increased stress on the repaired stifle, the repair may be protected with a bandage or splint for the first 2 to 4 weeks. If the stifle is not bandaged, immediate PROM helps prevent joint contracture, promote cartilage homeostasis, and stimulate scar formation along normal lines of stress. If the stifle is bandaged postoperatively, the goal after bandage removal is to eliminate joint stiffness and re-establish range of motion with passive and active exercises. Therapeutic ultrasound with simultaneous stretching may also be beneficial. Weight-bearing activities are encouraged with weight shifting, slow leash walks, and treadmill walking. Aquatic therapy may also be helpful. Appropriate challenges to the healing tissues will enhance tissue remodeling and strengthening. Endurance and strengthening activities may be initiated between 4 and 6 weeks. A near full return to activities should be achieved by 12 to 16 weeks. The prognosis for stifle luxation is fair.

Long-term problems include decreased range of motion, chronic instability, and ongoing osteoarthritis.

Hock shear injuries

Most luxations of the tarsocrural joint occur with concomitant damage of one or both malleoli, the site of collateral ligament insertion. Subluxation can occur with rupture or avulsion of the collateral ligaments. Surgical repair may include imbrication, suturing, reattaching the ligaments, or replacing the ligaments with a prosthetic collateral ligament technique. In some cases, an external fixator may be applied as the primary repair [16]. There are often open wounds that must be treated. Ligament repairs are protected during healing by immobilizing the joint in a cast, splint, or external fixator for 3 weeks. Ligament repairs are generally not able to withstand full weight-bearing stresses for several weeks; however, the ligaments fail to gain as much strength if the joint is rigidly immobilized for 6 weeks when compared with ligaments of joints that are not immobilized beyond 3 weeks [17]. After the cast or external fixator is removed, remobilization of adjacent joints, weight-bearing exercises, and muscle reconditioning are begun. Active or passive therapeutic exercises that place varus or valgus stresses on the collateral ligaments should be avoided.

Arthrodesis may be indicated for shear injuries if the degree of tissue loss makes joint reconstruction impossible. Hyperextension injuries that result in subluxation or luxation of the tarsometatarsal joint, or the proximal or distal intertarsal joints, also require arthrodesis for a good outcome [18]. Arthrodesis is performed by application of internal or external fixation. If internal fixation is used, the distal limb is supported by a splint or cast for 6 to 8 weeks or until there is radiographic evidence of fusion. Remobilization of adjacent joints, weight-bearing exercises, and muscle reconditioning are begun after the cast has been removed. The digits should also undergo mobilization and PROM techniques following tarsal arthrodesis.

Metacarpophalangeal, metatarsophalangeal, and phalangeal luxation

Metacarpophalangeal, metatarsophalangeal, and phalangeal luxations can be treated by repair of the collateral ligaments and joint capsule. After surgery, the foot is splinted for 2 to 3 weeks. It is beneficial to change the splint once weekly to perform PROM exercises on the distal joints. After the splint has been permanently removed, range of motion exercises are continued. Limited weight-bearing activities are initiated and gradually increased over another 3 weeks.

Other options for metacarpophalangeal, metatarsophalangeal, and phalangeal luxations include arthrodesis of the joint or amputation of the digit. Arthrodesis is a better choice if a high level of function is required, such as racing. Postoperatively, the foot is splinted until there is radiographic evidence of fusion. Weekly splint changes with PROM of the other distal joints may be beneficial.

Joint Diseases
Osteoarthritis

Osteoarthritis may also be termed *osteoarthrosis* or *degenerative joint disease*. Joint health deterioration typically occurs secondary to joint incongruity, instability, or some other disruption of the articular cartilage. Mechanical and biochemical changes result in decreased cartilage resiliency, cartilage thinning, subchondral sclerosis, synovitis, and osteophyte formation. Clinical signs include joint pain, crepitus, and stiffness. Normal range of motion may be lost owing to joint surface incongruity, muscle spasm and contracture, periarticular fibrosis, or mechanical block from osteophytes or joint mice. The joint may be enlarged owing to synovitis, synovial effusion, osteophytes, or periarticular fibrosis. The pain and stiffness may lead to lameness or decreased activity and loss of muscle mass and strength.

The goals of treating osteoarthritis are to manage pain, maintain function and range of motion, and maintain or regain normal activity. These goals are primarily accomplished by means of weight management, therapeutic exercise, and medications. Weight reduction is essential for obese patients. Weight reduction alone can cause a significant improvement in clinical signs in dogs with hip dysplasia that are more than 10% above their ideal body weight [19]. A controlled, low-impact exercise program alone has been shown to improve pain and overall function scores in geriatric dogs with osteoarthritis [20]. Regularly performed low-impact exercise, such as leash walking, walking in water, or swimming, helps to maintain muscle strength and joint function while minimizing joint stresses. Bursts of vigorous activity, such as running or jumping, may exacerbate inflammation and should be minimized. Certain activities may be used to target specific muscle groups. Repeated sit-to-stand exercises or walking up stairs help to strengthen the hind limb muscles. Exercise sessions should be challenging but should not result in increased pain. The exercise program must be tailored to the individual and adjusted to account for the fluctuations in clinical signs that are typically seen with osteoarthritis.

Other techniques and modalities may be used to enhance the exercise program. In animals with severe muscle loss and weakness, NMES may be used for muscle strengthening. Passive and active exercises are used to improve joint range of motion and promote cartilage metabolism and diffusion of nutrients. Passive stretching alone can improve range of motion in dogs with osteoarthritis [21]. Joint mobilization may also help improve joint motion and health and reduce pain. Hot packs, therapeutic ultrasound, or massage may be useful to reduce pain associated with muscle spasms and to decrease joint stiffness. These modalities can also be used to increase blood supply to the muscle in preparation for an exercise session. TENS has been shown to be of benefit in dogs with osteoarthritic pain [22]. Extracorporeal shock wave therapy also shows promise as a method to decrease pain in dogs with osteoarthritis; however, the number of cases reported is limited [23,24]. Cryotherapy can be used to reduce acute inflammatory episodes associated with overuse or postexercise inflammation.

Numerous drugs and substances are promoted for the treatment of osteoarthritis. Slow-acting, disease-modifying osteoarthritic agents (DMOAs), or chondroprotective agents, have the potential to improve joint health by stimulating cartilage metabolism and hyaluronan synthesis, inhibiting periarticular fibrin formation, and inhibiting catabolic enzymes. Some of these agents may also function as anti-inflammatory agents or free radical scavengers. Injectable hyaluronic acid or polysulfated glycosaminoglycan (Adequan) may be of benefit for some arthritic patients [25,26]. Oral glucosamine and chondroitin sulfate may have a synergistic effect benefiting dogs with osteoarthritis [27]. S-adenosylmethionine (SAMe) appears to be effective in humans with osteoarthritis. The oral forms of DMOAs, known as neutraceuticals, are not regulated as drugs; therefore, there may be considerable variation in product content and quality. Although several compounds are marketed as being effective in the treatment of osteoarthritis, they have not been proven effective by scientific studies. Although the efficacy of most DMOAs is still unclear, the risk of adverse side effects appears to be low.

NSAIDs may be used as needed for pain management and to treat chronic inflammation or episodes of acute inflammation. It is advisable to maintain the lowest effective dose to minimize the risks of adverse side effects. The efficacy of NSAIDs varies between individuals; therefore, if the patient is not responding well to one NSAID, another may be more effective [28]. It is advisable to stop one NSAID completely before starting another. Additional analgesics may be needed in severely affected patients. Although corticosteroids are excellent anti-inflammatory drugs, they should be avoided for chronic use [29].

Lifestyle modifications may be beneficial for some patients with osteoarthritis [30]. Patients should be housed in a warm dry area with good footing and provided with a padded area for sleeping. Stair climbing and jumping may be minimized by the use of ramps. Table 2 summarizes the goals of treatment in the rehabilitation of joints with osteoarthritis.

Osteochondritis dissecans

Osteochondrosis is a developmental disease affecting the cartilage in medium and large breed dogs. Abnormal endochondral ossification of the deep layers of articular cartilage results in focal areas of thickened cartilage that are prone to injury. In the absence of excessive stress, the lesion may heal. Further stress on the cartilage may result in a cartilage flap. This condition is termed *osteochondritis dissecans*. It has been described in various joints of the dog but most commonly occurs in the shoulder joint.

Dogs typically have mild-to-moderate lameness between 4 and 9 months of age. Atrophy of the muscles may be apparent in the affected limb if the dog has been lame for several weeks. Pain may be elicited on flexion or extension of the affected joint. Dogs with hock and elbow osteochondritis dissecans may have signs of osteoarthritis, such as joint effusion, thickening of the periarticular soft tissues, decreased range of motion, and crepitus. Radiographs may demonstrate a defect in the subchondral bone under the cartilage flap. In some cases,

Table 2
Rehabilitation of joints with osteoarthritis

Goals	Treatment
Reduce joint stresses	Dietary counseling and exercise program to achieve and maintain lean body weight
	Lifestyle changes, such as ramps instead of steps or jumping
	Encourage controlled, low-impact activities
Strengthen periarticular muscles	Controlled, low-impact exercise (walking or aquatic exercise)
	NMES if too weak or painful for active exercise
Maintain or improve joint range of motion	PROM
	Active range of motion—therapeutic exercise (walking or aquatic)
	Joint mobilization
Maintain or improve cartilage health	PROM
	Weight-bearing exercise with low impact (walking or aquatic)
	DMOAs
Limit inflammation	NSAIDs to treat chronic or acute inflammation
	Cryotherapy for episodes of acute inflammation
	Limit high-impact or uncontrolled activities
Pain management	NSAIDs and other analgesics as needed
	Cryotherapy, hot packs, therapeutic ultrasound, or massage for muscle spasms

especially those affecting the elbow or hock, the diagnosis may be difficult and best made by CT or arthroscopy.

Surgery is generally the treatment of choice in dogs with clinical signs [31]. It is performed via arthrotomy or arthroscopy to remove the defective cartilage and to forage or curettage the bed of the lesion. This procedure encourages vascular ingrowth and healing by the formation of fibrocartilage. After surgery, NSAIDs, cryotherapy, PROM, and controlled leash walks are instituted for the first 2 to 4 weeks. After this initial healing period, the duration of the leash walks is progressively intensified. In addition, treadmill walking and swimming may be initiated. By 6 weeks, light jogging can usually be started [30]. Seroma formation is a common complication after shoulder surgery but is usually self-limiting and resolves with rest. If shoulder seroma is observed, the activity level should be reduced until it resolves. Long-term management of osteochondritis dissecans is focused on limiting or treating osteoarthritis. Table 3 summarizes the goals of joint rehabilitation after surgery for osteochondritis dissecans.

Table 3
Joint rehabilitation after surgery for osteochondritis dissecans

Goals	Treatment
Control inflammation	Cryotherapy immediately after surgery or after exercise
Maintain or improve range of motion	PROM or stretching
Control pain	NSAIDs for first few weeks, as needed
Strengthen muscle	Begin with controlled slow leash walking and progress to jogging or swimming

The long-term prognosis for osteochondritis dissecans in the shoulder is excellent in most cases [32]. The prognosis for disease affecting the elbow is good if surgery is performed before osteoarthritis is advanced but is more guarded than for disease affecting the shoulder. The prognosis for osteochondritis dissecans affecting the stifle and hock tends to be guarded, because osteoarthritis usually progresses even after surgery.

Elbow dysplasia
Elbow dysplasia includes a fragmented medial coronoid process, ununited anconeal process, and osteochondritis dissecans. Dogs with elbow dysplasia usually have only one of the three conditions. Elbow incongruity may also be present. Elbow dysplasia usually occurs in large or giant breeds of dogs. Affected dogs typically have bilateral problems, although one elbow may be more severely affected.

Fragmented medial coronoid process. Dogs with a fragmented medial coronoid process have a mild-to-moderate weight-bearing lameness that is usually noted between 5 and 9 months of age. Physical examination findings include pain on flexion and extension of the elbow, pain on palpation of the medial aspect of the joint, and palpable joint effusion. In dogs older than 11 months, crepitus, decreased range of motion, and general joint thickening may be evident. Radiographs often show degenerative changes in the joint, but the actual lesion may not be seen. In many cases, CT or arthroscopy is needed to make a definitive diagnosis.

Treatment is removal of the fragmented medial coronoid process via arthrotomy or arthroscopy. Postoperatively, activity is limited for 2 to 4 weeks. The prognosis is good if the medial coronoid process is removed before there is advanced osteoarthritis. Osteoarthritis will progress regardless of treatment, but the changes are more severe in untreated cases. If the osteoarthritis is severe at the time of diagnosis, the value of surgical treatment is questionable. These dogs may be managed by conservative treatment for the osteoarthritis [33]. In all cases, rehabilitation is directed toward treatment of osteoarthritis.

Ununited anconeal process. An ununited anconeal process is a failure of the anconeal process of the ulna to fuse properly with the olecranon by 5 months of age and is apparent on a flexed lateral radiograph [33]. Instability of the anconeal process causes inflammation and eventual osteoarthritis. The dog usually has a weight-bearing lameness. Decreased range of motion and joint effusion may be apparent on palpation.

Treatment options include surgical removal of the anconeal process, screw fixation, or osteotomy of the proximal ulna to relieve joint incongruity and allow healing of the anconeal process. Regardless of the treatment, osteoarthritis progresses; therefore, continued treatment is directed toward managing osteoarthritis.

If the ununited anconeal process is treated by screw fixation, the rehabilitation program should have a slower progression of weight-bearing activities until there is radiographic evidence of healing. This period may take as long as 12 weeks in some cases. If the ununited anconeal process is treated by removal, the rehabilitation program may progress more rapidly, as dictated by the degree of joint effusion, pain, range of motion, and weight bearing. Immediately after surgery, PROM, aquatic therapy, and light leash walks are recommended. Cryotherapy and NSAIDs may be used as needed to control inflammation and pain.

Elbow incongruity. Asynchronous growth of the radius and ulna can cause elbow incongruity in chondrodystrophoid dogs and is usually evident by 4 to 5 months of age. The ununited anconeal process and fragmented medial coronoid process have been associated with elbow incongruity, although they can occur in the absence of incongruity. Traumatic closure of a radial or ulnar physis also leads to asynchronous growth with elbow subluxation and an angular limb deformity.

Surgical options to improve congruity include corrective osteotomy or ostectomy of the radius or ulna, and may involve stabilization with a bone plate or external fixator. The prognosis is worse if the incongruency is severe and if the animal is older than 9 months [34].

After surgery, normal range of motion of the joints proximal and distal to the repair should be maintained. Pain and edema may be controlled by NSAIDs and cryotherapy. If the goal was to lengthen the limb following surgery, increased tension on the soft tissues may result in decreased range of motion, joint stiffness, and lameness. In these cases, therapeutic ultrasound with simultaneous stretching and range of motion activities may be helpful. As bone healing progresses, more aggressive weight-bearing exercises may be initiated.

Elbow incongruity invariably results in some degree of osteoarthritis of the elbow. Some dogs may not present for rehabilitation until they have end-stage osteoarthritis. Regardless, rehabilitation is directed toward managing osteoarthritis to maintain an acceptable quality of life.

Hip dysplasia

Hip dysplasia is an abnormal development of the hip joint, usually bilateral, that occurs primarily in medium and large breed dogs. The causes are multifactorial and include genetic predisposition, a rapid growth rate, and diet. The hips develop instability between 4 and 12 months of age. At this stage, the dog may exhibit difficulty rising, a decreased activity level, a "bunny-hopping" gait, and loss of muscle mass in the hindquarters. At this point, the diagnosis is made by palpation of joint laxity (subluxation). Radiographs may appear normal, although some degree of subluxation may be evident. As the disease progresses, periarticular fibrosis causes some joint stability, and the pain may be significantly decreased. With further progression of the disease, osteoarthritis results in pain, crepitus, decreased range of motion, a waddling gait, and reluctance to stand. Thigh and hip muscles atrophy, and shoulder muscles may hypertrophy because the body weight is shifted toward the forelimbs. Radiographs show varying degrees of osteoarthritis with remodeling of the femoral head and acetabulum. The rate of progression of hip dysplasia varies between individuals and is difficult to predict. Some dogs may have degenerative changes by 1 year of age, whereas many individuals develop advanced osteoarthritis in midlife or later.

In young dogs, several surgical procedures are designed to change the joint alignment to improve joint stability and slow the progression of osteoarthritis. The most common of these procedures are the triple pelvic osteotomy and juvenile pubic symphysiodesis. Triple pelvic osteotomy is performed on dogs that show early signs of hip dysplasia and joint laxity but have not progressed to the point of having significant radiographic evidence of osteoarthritis. Most dogs that fit these criteria are between 4 and 10 months of age. They usually have atrophy of the gluteal and thigh muscles. The technique involves making three osteotomies to change the orientation of the acetabulum. A bone plate is used to stabilize the ilium. Postoperatively, activity is restricted for 4 to 6 weeks to allow for bone healing. Cryotherapy, NSAIDs, PROM, and assisted ambulation for 2 weeks, followed by controlled low-impact therapeutic exercises, are indicated. After adequate bone healing has occurred, the focus of rehabilitation is to strengthen muscles of the hindquarters. Strengthening activities should parallel bone healing and tissue strength.

Juvenile pubic symphysiodesis is performed in dogs between 16 and 18 weeks of age that are considered to be at risk for hip dysplasia. The pubic symphysis is surgically damaged, causing it to fuse and alter pelvic growth. These puppies are often clinically normal, and the surgical trauma is minimal. The focus of rehabilitation is to promote muscular development of the hind limbs with low-impact exercise.

Dogs with mild or intermittent signs of hip dysplasia may be treated by conservative methods to limit the progression of osteoarthritis. These methods include a combination of NSAIDs, DMOAs, diet, and exercise and are discussed in the previous section on osteoarthritis. For dogs with pain that is not adequately managed by conservative methods, two salvage surgical options exist: total hip replacement or femoral head and neck ostectomy. Both procedures eliminate the normal joint, eliminating the pain. In general, total hip replacement is not an option after femoral head ostectomy has been performed. Rehabilitation after femoral head and neck ostectomy has been discussed previously in the section on excision arthroplasty.

Total hip replacement involves replacing the acetabulum with an acetabular prosthesis. The femoral head is removed, and a femoral prosthesis is implanted in the medullary canal of the femur. Most commonly, the prostheses are secured with bone cement, but some systems do not use cement. In the initial postoperative period, NSAIDs, cryotherapy, and gentle PROM are indicated. The most common postoperative complication is hip luxation; therefore, muscle strengthening is important, especially because there is often pre-existing muscle atrophy. Close confinement is enforced for the first postoperative month when the dog is unsupervised. During early ambulation, the dog is supported with a sling to prevent abduction of the limb and dislocation of the prosthesis. Muscle strengthening can be achieved using controlled walking, treadmill activity, and sit-to-stand exercises. The duration of these activities is gradually increased during the first 2 months. Balance and proprioception re-education may also be important. Dogs are restricted to leash walking, with no running or jumping for the first 3 postoperative months to reduce the chances of implant loosening or dislocation. The prognosis is good to excellent in most cases. A deterioration in limb use may signal loosening of the implant or the onset of another problem, such as a cranial cruciate ligament rupture.

Legg Calve Perthes

Legg Calve Perthes disease is noninflammatory aseptic necrosis of the femoral head and neck that occurs in small breed dogs. The etiology is unknown, although a genetic component has been identified in some breeds. Dogs usually develop lameness between 6 and 10 months of age and experience pain with hip manipulation. With chronic lameness, there is muscle atrophy of the hip and thigh muscles. Radiographs show deformation of the femoral head and neck with joint incongruity. In some cases, there may be advanced osteoarthritis or fractures secondary to collapse of the femoral head and neck. If the condition is diagnosed early, a non–weight-bearing sling may be used for 3 to 4 weeks [35]; however, the treatment of choice is generally femoral head and neck ostectomy. The prognosis is good provided appropriate rehabilitation is performed beginning immediately after surgery (discussed in the section on excision arthroplasty).

Patellar luxation

Although patellar luxations may be traumatic in origin, they are most commonly related to abnormalities in hind limb conformation. Medial luxations are more common than lateral luxations in all dog breeds and in cats. Concurrent cranial cruciate ligament rupture is present in 15% to 20% of middle-aged and older dogs with chronic patellar luxation [34]. Patellar luxations are classified from grade 1 to 4, with grade 4 being the most severely affected. The classifications are based on the degree of clinical signs, ease of patellar luxation and reduction, and severity of bony abnormalities. Surgery is indicated when gait abnormalities or lameness are present.

Surgical correction of patellar luxations usually requires reconstruction of soft tissues and bone to realign the quadriceps mechanism. In almost all cases, the tibial crest is transposed and pinned. A technique to deepen the trochlear groove (trochleoplasty) is also used in most cases, as well as a capsulectomy or imbrication of the soft tissues on the redundant side. After surgery, the tissues must be allowed to heal before vigorous rehabilitation begins, particularly if the tibial crest is transposed. During the first few weeks, cryotherapy and NSAIDs may be used for inflammation. Active use of the limb is encouraged, but initial activity should be limited to short leash walks, and jumping is not allowed. PROM is beneficial for joint resurfacing and cartilage healing, especially if a trochleoplasty is performed [36]. Small breed dogs in particular are sometimes reluctant to bear weight on the affected limb, even in the absence of apparent pain or complications. In these cases, weight-shifting activities or swimming may be instituted to encourage limb use. After several weeks, strengthening exercises may be initiated. Motion should be limited to the sagittal plane to avoid undue stress on the repair; therefore, activities that involve turning or pivoting, such as figure-of-eights and weaving through vertical poles, should be avoided. The prognosis is generally fair to good for grades 2 and 3 luxations but guarded for grade 4 luxations.

Cranial cruciate ligament rupture

Acute rupture of the cranial cruciate ligament results in gross instability of the stifle and is often accompanied by a sudden non–weight-bearing lameness, which may improve gradually over the first few weeks. Alternatively, the ligament may sustain a partial rupture, causing less obvious instability and lameness. In both cases, degenerative joint changes are initiated at the time of the rupture and progress with time. The cause of cranial cruciate ligament rupture may be acute trauma or, more commonly, chronic degeneration of the ligament. Joint instability invariably leads to progressive osteoarthritis with deterioration of limb function.

Damage to the caudal pole of the medial meniscus often occurs as a result of joint instability. Damage to the meniscus rarely occurs as an isolated injury but may be seen in approximately 45% of patients with rupture of the cranial cruciate ligament [37]. In some cases, the meniscus may be normal at the time of the initial surgery for cranial cruciate ligament rupture but become damaged at some time in the future. Clinical signs of a meniscal tear may include lameness, reduced limb use, or an audible click during joint motion. Partial or total meniscectomy via arthrotomy or arthroscopy is used to treat meniscal tear. If the meniscus is damaged, osteoarthritis may progress more rapidly, or the animal may have reduced function. The rehabilitation program after meniscectomy is dictated by the procedure used to stabilize the joint but may be accelerated if the meniscectomy is performed some time after a stifle stabilization procedure.

Cruciate ligament rupture is diagnosed by palpating cranial drawer motion (cranial subluxation of the tibia). In acute cases, joint effusion may be evident.

In chronic cases, drawer motion may be difficult to elicit, and the periarticular tissues may be thickened, particularly on the medial aspect of the stifle. Radiographs may be used to confirm the presence of joint effusion, assess the severity of any degenerative changes, and rule out other problems.

Conservative treatment by strict confinement for 4 to 8 weeks may be attempted in small dogs; however, surgery is generally accepted as the treatment of choice, regardless of dog size. Many surgical techniques have been described to treat cranial cruciate ligament rupture, but none have been proven to stop the progression of osteoarthritis. The surgical procedures can be classified as extracapsular, intracapsular, or tibial osteotomy.

Extracapsular procedures stabilize the joint by transposition of the patient's own tissues or securing a synthetic material (usually suture) external to the joint capsule. Because the joint is stabilized by periarticular fibrosis within 8 to 10 weeks, breakdown of the suture several months postoperatively does not affect joint stability. Physical rehabilitation of animals undergoing extracapsular techniques begins in the immediate postoperative period with cryotherapy, NSAIDs, and PROM. Controlled leash walks and active use of the limb are encouraged within 1 day. Treadmill walking can be used to encourage weight bearing. Aquatic therapy can begin 1 week postoperatively if the incision is sealed and has no drainage or discharge. PROM is continued with an emphasis on stifle extension. Hind limb muscles can be strengthened by stair climbing, uphill walking, sit-to-stand exercises, or pulling a cart. As strength and endurance improve, the duration and intensity of the exercises can increase to include jogging, controlled ball playing, and swimming. Explosive activity such as jumping is not allowed for the first 3 months to avoid failure of the stabilization, especially tearing of the suture through the femorofabellar ligament if a suture has been passed around the fabella.

Intracapsular procedures replace the cruciate ligament in a nearly anatomic position with a graft, synthetic material, or a combination of these materials. Biologic tissues undergo a period of weakness until the tissue revascularizes and gains additional strength. It may take months for the graft to regain sufficient strength to function as a cranial cruciate ligament. Physical rehabilitation of animals undergoing intracapsular techniques includes cryotherapy and NSAIDs to reduce pain and inflammation. The rehabilitation program must consider the material used for the surgery. Autografts and allografts are generally strong when initially placed but stretch under tension. The tissue becomes weaker over the next 2 to 20 weeks while revascularization and incorporation occur. Ultimate tissue strength is achieved following biointegration of the graft. The rehabilitation program can be similar to that for extracapsular repair but should not progress as rapidly because of the limited graft strength. In some cases, intracapsular repairs are combined with an extracapsular repair. In these cases, rehabilitation may progress at the rate for an extracapsular repair.

Although several tibial osteotomy techniques have been described, the most commonly used is the tibial plateau leveling osteotomy. The theory behind the osteotomy techniques is to alter the joint biomechanics to eliminate abnormal stifle motion. The tibial plateau leveling osteotomy is performed by making an osteotomy in the proximal tibia, rotating the proximal tibia to create a more level joint surface, and stabilizing it with a bone plate until the bone has healed. Patellar desmitis is a common complication that is seen in the first postoperative month and is identified by pain on palpation of the patellar tendon at its insertion on the tibial crest. Another complication is avulsion of a portion of the tibial crest. Because of these potential complications, excessive stress on the patellar tendon should be avoided in the early postoperative period. The quadriceps muscle-patellar tendon unit should be maintained in a relatively shortened position to reduce forces on the tibial crest. Excessive flexion of the stifle during weight bearing should be avoided. Such flexion occurs during jumping, running, stair climbing, or walking in a crouched position. The therapist must watch for these complications and adjust the treatment protocol if they occur. The complications can usually be managed by rest, NSAIDs, and cryotherapy. After the tissues have begun to heal and remodel, a more gradual increase in activity level can be instituted, usually by 3 to 4 weeks. The osteotomy site must be given adequate time to heal (3 to 6 weeks) to prevent complications related to bone healing and implant failure. Aquatic therapy is helpful to reduce weight-bearing stresses on the repair. As the osteotomy site heals, gradual increased use of the leg is begun.

The prognosis for cranial cruciate ligament rupture is variable. In humans, a trend toward more aggressive rehabilitation has shown improved outcomes following surgery for cruciate rupture [38]. Postoperative rehabilitation programs for cranial cruciate ligament surgery in dogs improve joint range of motion, reduce muscle spasms, and improve weight bearing and overall joint function [39,40]. Dogs treated only with NMES after surgery on the cranial cruciate ligament had improved lameness scores, increased thigh circumference, and decreased radiographic changes when compared with untreated dogs [41]. The focus of rehabilitation in most cases is on improving stifle extension and increasing mass of the quadriceps, biceps femoris, and semimembranosus muscles [42]. Some dogs will recover with near-normal function, whereas others have moderate-to-severe osteoarthritis requiring long-term management.

TENDONS

A strain is a tear or rupture of some part of the muscle-tendon unit. The point of damage may be the tendon, muscle-tendon junction, muscle, or attachment sites. Tendons heal with scar tissue, similar to other soft tissues; however, it is undesirable for a tendon to heal with adhesions to the surrounding tissue. Optimal healing results in minimal scar tissue and adhesions to allow tendon gliding. The surgeon can promote optimal healing by attention to gentle tissue handling, aseptic technique to prevent contamination, and proper hemostasis. Flexor tendons usually require more gliding function than extensor tendons. After tendon surgery, active motion should be limited to allow the tendon to develop a blood supply from surrounding tissue and begin healing with minimal collagenous adhesions. PROM can be started after 3 weeks of rest. Gentle tendon motion will promote remodeling of the peritendinous scar, which allows the tendon to glide [17]. At this point, the tendon is still not strong enough to withstand active motion and full weight bearing, but rigid immobilization is not desirable because it will prevent an increase in tensile strength. Between 3 and 6 weeks, exercise should be limited, and a cast or splint may be used to protect the tendon from excess stress when not performing rehabilitation activities. By 6 weeks, the tendon has not attained full strength but should be strong enough to support full weight while walking [17]. The tendon may continue to increase slowly in strength for a year or more.

Biceps Tenosynovitis

Biceps tenosynovitis causes forelimb lameness in medium and large breed dogs. It is thought to be caused by direct trauma, indirect trauma, or overuse. The initial irritation may affect the tendon or the synovial membrane, but the result is inflammation of both structures. Adhesions between the tendon and sheath can limit motion and cause pain [43]. Pain occurs during tendon gliding; therefore, there is minimal or no change in weight bearing during the stance phase of gait. The lameness is usually insidious in onset, intermittent, and worsens with exercise. Chronic cases will have shoulder muscle atrophy. Pain is not a consistent finding but may be elicited on palpation of the tendon during flexion of the shoulder and simultaneous extension of the elbow to place additional tension on the biceps tendon. Radiographs may demonstrate mineralization of the bicipital tendon, osteophytes in the intertubercular groove, or other degenerative changes. The diagnosis can be difficult and is sometimes made by diagnostic ultrasound, MRI, or observation during arthroscopy.

In acute cases, the goal is to reduce inflammation. Rest and NSAIDs are used. Rest should be enforced for 4 to 6 weeks. Intra-articular steroids may be helpful if there are no mechanical causes such as joint mice. In addition, pulsed mode 3.3-MHz therapeutic ultrasound may be used over the tendon and musculotendinous junction [30]. The ultrasound should not result in significant tissue temperature increase, and the patient should be monitored for pain. Cryotherapy may also be prescribed to reduce inflammation. Fifty percent to 66% of dogs respond to medical therapy [34,44]; however, the response is often unsatisfactory, or signs recur with active exercise.

Surgical treatment is recommended for dogs that do not respond to medical treatment. Surgical techniques include transposition of the tendon to the proximal humerus or arthroscopic tendon release [44,45]. Postoperatively, activity is limited to short leash walks for 3 weeks. Cryotherapy and PROM are also used during this time. After the initial 3 weeks, gradual strengthening of the biceps and brachialis muscle is begun. Strengthening may be accomplished by NMES of the biceps and brachialis muscle, aquatic therapy, and treadmill activity. Cryotherapy may be needed to minimize postexercise inflammation. Most surgically treated dogs regain normal function and gait [34,44].

Supraspinatus Tendon Mineralization

Mineralization of the supraspinatus tendon may cause mild-to-moderate lameness in medium and large breed dogs. The presence of mineralization can also be asymptomatic. The etiology is unknown. Palpation of the area is usually not painful. Diagnosis is made by observing mineralization on radiographs and ruling out other conditions that could cause forelimb lameness. Medical treatment includes rest, NSAIDs, cryotherapy, and PROM exercises [30]. Therapeutic ultrasound has been used in humans to treat the deposits and may be beneficial for dogs [30]. Surgical excision of the mineralized tissue may be performed in some cases [46]. After surgery, a carpal flexion bandage may be applied for 2 weeks to prevent weight bearing. Activity is limited for an additional 2 to 3 weeks. Swimming may cause too much tendon stress and is not advised for several months. The prognosis is good, with total recovery in 6 to 8 weeks.

Infraspinatus Contracture

Infraspinatus contracture causes a mild weight-bearing lameness in hunting or working dogs. The cause is hypothesized to be acute muscle trauma, which results in incomplete rupture of the infraspinatus muscle and resultant fibrotic contracture. Replacement of muscle fibers by fibrous tissue occurs over days to weeks. The elbow is held in adduction and the foot in abduction. The scapulohumeral joint cannot fully extend. The limb circumducts as it is advanced during the stride.

Physical rehabilitation may be beneficial if the condition is diagnosed early. Continuous therapeutic ultrasound with stretching exercises may help to lengthen contracted tissues, but the degree of contracture is usually so severe at the time of diagnosis that it is difficult to improve the condition with nonsurgical techniques [30]; therefore, the treatment of choice is surgical transection of the infraspinatus tendon and associated fibrous tissue [47]. Normal activity is resumed 2 weeks after surgery, and the prognosis is good.

Postoperatively, full weight bearing is allowed, but activity should be restricted for the first few weeks. Uncontrolled activity may cause tissue damage and recurrence of fibrous tissue [30]. PROM exercises to the joints of the forelimb several times daily maintain joint range of motion and promote normal alignment of the healing tissues [30]. Lateral hopping exercises may help strengthen other surrounding supporting muscles. Cryotherapy can be used to reduce inflammation after exercise. When there is significant disuse atrophy of the forelimb muscles, general conditioning exercises for the limb are used to return the muscle gradually to normal size and strength. Conditioning exercises include walking, wheel barrowing, and aquatic therapy. NMES may be used if the atrophy is severe and the dog is too weak to use the leg well.

Tendon of the Long Digital Extensor Muscle

Avulsion of the tendon of the long digital extensor muscle is a rare condition that occurs in young dogs. Clinical signs include joint effusion and pain in the craniolateral aspect of the joint. If not treated, osteoarthritis and chronic low-grade lameness may result. Treatment involves reattachment of the avulsed fragment of bone or removing the fragment and attaching the tendon to the proximal tibia or joint capsule. If the bony fragment is reattached, time is allowed for union before starting aggressive rehabilitation. In the initial postoperative period, pain and inflammation are resolved with NSAIDs and cryotherapy. Limited weight bearing with muscle re-education and proprioceptive training are instituted as the fracture heals. If the fragment is excised and the tendon reattached, weight-bearing controlled activity can be started soon after surgery. The prognosis is good if surgical treatment is performed before osteoarthritis is apparent.

Luxation of the proximal tendon of the long digital extensor muscle may cause mild to marked lameness and a clicking sound. Surgical treatment involves suturing of the retinacular support.

Flexor Tendon Contracture

Contracture is a shortening of the tendon-muscle unit that is caused by a lack of active muscle contraction. Most cases of contracture involve the flexor tendons. After immobilization or prolonged disuse, the flexor tendons may undergo contracture. The result is limited extension of the joints distal to the elbow or tarsus, which can impair the gait. One example is contracture of the tendons following cast application to a forelimb. Methods of lengthening and stretching the contracted tendon-muscle units include 3.3-MHz therapeutic ultrasound or hot packs, manual stretching exercises, and massage. If stretching is too aggressive, it may cause tearing of soft tissues or bone fractures. The goal is to stretch and realign the tissues without damaging them. Various surgical techniques are available to lengthen tendon in cases of severe contracture. In some cases, a tenotomy may be performed. If the contracture is not severe, splinting with the tendon in tension and stretching activities may lengthen the tendon-muscle unit.

Achilles Rupture

The common calcanean (Achilles) tendon consists of three tendons that insert on the tuber calcanei: the gastrocnemius; the common tendon of the biceps femoris, semitendinosus, and gracilis muscles; and the tendon of the superficial digital flexor muscle. Rupture of the common calcanean tendon can occur at the musculotendinous junction, the midsubstance, or near the tendon's insertion on the tuber calcanei. The tendon may be injured by sharp penetrating trauma or chronic repetitive use. Chronic stretching and tearing may also occur and may be the result of tendon degeneration, especially in Doberman Pinschers. If the tendon is avulsed, the end may be palpable 2 to 3 cm proximal to the tuber calcaneus. The distal end of the tendon becomes enlarged and firm as fibrous tissue develops. Radiographs are helpful to identify any avulsion fractures. If the tendon is avulsed, it may be sutured to bone tunnels in the calcaneus. A large bone fragment avulsion may be repaired with a pin and tension band. The tendon is usually sutured primarily in cases of ruptures at the musculocutaneous junction or midtendon. Partial tendon ruptures may be managed by a cast or splint.

After tendon surgery, the hock is immobilized in a normal standing angle to prevent tension on the repair. Three or more weeks of immobilization may be accomplished with a splint, cast, positional screw, or external fixator. Rigid fixation should be used for the shortest time necessary. Early weight bearing and joint movement create stress on the reconstructed tissue to promote parallel collagen alignment in the repaired tendon and increased early tendon strength [48,49]. External skeletal fixators may be applied with a hinge to allow limited motion. External fixators may also provide progressive loading of the tendon by performing a staged removal [49]. After 3 weeks, restricted active motion can be started.

Pulsed 3.3-MHz therapeutic ultrasound may be used to stimulate collagen repair. After the period of immobilization, ultrasound or hot packs may be used to warm the tissues before stretching [50]. Tendon strength and joint flexion may improve over several months to a year. During this time, explosive motion that places large tension forces on the tendon (eg, jumping) should be avoided. The long-term prognosis is fair to good. The condition may occur bilaterally in dogs with spontaneous rupture of the Achilles tendon.

Superficial Digital Flexor Tendon Luxation

The tendon of the superficial digital flexor muscle may luxate medially or laterally from its location as it crosses the calcaneus. It is a traumatic injury, but dysplasia of the tuber calcanei may be a predisposing factor in some cases [51]. Luxation of the tendon may be palpated while the hock is flexed and extended. Treatment is surgical repair of the torn retinaculum. The healing tissues are protected by immobilization of the hock in a splint for 2 to 3 weeks. After the splint has been removed, range of motion and weight-bearing exercises are begun. Tissue mobilization may be applied to the area to prevent fibrosis of the tendon, which could limit motion of the digits. The prognosis is good if the repair is done early. Chronic tendonitis and bursitis may worsen the prognosis.

Superficial and Deep Digital Flexor Tendons

Laceration or avulsion of superficial or deep digital flexor tendons is a traumatic injury. Avulsion or laceration of tendon at its insertion on P2 and P3 results in abnormal toe carriage. The tendons may be reattached or repaired for cosmetic reasons and for improved athletic function. Postoperatively, the foot is immobilized in a splint for 2 to 3 weeks.

Weekly splint changes with range of motion exercises of adjacent joints should be performed if possible. The splint should be removed within 3 weeks of the injury, because prolonged immobilization may delay healing and weaken the repaired tissue; however, restricted activity must be enforced, because running or jumping could place catastrophic stress on the healing tissues and result in failure. After time has permitted initial healing, the goal of rehabilitation is to restore range of motion and strength. If there is contracture of muscles or tendons, 3.3-MHz continuous mode therapeutic ultrasound or hot packs with simultaneous stretching are indicated.

References

[1] Heinrichs K. Superficial thermal modalities. In: Millis DL, Levine D, Taylor RA, editors. Canine rehabilitation & physical therapy. St Louis: Saunders; 2004. p. 277–88.

[2] Hellyer PW, Fails AD. Pain management for the surgical patient. In: Slatter D, editor. Textbook of small animal surgery. 3rd edition. Philadelphia: Saunders; 2003. p. 2503–15.

[3] Cook JL, Tomlinson JL, Reed AL. Fluoroscopically guided closed reduction and internal fixation of fractures of the lateral portion of the humeral condyle: prospective clinical study of the technique and results in ten dogs. Vet Surg 1999;28:315–21.

[4] Palmoski M, Perricone E, Brandt KD. Development and reversal of proteoglycan aggregation defect in normal canine knee cartilage after immobilization. Arthritis Rheum 1979;22: 508–17.

[5] Liptak JM, Simpson DJ. Successful management of quadriceps contracture in a cat using a dynamic flexion apparatus. Veterinary Comparative Orthopaedics and Traumatology 2000;13:44–8.

[6] Aron DN, Crowe DT. The 90–90 flexion splint for prevention of stifle joint stiffness with femoral fracture repairs. J Am Anim Hosp Assoc 1987;23:447–54.

[7] Millis DL, Lewelling A, Hamilton S. Range-of-motion and stretching exercises. In: Millis DL, Levine D, Taylor RA, editors. Canine rehabilitation & physical therapy. St Louis: Saunders; 2004. p. 228–43.

[8] Marti JM, Miller A. Delimitation of safe corridors for the insertion of external fixator pins in the dog. 1. Hindlimb. J Small Anim Pract 1994;35:16–23.

[9] Marti JM, Miller A. Delimitation of safe corridors for the insertion of external fixator pins in the dog. 2. Forelimb. J Small Anim Pract 1994;35:78–85.

[10] Levine D, Rittenberry L, Millis DL. Aquatic therapy. In: Millis DL, Levine D, Taylor RA, editors. Canine rehabilitation & physical therapy. St Louis: Saunders; 2004. p. 264–76.

[11] Jackson AM, Millis DL, Stevens M, et al. Joint kinematics during underwater treadmill activity. In: Proceedings of the 2nd International Symposium on Rehabilitation and Physical Therapy in Veterinary Medicine. Knoxville (TN): University of Tennessee; 2002. p. 191–2.

[12] Marsolais GS, McLean S, Derrick T, et al. Kinematic analysis of the hind limb during swimming and walking in healthy dogs and dogs with surgically corrected cranial cruciate ligament rupture. J Am Vet Med Assoc 2003;222(6):739–43.

[13] Grisneaux E, Dupuis J, Pibarot P, et al. Effects of postoperative administration of ketoprofen or carprofen on short- and long-term results of femoral head and neck excision in dogs. J Am Vet Med Assoc 2003;223:1006–12.

[14] Carberry CA, Harvey HJ. Owner satisfaction with limb amputation in dogs and cats. J Am Anim Hosp Assoc 1987;23:227–32.

[15] Willer RL, Johnson RA, Turner TM, et al. Partial carpal arthrodesis for third degree carpal sprains: a review of 45 carpi. Vet Surg 1990;19:334–40.

[16] Diamond DW, Besso J, Boudrieau RJ. Evaluation of joint stabilization for treatment of shearing injuries of the tarsus in 20 dogs. J Am Anim Hosp Assoc 1999;35(2): 147–53.

[17] Montgomery RD. Healing of muscle, ligaments, and tendons. Semin Vet Med Surg (Small Anim) 1989;4(4):304–11.

[18] Piermattei DL, Flo GL. Fractures and other orthopedic injuries of the tarsus, metatarsus, and phalanges. In: Piermattei DL, Flo GL, editors. Brinker, Piermattei, and Flo's handbook of small animal orthopedics and fracture repair. Philadelphia: WB Saunders; 1997. p. 607–55.

[19] Impellizeri JA, Tetrick MA, Muir P. Effect of weight reduction on clinical signs of lameness in dogs with hip osteoarthritis. J Am Vet Med Assoc 2000;216:1089–91.

[20] Hudson S, Hulse D. Benefit of rehabilitation for treatment of osteoarthritis in senior dogs. In: Proceedings of the 3rd International Symposium on Rehabilitation and Physical Therapy in Veterinary Medicine. Raleigh (NC): North Carolina State University; 2004. p. 235.

[21] Crook TC. The effects of passive stretching on canine joint motion restricted by osteoarthritis in vivo. In: Proceedings of the 3rd International Symposium on Rehabilitation and Physical Therapy in Veterinary Medicine. Raleigh (NC): North Carolina State University; 2004. p. 207.

[22] Johnston KD, Levine D, Price MN, et al. The effects of TENS on osteoarthritic pain in the stifle of dogs. In: Proceedings of the 2nd International Symposium on Rehabilitation and Physical Therapy in Veterinary Medicine. Knoxville (TN): University of Tennessee; 2002. p. 199.

[23] Francis DA, Millis DL, Evans M, et al. Clinical evaluation of extracorporeal shockwave therapy for the management of canine osteoarthritis of the elbow and hip joints. In: Proceedings of the 31st Veterinary Orthopedic Society. Okemos (MI): Veterinary Orthopedic Society; 2004. p. 13.

[24] Adamson CP, Taylor RA. Preliminary functional outcomes of extracorporeal shockwave therapy on ten dogs with various orthopedic conditions. In: Proceedings of the 2nd International Symposium on Rehabilitation and Physical Therapy in Veterinary Medicine. Knoxville (TN): University of Tennessee; 2002. p. 195.

[25] Todhunter RJ, Lust G. Polysulfated glycosaminoglycan in the treatment of osteoarthritis. J Am Vet Med Assoc 1994;204:1245–51.

[26] Kuroki K, Cook JL, Kreeger JM. Mechanisms of action and potential uses of hyaluronan in dogs with osteoarthritis. J Am Vet Med Assoc 2002;221:944–50.

[27] Anderson MA. Oral chondroprotective agents. Part I. Common compounds. Comp Cont Educ Pract Vet 1999;21:601–9.

[28] McLaughlin RM. Management of chronic osteoarthritic pain. Vet Clin North Am Small Anim Pract 2000;30:933–49.

[29] Johnston SA, Budsberg SC. Nonsteroidal anti-inflammatory drugs and corticosteroids for the management of canine osteoarthritis. Vet Clin North Am Small Anim Pract 1997;27:841–61.

[30] Levine D, Taylor RA, Millis DL. Common orthopedic conditions and their physical rehabilitation. In: Millis DL, Levine D, Taylor RA, editors. Canine rehabilitation & physical therapy. St Louis: Saunders; 2004. p. 355–87.

[31] Trostel CT, McLaughlin RM, Pool RR. Canine lameness caused by developmental orthopedic diseases: osteochondrosis. Comp Cont Educ Pract Vet 2002;24:836–54.

[32] Rudd RG, Whitehair JG, Margolis JH. Results of management of osteochondritis dissecans of the humeral head in dogs: 44 cases (1982 to 1987). J Am Anim Hosp Assoc 1990;26:173–8.

[33] Trostel CT, McLaughlin RM, Pool RR. Canine lameness caused by developmental orthopedic diseases: fragmented medial coronoid process and ununited anconeal process. Comp Cont Educ Pract Vet 2003;25:112–20.

[34] Piermattei DL, Flo GL. Brinker, Piermattei, and Flo's handbook of small animal orthopedics and fracture repair. 3rd edition. Philadelphia: WB Saunders; 1997.

[35] Gibson KL, Lewis DD, Pechman RD. Use of external coaptation for the treatment of avascular necrosis of the femoral head in a dog. J Am Vet Med Assoc 1990;197:868–70.

[36] Roush JK. Canine patellar luxation. Vet Clin North Am Small Anim Pract 1993;23(4):855–68.

[37] Lampman TJ, Lund EM, Lipowitz AJ. Cranial cruciate disease: current status of diagnosis, surgery, and risk for disease. Vet Comp Orthop Traumtol 2003;16(3):122–6.

[38] Wilk KE, Reinold MM, Hooks TR. Recent advances in the rehabilitation of isolated and combined anterior cruciate ligament injuries. Orthop Clin North Am 2003;34(1):107–37.

[39] Marsolais GS, Dvorak G, Conzemius MG. Effects of postoperative rehabilitation on limb function after cranial cruciate ligament repair in dogs. J Am Vet Med Assoc 2002; 220(9):1325–30.

[40] Bockstahler B, Grosslinger K, Lendi S, et al. The effect of physical therapy on postoperative rehabilitation of dogs after cranial cruciate ligament repair. In: Proceedings of the 2nd International Symposium on Rehabilitation and Physical Therapy in Veterinary Medicine. Knoxville (TN): University of Tennessee; 2002. p. 201–2.

[41] Johnson JM, Johnson AL, Pijanowski GJ, et al. Rehabilitation of dogs with surgically treated cranial cruciate ligament-deficient stifles by use of electrical stimulation of muscles. Am J Vet Res 1997;58(12):1473–8.

[42] Millis DL, Levine D, Mynatt T, et al. Changes in muscle mass following transection of the cranial cruciate ligament and immediate stifle stabilization. In: Proceedings of the 27th Annual Conference of the Veterinary Orthopedic Society. Okemos (MI): Veterinary Orthopedic Society; 2000. p. 3.

[43] Lincoln JD, Potter K. Tenosynovitis of the biceps brachii tendon in dogs. J Am Anim Hosp Assoc 1984;20:385–92.

[44] Stobie D, Wallace LJ, Lipowitz AJ, et al. Chronic bicipital tenosynovitis in dogs: 29 cases (1985–1992). J Am Vet Med Assoc 1995;207(2):201–7.

[45] Wall CR, Taylor R. Arthroscopic biceps brachii tenotomy as a treatment for canine bicipital tenosynovitis. J Am Anim Hosp Assoc 2002;38(2):169–75.

[46] Laitinen OM, Flo GL. Mineralization of the supraspinatus tendon in dogs: a long-term follow-up. J Am Anim Hosp Assoc 2000;36:262–7.

[47] Bennett RA. Contracture of the infraspinatus muscle in dogs—a review of 12 cases. J Am Anim Hosp Assoc 1986;22(4):481–7.

[48] King M, Jerram R. Achilles tendon rupture in dogs. Comp Cont Educ Pract Vet 2003;25(8): 613–20.

[49] Sivacolundhu RK, Marchevsky AM, Read RA, et al. Achilles mechanism reconstruction in four dogs. Vet Comp Orthop Traumatol 2001;14(1):25–31.

[50] Loonam J, Millis DL, Stevens M, et al. The effect of therapeutic ultrasound on tendon healing and extensibility. In: Proceedings of the 30th Veterinary Orthopedic Society. Okemos (MI): Veterinary Orthopedic Society; 2003. p. 69.

[51] Reinke JD, Mughannam AJ. Lateral luxation of the superficial digital flexor tendon in 12 dogs. J Am Anim Hosp Assoc 1993;29(4):303–9.

Vet Clin Small Anim 35 (2005) 1389–1409

VETERINARY CLINICS
SMALL ANIMAL PRACTICE

Rehabilitation for the Neurologic Patient

Natasha Olby, Vet MB, PhD[a],*, Krista B. Halling, DVM[b],
Teresa R. Glick, PT[c]

[a]Department of Clinical Sciences, College of Veterinary Medicine,
North Carolina State University, 4700 Hillsborough Street, Raleigh, NC 27606, USA
[b]Department of Clinical Studies, Ontario Veterinary College, University of Guelph,
Guelph, Ontario, Canada N1G 2W1
[c]Department of Small Animal Clinical Sciences, University of Tennessee,
C247 Veterinary Teaching Hospital, 2407 River Drive, Knoxville, TN 37996-4544, USA

Neurologic disease presents a unique circumstance in which physical therapy has a critical role in maintenance and recovery of function. Dysfunction of the nervous system can cause loss of motor and autonomic function and a range of sensory abnormalities, including loss of sensation (analgesia), abnormal sensations (paresthesia), and heightened sensitivity to stimuli (hyperesthesia). The secondary effects of these problems can be as debilitating and serious as the primary injury. For example, an animal with a peripheral neuropathy may develop muscle contractures that preclude any chance of recovery of function, and the sequelae to recumbency such as decubital ulcers and aspiration pneumonia may be fatal.

A properly designed rehabilitation program should be an important component of the treatment plan of animals with neurologic disease. Such a program should be designed in conjunction with appropriate treatment of the underlying problem and after special consideration of the origin of the neurologic problem (eg, central [CNS] versus peripheral nervous system [PNS], upper or lower motor neuron disease), the severity of the signs, the cause of the signs, their anticipated progression, and the needs of the owner and the pet. This article describes the pathophysiology of injury and recovery in the CNS and PNS, assessment of the neurologic patient, data on the prognosis and expected course of recovery for a variety of different diseases, and rehabilitation exercises appropriate for neurologic patients.

*Corresponding author. *E-mail address:* natasha_olby@ncsu.edu (N. Olby).

0195-5616/05/$ – see front matter
doi:10.1016/j.cvsm.2005.08.004

ACUTE SPINAL CORD INJURY

Pathophysiology

The most common causes of acute spinal cord injury in dogs and cats include acute (Hansen type 1) intervertebral disk herniations, traumatic injuries (causing spinal fractures and luxations or hyperextension injuries), and vascular events such as fibrocartilaginous emboli (FCE). The types of injury caused to the spinal cord include concussion, compression, laceration, and ischemia (Table 1). The primary injury, whether mechanical or vascular in origin, initiates a cascade of events that causes progressive reduction of perfusion and neuronal necrosis [1]. Most of this secondary tissue damage occurs over the 48 hours subsequent to the injury. Most acute spinal cord injuries are self-limiting (eg, fibrocartilaginous embolism) or can be treated surgically (eg, decompression of herniated disk material). The goal is to maximize the functional recovery mediated by spared neural tissue.

Recovery of function in the CNS does not occur by regeneration of neural tissue but rather by the surviving tissue taking on the functions of those axons that have been damaged [2]. So-called "complete" lesions that physically transect the spinal cord tend to cause permanent paralysis, whereas if there is any tissue still crossing the site of a lesion, there is a potential for recovery. This functional plasticity can be enhanced by performing suitable rehabilitative exercises.

One must distinguish between the types of neural tissue that have been injured to predict the expected recovery and to design the most appropriate rehabilitation program. Vascular and pure concussive injuries tend to cause maximum damage to the spinal cord gray matter, killing neuronal cell bodies [3]. If this occurs at a site of functionally important motor neurons (eg, the fourth and fifth lumbar spinal cord segments giving rise to the femoral nerve), the results are devastating. If the injury occurs at the level of the thoracolumbar junction, where the motor neurons innervate the abdominal wall, there is little functional effect. If the vascular or concussive lesion is extensive, the surrounding white matter tracts are also affected, but a subpial rim of axons are often spared [3]. This observation is important when considering the prognosis. Animals with vascular spinal cord injuries often show a sudden and dramatic improvement over the first week. Initially, a zone of edema surrounding the infarcted area of the spinal cord prevents conduction of action potentials. This edema resolves quickly, allowing a return to function to these areas.

Table 1
Tissue trauma associated with common neurologic problems in dogs

Type of injury	IVDD	Fracture/luxation	FCE
Concussion	+	+	−
Compression	+	+	−
Laceration	−	+	−
Ischemia	+	+	+

Abbreviations: FCE, fibrocartilaginous embolism; IVDD, intervertebral disk disease.

By contrast, compressive lesions are more likely to affect the white matter tracts by damaging myelin, deforming ion channels, obstructing blood flow, and ultimately disrupting axons [4]. Surgical decompression of the spinal cord can cause a dramatic reversal of signs if axonal loss and myelin damage are not significant. Damaged myelin takes time to recover, but remyelination of axons in the CNS can occur, leading to recovery of function. If axons have been disrupted, which is common in chronic compressive lesions, the potential for recovery of function is decreased.

Acute intervertebral disk herniations cause compression and concussion of the spinal cord in varying degrees, producing a mixed white and gray matter lesion [5]. The extent of damage can range from minor, with little loss of actual neural tissue and an expectation of full recovery, to extremely severe, effectively causing a complete spinal cord transection.

Lacerations, most commonly seen in traumatic injuries, have more serious implications because the neural tissue is actually disrupted, producing a truly complete injury. The prognosis for recovery from this type of injury tends to be more guarded for animals presenting with a functionally complete spinal cord lesion.

In some cases, surgical treatment of the primary disease may not be completed owing to financial constraints of the owner or other health issues. For example, following a traumatic injury that causes a spinal fracture, the animal may have severe cardiac arrhythmias that preclude prolonged anesthesia, or the owner may not be able to afford surgical stabilization. In such cases, recovery may be possible with rehabilitation as long as further injury does not occur. The main mechanisms for further injury include instability causing repeated spinal cord concussion and compression and severe persistent compression of the spinal cord. Of these, spinal instability can be addressed by suitable external splinting and management of the animal, but the physical therapist should always be aware of the potential for causing further damage in such cases. One must also consider the effect of ongoing compression of nerve roots as they exit intervertebral foraminae. Nerve root compression can cause severe pain and may be a limiting factor in the management of such cases.

Assessment

Several important questions must be answered by the patient assessment.

- All systems should be reviewed and all health problems identified, including coexisting orthopedic problems.
- The neurologic lesion must be localized accurately to one (or more in the case of trauma) of four different regions of the spinal cord: the first to fifth cervical spinal cord, the sixth cervical to second thoracic spinal cord, the third thoracic to third lumbar spinal cord, and the fourth lumbar to the third sacral spinal cord (Table 2).
- The severity of the lesion must be assessed. The particular parameters to evaluate for the different localizations to generate the necessary information are listed in Table 3.
- The degree of hyperesthesia should be assessed and the potential source of pain identified (eg, postoperative pain, muscle spasticity, nerve root entrapment).

Table 2
Localization of spinal cord lesions in dogs

Lesion localization	Motor function	Thoracic limb reflexes and muscle tone	Pelvic limb reflexes and muscle tone
C1-5	Tetraparetic–plegic	Normal to increased	Normal to increased
C6-T2	Tetraparetic–plegic Thoracic limb gait may be short and stilted	Decreased to absent	Normal to increased
T3-L3	Paraparetic–plegic	Normal	Normal to increased
L4-S3	Paraparetic–plegic	Normal	Decreased to absent

The specific components to evaluate to determine the prognosis and to design an appropriate rehabilitation program are described in the following sections.

Gait
The animal's gait should be classified as ambulatory versus nonambulatory paretic (tetra-, para-, mono-, or hemiparetic). If the animal is nonambulatory, complete paralysis (-plegia) must be distinguished from nonambulatory paresis for prognostic purposes. Scales to score the severity of pelvic limb paresis have been developed. The scale used most commonly to determine the prognosis at the time of injury grades deficits from 0 to 5 [6] where 0 is normal, 1 is hyperesthesia only, 2 is paraparesis and ataxia, 3 is paraplegia, 4 is paraplegia with urinary incontinence, and 5 is paraplegia with loss of deep pain perception. A more extensive scale has been developed to score the extent of recovery in more detail for the purposes of comparing the efficacy of different treatments [7,8].

Deep pain perception
An evaluation of deep pain perception is central when evaluating paraplegic animals. This evaluation is performed correctly by placing the animal in lateral

Table 3
Assessment of the severity of spinal cord lesions in dogs

Parameters to assess	C1-5	C6-T2	T3-L3	L4-S3
Ambulatory versus nonambulatory	+	+	+	+
Paretic versus plegic	+	+	+	+
Respiratory pattern/ arterial blood gas	+	+	−	−
Deep pain perception	+/−[a]	+, must evaluate medial and lateral digits	+	+, must evaluate medial and lateral digits

+, must evaluate; −, not pertinent.
[a]It is unusual for animals to survive if they have a severe enough C1-5 lesion to cause loss of deep pain perception.

recumbency or holding it off the ground in a position in which it is comfortable. Pressure is applied to the bone of the digits using hemostatic forceps gently at first to stimulate a withdrawal reflex, and then the pressure is increased (the aim is to stimulate the periosteum) until a conscious response is elicited. Deep pain perception is believed to be mediated by small diameter, polysynaptic, diffuse pathways in the spinothalamic and priopriospinal tracts that lie deep within the white matter. As such, a serious injury must occur to interrupt conscious perception of pain. At the time of an acute injury, loss of deep pain perception indicates a functional spinal cord transection. Nevertheless, it does not mean that there is anatomic transection, and, in the long term, loss of deep pain perception does not necessarily imply a complete spinal cord lesion [9].

Tetraplegia with loss of deep pain perception is an unusual presentation because cervical spinal cord injuries severe enough to cause loss of deep pain perception will also cause paralysis of the respiratory muscles and loss of sympathetic tone to the heart, with most patients dying before they reach the veterinarian. The exceptions to this are severe gray matter lesions of the brachial intumescence (usually the result of FCE) that can cause loss of deep pain perception in one or both thoracic limbs while deep pain perception is preserved in the pelvic limbs.

Respiratory function

The most severe and potentially life-threatening grade of cervical injury causes tetraplegia with compromise of respiratory function. It is vital that respiratory function is evaluated in any tetraplegic animal and that hypoventilation or other respiratory compromise (such as aspiration pneumonia) is identified before embarking on exercises that may exacerbate the problem. For example, the weight of water in a hydrotherapy bath may cause decompensation of an animal that is hypoventilating.

Prognosis and Recovery

If the underlying spinal cord disease has been addressed and is not ongoing, any animal that has intact deep pain perception in its affected limbs has the potential to recover useful function.

Paraparesis

For the paraplegic animal, the best prognostic guide is the presence of deep pain perception. Extensive information exists about the prognosis for and rate of recovery of animals that have suffered an acute intervertebral thoracolumbar disk herniation. One study showed a direct relationship between the rate of recovery and body weight and age [9]. A relatively high percentage of dogs that recovered from paraplegia with loss of deep pain perception had persistent mild urinary (32%) or fecal continence (41%). The same study looked at the long-term recovery of dogs with disk herniations that did not regain deep pain perception. Approximately 40% of these dogs recovered apparently voluntary motor function and tail wag, although they did not recover deep pain perception or continence. The mean time to recovery of motor function was just over

9 months, and one dog took 18 months. The recovery of a voluntary tail wag preceded the recovery of pelvic limb function and in most cases was present within a month of injury, serving as a useful prognostic indicator. This motor function is hypothesized to be mediated by surviving subpial axons [9].

Less information is available on the exact course of recovery of dogs that have sustained FCE or traumatic injuries. The most accurate prognostic indicator for both types of injury is the presence of deep pain perception. All dogs with intact deep pain perception have the ability to recover from these injuries unless there is ongoing damage. For example, if a dog with a spinal fracture remains unstable, it could deteriorate to a paraplegic condition with loss of deep pain perception. Some work has been done on the prognosis of dogs with spinal fractures and loss of deep pain perception. If there is displacement of the vertebrae at the time of injury, it is extremely unlikely that there will be recovery of function. If the vertebrae are not displaced, the odds of a recovery of function are improved, although they do not reach the 50% chance of recovery noted with disk herniations [9]. The recovery from FCE is notable in that there can be a rapid improvement in the first 7 to 10 days after injury. This observation probably reflects the fact that the lesion often centers on gray matter, with a zone of surrounding edema affecting the white matter.

There has been much discussion of the phenomenon of "spinal walking." This behavior develops in rodents and cats following surgical transection of the spinal cord and has been postulated to occur in dogs. Nevertheless, in one of the author's (NJO) experience, dogs with traumatic spinal cord injuries in which there is significant displacement of vertebrae and loss of deep pain perception (ie, suggesting an anatomic transection of the spinal cord) do not recover useful motor function despite prolonged efforts at rehabilitation, although they develop pronounced reflex movements in their pelvic limbs. A group of dogs will recover motor function (albeit, disconnected and crude) without recovery of deep pain. These dogs invariably have sustained a disk herniation and have a voluntary tail wag (ie, it occurs when they see their owner). It is likely that these dogs have some intact axons running across their lesion, and that the dogs are more similar to humans in that they do not develop useful spinal walking.

Tetraparesis

There is far less objective information on the rate of recovery of tetraparetic dogs from different types of injury. In general, the involvement of all four legs can make rehabilitation more difficult; therefore, the course of recovery may be more protracted. As noted previously, it is extremely unusual to encounter an acutely injured tetraplegic patient with loss of deep pain perception in all four legs. If one did encounter such a case, the animal would be unlikely to survive. Any animal with hypoventilation as a result of its injury carries a poor prognosis unless it can be mechanically ventilated.

Rehabilitation

The goals of a rehabilitation program for acute spinal cord disease include reducing postoperative and muscular pain, maintaining joint range of motion, reducing the development of muscle atrophy, and restoring neuromuscular function. These goals can be achieved through a rehabilitation program that incorporates exercise, functional activities, and therapeutic modalities (Table 4) [10,11].

Passive and Reflexive Exercises

Passive exercises should be performed in neurologic patients who lack voluntary movement or strength or whose proprioceptive deficits preclude a normal gait.

Passive range of motion

Placing each joint through a normal range of motion will help maintain joint health in patients who have deficits in voluntary movement [12]. Passive range

---

Table 4
Guidelines for rehabilitation activities for patients with cervical or thoracolumbar spinal cord disease

Step 1: Immediately postoperatively (neurologic stages 1 and 2)
• Cold-packing the incision
• Range of motion exercises
• Massage of limb muscles
• Nursing care
    Provide soft, padded, and dry bedding
    Turn patient at least every 4 hours to prevent decubital ulcers, every 2 hours in ideal situations
    Keep patient clean and dry
    Water and food easily accessible
    Bladder and bowel care
• Assess feet and bony prominences for ulcers or abrasions; protective boots may be used if needed
Step 2: Able to support weight (no limb movements) (neurologic stage 3)
• Passive range of motion exercises
• Standing exercises
• Standing in water
• Neuromuscular stimulation
Step 3: Initial limb movements (neurologic stage 4)
• Passive range of motion exercises
• Standing exercises
• Pregait and weight-shifting activities
• Walking (treadmill, dry land), depending on level of assistance required
• Swimming (with support)
• Neuromuscular stimulation
Step 4: Good limb movements (neurologic stage 4)
• Passive range of motion exercises
• Sit-to-stand exercises
• Balance and coordination exercises
• Walking (treadmill, dry land, sand, snow)
• Swimming (with support)
Step 5: Near-normal gait (neurologic stage 5)
• Balance and coordination exercises
• Walking (longer duration, up inclines or stairs)
• Swimming

of motion (PROM) exercises will not improve strength or muscle mass; active range of motion is necessary to stimulate muscle tissue. PROM should be performed with the patient lying in lateral recumbency on a well-padded surface. The uppermost limbs should be put through gentle flexion and extension of each joint within the patent's comfort zone. In patients with spinal cord injury, there is usually increased muscle tone or spasticity. To overcome this tone, one should avoid placing his or her hands on the bottom of the patient's foot (which may elicit an extensor reflex). Placing graded pressure behind the stifle or in front of the elbow can relax the tone. In severe cases of increased tone, gently flexing the digits may decrease extensor tone. Once each joint has been put through 15 to 20 cycles, each limb may be put through bicycling movements for another 15 to 20 repetitions. The patient is then flipped and the exercise repeated on the contralateral limbs. This exercise should be performed three to four times per day until the patient can ambulate.

Flexor reflex stimulation

In patients with upper motor neuron deficits, elicitation of a withdrawal reflex in the forelimb or hind limb causes active flexion of the elbow and carpal joints or stifle and tarsal joints, respectively, thereby improving muscle tone. This exercise is performed by placing the patient in lateral recumbency and pinching the interdigital skin of the upper limb. As the reflex causes the limb to retract actively, resistance is achieved by the therapist holding the foot, creating a gentle "tug-of-war" in which the patient is pulling more forcefully to withdraw the limb from the therapist's grip. This exercise should be performed for three to five repetitions per limb, three to four times per day.

Patellar (extensor) reflex stimulation

Similar to the flexor reflex, stimulation of the patellar reflex will enhance muscle tone and strength in patients with weak or intact femoral nerves. This exercise should be performed in patients with upper motor neuron deficits to take advantage of their normal to hyperactive extensor reflex. To stimulate contraction of the quadriceps muscles, the patient is placed in a standing position with the hind feet placed squarely on the ground. The animal may require assistance to maintain this position. The patient's hind end is then gently raised (enough to lift their toes off the ground) and lowered, such that the animal is required to support their body weight as their hind end is lowered to the ground. The patient may be kept in a standing position until they start to collapse; at this point, the animal is supported and returned to a standing position. Alternatively, the extensor reflex can be evoked by the therapist placing his or her hand on the bottom of the patient's foot and pressing toward the body. This should be repeated 15 to 20 times, and the exercise performed two to three times per day.

Active Exercises

These activities are designed to improve muscle strength, neuromuscular balance, and coordination in patients who have at least some voluntary movement of their limbs. In patients with acute disease, loss of neuromuscular function will be of greater importance than muscle atrophy, and the choice of rehabilitation activities will reflect this. In humans with traumatic spinal cord injury, early (within 2 weeks of injury) intervention with resistance training has been shown to improve motor activities and function [13,14].

Sit-to-stand exercises

The sit-to-stand exercise strengthens stifle and hip extensor muscles and is indicated in patients with enough motor activity and strength to stand up with minimal to no assistance. The patient is placed in a sitting position and prompted to stand up on all four limbs. This activity should be repeated three to five times and performed two to three times per day until near-normal movements and gait have been restored. It may be performed before other active exercises; however, if the patient appears too fatigued, the activities should staggered.

Assisted walking

When some voluntary movement is present, having the patient perform several short walks per day will improve muscle strength and neuromuscular coordination. A padded sling (commercially available or one home-made from a stockinette or Vetrap bandaging material) should be used to support the hindquarters as necessary. If recovery is anticipated to be prolonged, a cart or counterbalance wheelchair can be used to facilitate ambulation. Non-slip flooring is ideal to encourage proprioceptive recognition and appropriate limb placement. Commercially available booties may provide additional traction. A land or underwater treadmill may also be used. Treadmill walking has been shown to encourage a consistent and symmetric gait in humans with hemiplegia [15], and buoyancy from an underwater treadmill or pool will help to support the patient's body weight [16]. The patient should be walked slowly for 2 to 5 minutes depending on their ability. It is best to stop before the patient has fatigued, performing multiple short walks per day rather than one or two longer ones.

Ambulation activities

Once the patient is able to walk, even with residual proprioceptive deficits, some resistance may be added to improve muscle condition. This resistance may involve walking up a sturdy incline, briskly in an underwater treadmill, with resistive exercise bands, on sand, or through snow. The depth of water, sand, or snow will influence the amount of resistance against which the patient must work. For underwater activities in postoperative patients, one of the authors (KBH) recommends waiting 7 to 14 days following surgery and confirming that the surgical wound has healed. As is true for assisted walking, resistive walking should be limited to 2 to 5 minutes as dictated by the patient's fatigue level. It may be performed daily to every other day until a normal gait has been restored.

Swimming

Aquatic therapy can be beneficial by minimizing weight-bearing forces [16] and allowing the patient to improve joint range of motion [17] and muscle strength.

In human patients with spinal cord injury, water exercises have been demonstrated to decrease muscle spasticity and improve strength [18]. Because swimming can result in forceful muscular contractions, one of the authors (KBH) recommends that this activity be delayed in postoperative neurosurgical patients for the first 4 to 6 weeks until the tissues adjacent to the laminectomy or pediculectomy site have sufficiently healed. Walking in an underwater treadmill may be performed in the interim.

When swimming a patient with neurologic disease, the animal must be supported at all times using manual assistance or a life preserver. For small breed dogs, the swimming pool may consist of a bathtub filled deep enough such that the patient cannot touch the bottom. The water temperature should be 25 to 30°C (77–86°F) to maximize patient comfort during exercise. Larger dogs require a commercial or home-based swimming pool (preferably 1.5 m wide × 2.5 m long × 1.2 m deep (5′ wide × 8′ long × 4′ deep). An underwater treadmill with a jet current may also be used to allow swimming. Patients may be fatigued easily; therefore, swimming should be limited to 2 to 5 minutes every other day.

Balance and coordination exercises

Several exercises will improve balance and coordination, especially in patients who have voluntary movement with severe proprioceptive deficits. Neuromuscular weakness may necessitate that the therapist support the patient during these activities. A simple coordination exercise entails having the patient in a standing position and lifting a limb off the ground. This lifting requires the patient to adjust and redistribute weight to the other limbs. This exercise may be performed on each limb on an alternating basis. Treats may be placed on the floor in front of the patient to encourage weight shifting as the patient reaches for the treat.

Several commercial or homemade objects may also be used for this purpose. Balance balls are large-diameter exercise balls that the patient can be placed on and supported while alternately being rolled onto their front and hind limbs. A balance board is a rectangular piece of plywood with a narrow rod running along the bottom. The board tips in a lateral or cranial-caudal direction when the patient stands on it, depending on the orientation of the rod. Cavaletti rails are horizontal bars that are elevated such that the patient must pick the limbs up to clear the rods. Having the patient walk across or stand on a foam mattress may also be performed to improve balance and coordination.

Balancing and coordination activities may be incorporated into regular walking activities. For example, the patient can spend part of the time negotiating Cavaletti rails or walking over a foam mattress. These exercises should be continued until the patient has a normal or near-normal gait.

Therapeutic Modalities

Cold-packing

Pain from acute postoperative inflammation may be alleviated by the administration of cryotherapy [19]. For the first 2 days following surgery, a cold pack placed in a moist towel can be applied to the surgical incision for 10 to 15 minutes. This application may be repeated every 4 hours during the inflammatory period. One should closely monitor patients if moist towels are used during the recovery from anesthesia or sedation (use dry towels in sedated animals). Continued inflammation (pain, redness, and swelling) of the surgical site beyond 48 hours may be indicative of an infection and should be assessed appropriately and managed.

Therapeutic ultrasound

The application of therapeutic ultrasound to soft tissues helps alleviate pain while improving tissue blood supply and healing (speed). Ultrasound may be beneficial for epaxial muscles that are experiencing muscle spasms. Its use is contraindicated over an exposed spinal cord, and continuous mode ultrasound is not recommended in postoperative neurosurgical patients. In nonsurgical patients with acute spinal cord disease and neuromuscular spasm, ultrasound may be applied to the epaxial muscles to help manage pain and muscle spasm.

Neuromuscular stimulation

The application of neuromuscular electrical stimulation (NMES) in patients with acute spinal cord disease may be beneficial to increase tissue perfusion, decrease pain, and delay the onset of disuse muscle atrophy [20,21]. In patients with lower motor neuron disease, stimulation of the affected muscle groups will delay the onset and severity of neurogenic muscle atrophy.

The use of electrical stimulation is preferred for muscle groups that are not already experiencing spasms. It is contraindicated over surgical sites following a laminectomy or pediculectomy until adequate healing has taken place. NMES should be applied to the muscle groups of affected limbs once a day for 15 minutes each until the patient is ambulating with mild-to-moderate ataxia.

CHRONIC SPINAL CORD INJURY
Pathophysiology

Chronic spinal cord diseases are a common and insidious problem in older dogs of large and small breeds. They usually result from degenerative changes of the vertebrae and their associated soft-tissue structures. Examples include cervical spondylomyelopathy ("wobbler" syndrome in all of its forms), Hansen type II intervertebral disk disease of the thoracolumbar and cervical spine, spinal malformations such as atlantoaxial subluxation and spinal stenosis, and cystic diseases such as subarachnoid cysts and syringohydromyelia. Degenerative lumbosacral disease primarily affects peripheral nerves of the cauda equina and is discussed in the section on peripheral neuropathies. Neoplastic disorders also cause chronic compression, and, if the underlying cancer is slow growing or has been treated definitively, rehabilitation should have an important role in the treatment plan.

In general, chronic compressive diseases produce neurologic damage by compressing neural tissue, causing demyelination, deforming axonal membranes, and eventually killing axons [4,22,23]. Recovery will be enhanced by decompression of the spinal cord if this is viable without causing a dramatic deterioration in signs. Nevertheless, histopathology of chronic compressive diseases such as caudal cervical spondylomyelopathy shows that there is significant gray matter damage [3,23]. This damage may reflect compression of the blood supply to the spinal cord and may also be the result of small concussive injuries to the spinal cord as the spine moves caused by the hypertrophied soft tissue, such as annulus fibrosus, or the hypertrophied bone, such as articular facets. There is potential benefit from strengthening the spinal musculature to minimize any sudden movements and to maintain a normal range of motion in the spine.

Assessment

The approach for assessing the chronically paretic animal is identical to that for the acutely paretic animal. Identification of other chronic conditions such as degenerative joint disease of the stifle joints is extremely important, and long-term secondary effects of the neurologic disease should be noted (eg, chronic urinary tract infections owing to impaired urination). Hyperesthesia may be a significant problem in these patients, in particular in animals with cervical disease. The severity and possible causes of that hyperesthesia should be determined. In addition, owing to the chronicity of the signs, any significant muscle atrophy should be documented and taken into account when designing the rehabilitation program.

Prognosis and Recovery

The expectations and therapeutic goals for recovery are different when dealing with chronic versus acute spinal cord injuries. First, the spinal cord lesion usually results from some underlying often poorly understood structural abnormality of the spinal cord or vertebral column. For example, although wobbler syndrome is postulated to result from underlying instability of the cervical spine, it is difficult to demonstrate instability in radiographic or biomechanical studies. Although the spinal cord may be decompressed surgically and stabilized, this may not correct the abnormality that triggered the problem, or it may change the dynamics of the adjacent spine. A complete cure is unusual, and recurrence of signs is relatively common. As noted in the section on pathophysiology, the role of physical therapy in addressing the actual underlying spinal abnormality may be critical and is a field that needs to be developed. A second problem is that, with chronic spinal cord diseases, the gradual accumulation of damage allows the animal to compensate functionally; therefore, signs become evident once a large amount of irreversible damage is present. The anticipated recovery is not as rapid and complete when compared with that in acute spinal cord injuries. It is preferable to begin conservative or surgical treatment and rehabilitation while the animal is still ambulatory.

The outcome of the surgical management of caudal cervical spondylomyelopathy using a variety of procedures has been reported. In general, even if the animal is nonambulatory, approximately 80% of dogs will recover the ability to walk in the long term, although at least 20% of these recovered dogs will have a recurrence.

Rehabilitation

The goals of a rehabilitation program for chronic spinal cord disease include reducing postoperative and muscular pain, improving joint range of motion, correcting muscular atrophy, and restoring neuromuscular function. These goals can be achieved through a rehabilitation program that incorporates therapeutic modalities and exercise (see Table 4).

Passive and Reflexive Exercises

Passive exercises should be performed in neurologic patients who lack voluntary movement or strength, or whose proprioceptive deficits preclude a normal gait. In patients with chronic disease, joint range of motion will be determined by the chronicity and magnitude of the neurologic deficits. In these patients, baseline values for joint ranges of motion should be determined to establish which joints are the most compromised and will require preferential attention.

Passive range of motion

Placing each joint through a normal range of motion will help maintain joint health in patients who have deficits in voluntary movement and will help restore lost range of motion [12]. The methods for PROM have been described previously. Passive exercises will not improve strength or muscle mass. PROM in chronic patients should be performed three to four times per day until the patient is able to ambulate or has reached a recovery plateau.

Stretching

In joints that have lost range of motion, PROM activity should be combined with stretching exercises to help restore function in the affected joint. The affected joint and adjacent muscles should be prewarmed with a warm pack or massage. PROM should be performed to the joint. Upon reaching the respective endpoint of flexion and extension, the therapist should exert gentle traction to maintain the joint at the upper limit of flexion or extension, respectively. A gentle "bouncing" motion may be applied to assist in the breakdown of periarticular fibrous tissue. Following stretching, a cold pack can be applied to the joint if the patient experiences discomfort.

Flexor and patellar (extensor) reflex stimulation

Flexor and extensor reflex stimulation for patients with chronic neurologic disease is similar to stimulation in patients with acute neurologic disease. The stimulation should be performed 20 times, with two to three sessions per day.

Active Exercises

Active exercises are designed to improve muscle strength, neuromuscular balance, and coordination in patients who have at least some voluntary movement of their limbs. In patients with chronic disease, muscle atrophy may be almost as important as loss of neuromuscular function, and the rehabilitation protocol should address both of these conditions.

Sit-to-stand exercises

As described earlier, sit-to-stand exercises strengthen stifle and hip extensor muscles and are indicated in patients with enough motor activity and strength to stand up.

Assisted and resistive walking, swimming, balance, and coordination exercises

Assisted and resistive walking activities, swimming, balance, and coordination exercises are similar to the walking activities described for patients with acute neurologic problems. These activities are of particular importance in patients with chronic disease because of their potentially protracted recovery.

Therapeutic Modalities

Cold-packing, therapeutic ultrasound, and neuromuscular stimulation

Therapeutic modalities can be used in patients with chronic neurologic problems as described previously for the management of patients with acute neurologic problems. NMES helps recondition muscles atrophied from chronic disuse [21].

PERIPHERAL NERVE INJURY

Pathophysiology

Common causes of peripheral nerve injury include fractures (eg, the femoral fracture that damages the sciatic nerve), intramuscular injection (usually affecting the sciatic nerve), traumatic brachial plexus avulsion, and poor surgical technique. Vascular injuries can also occur, the most common of which is iliac thrombosis in cats causing a distal sciatic neuropathy, but thrombosis of the brachial artery can also cause thoracic limb monoparesis. Peripheral nerves differ from their CNS counterparts in that they regenerate at rates as fast as 1 mm a day [24]. Nerves must be in a Schwann cell environment for this regeneration to occur. Peripheral nerve injuries have three levels of severity [25] as follows:

- In neurapraxia, axonal conduction is lost without disruption of the axon. This injury usually results from compression, transient ischemia, or blunt trauma. Loss of conduction may be a result of myelin damage or insufficient energy to maintain axonal resting potential.
- In axonotmesis, the axon integrity is lost, but the endoneurium and Schwann cell sheath it lies within are still intact, providing the opportunity for regeneration back to the correct target. Successful regeneration may occur, particularly if the axon is damaged close to its target.
- In neurotmesis, the entire structure of the nerve is disrupted. The axon has the ability to regenerate but needs to find a Schwann cell sheath to do so, making it much more difficult. The prognosis for recovery from such injuries is guarded, even with surgical intervention.

In peripheral nerve injuries, one must consider sensation and muscle atrophy. Regenerating peripheral nerves, and indeed any disease causing a peripheral neuropathy, can cause unpleasant abnormal sensations (paresthesia) and hyperesthesia, both of which can result in self-mutilation. A sequela to denervation of a muscle is severe muscle atrophy, which over time may lead to muscle contracture and, in growing animals, to skeletal deformities.

Assessment

In the same manner as for spinal cord injuries, the exact location of the lesion and its severity must be determined by the neurologic examination. The muscles innervated by each nerve should be known [26]. It is also useful to refer to references depicting the cutaneous sensory zones of peripheral nerves [27,28]. Severity of the lesion is determined by assessing the level of motor function and assessing for deep pain sensation. Electrophysiologic evaluation of the muscles and nerves using electromyography (EMG) and nerve conduction velocity studies allows a more detailed description of the severity and course of the injury [29,30]. Muscles that are completely denervated develop spontaneous electrical activity when at rest, although such changes do not appear for at least a week after denervation of a muscle. Nerve conduction studies should be interpreted with care. Immediately after an injury, conduction may be lost across the site of injury, whereas the distal portion of the disrupted nerve can continue conducting for a period of hours to days. As nerves regenerate and sprout to innervate denervated muscles, the size of motor units increases; therefore, the size of motor unit potentials on EMG increases [30].

Prognosis and Recovery

As a rule, neurotmesis carries a poor prognosis unless immediate surgical intervention to reconnect the severed nerve occurs. Animals with axonotmesis or neurapraxia carry a better prognosis. Neurapraxia usually reverses within 2 weeks of injury, although damage to myelin slows recovery to 4 to 6 weeks. The recovery from axonotmesis is governed by the proximity of the injury from the target muscle, the severity of muscle atrophy, and the development of contractures. If the damage has occurred far from the target muscle (eg, at the brachial plexus), by the time the axon has regrown, severe muscle contractures could limit recovery.

Brachial plexus injuries tend to involve the caudal two thirds of the plexus (radial, median, ulnar, and lateral thoracic nerves and the sympathetic innervation of the head) or the complete plexus, although cranial plexus injuries have been reported [27]. It is easy to be misled when evaluating animals with caudal plexus injuries, because there is preservation of musculocutaneous function and elbow flexion. This function is not useful for recovery of the ability to bear weight and should not be used to determine the prognosis. Instead, it is important to test deep pain perception, particularly in the lateral digit [31]. The absence of deep pain in this digit implies severe radial nerve injury. If it does not reappear within 2 weeks of injury, the prognosis for recovery of useful motor function in that limb is guarded.

Rehabilitation

The goals of a rehabilitation program for patients with lower motor neuron injury include restoring and maintaining joint range of motion, improving muscle strength, restoring neuromuscular function, and preventing self-mutilation and trauma to the affected limb. The lack of spinal reflexes and corresponding muscle tone in these patients poses a unique challenge to their rehabilitation, and emphasis must be placed on restoration of muscle and joint function.

Passive and Reflexive Exercises

Because of the dysfunction of the spinal reflex arc in patients with lower motor neuron deficits, passive exercises should be performed in these patients until a near-normal gait is established.

Passive range of motion, stretching

These options are used in the same manner as in patients with acute and chronic neurologic problems. Patients with lower motor neuron deficits may benefit from stretching of affected and antagonist muscles. Loss of tone to antagonist muscle groups predisposes patients to joint contractures. Massage of a mildly contracted muscle group may also be beneficial in restoring its function and should be performed two to three times per day after prewarming the region.

Flexor and patellar (extensor) reflex stimulation

In patients with a sciatic nerve deficit, elicitation of a withdrawal reflex may not be possible. Nevertheless, progress should be monitored by serial evaluations of the spinal reflex arcs. In patients with weak or intact withdrawal reflexes, stimulation of the flexor reflex will improve muscle tone and neuromuscular coordination. Patients with femoral nerve injury require a lot of assistance to maintain this position. A balance ball (Swiss ball) may be used to support the trunk while slowly lowering the hind limbs to the ground. The patient's hind end is then gently raised (enough to lift their toes off the ground) and lowered, such that the animal is required to support their body weight as the hind end is lowered to the ground.

Radial nerve stimulation

Patients with mild radial nerve deficits will benefit from being challenged to bear weight on their forelimbs. Patients who lack any elbow or carpal extension (eg, brachial plexus avulsion) should not perform this activity until some extensor muscle tone is present. The exercise is performed by placing the patient in a standing position while supporting the trunk and forelimbs. With the animal's forefeet placed squarely on the ground, the amount of weight-bearing support is gradually reduced. When the patient starts to collapse in the forelimbs, the therapist supports the animal and returns the patient to a standing position. A balance ball or custom orthotics may similarly be used to support the patient. The exercise is repeated five times, two to three times per day.

Active Exercises

These activities are designed to improve muscle strength, neuromuscular balance, and coordination in patients who have at least some voluntary movement of their limbs. In certain patients with peripheral nerve disease affecting more than one limb, loss of neuromuscular function may preclude some of these activities.

Sit-to-stand exercises, assisted and resistive walking, and swimming
Patients with sciatic nerve deficits can often perform sit-to-stand exercises because they require active stifle extension but only passive stifle and tarsal flexion.

Balance and coordination exercises
Balance and coordination exercises benefit patients with peripheral nerve injuries. They are performed as described previously.

Therapeutic Modalities
Neuromuscular stimulation
The application of NMES in patients with peripheral nerve disease may delay the onset of neurogenic muscle atrophy and recondition the affected muscles [21,32,33]. When an affected muscle is completely denervated, electrical muscle stimulation is the modality of choice. Affected muscle groups should be stimulated once a day for 15 minutes each.

NEUROMUSCULAR DISEASE
Pathophysiology
Neuromuscular diseases include neuropathies, junctionopathies, and myopathies. The most common neuropathies that require rehabilitation include immune-mediated polyradiculoneuritis (also known as Coon Hound paralysis in dogs), infectious neuritis (eg, *Neospora caninum*), degenerative or toxic neuropathies (eg, either breed related or secondary to diabetes or insulinoma), and compressive neuropathies (eg, degenerative lumbosacral disease). Botulism is the most important junctional disorder that requires rehabilitation. There are many different myopathies, including infectious/inflammatory (immune-mediated polymyositis and protozoal myositis), degenerative (muscular dystrophy), and metabolic myopathies. A wide variety of pathologic processes occurs and needs to be considered carefully before designing a rehabilitation program. For example, an animal with X-linked muscular dystrophy may develop dramatic myonecrosis or myocardial failure after excessive exercise.

In general, diseases of the lower motor neuron cause dramatic and rapid muscle atrophy, and, over time, contractures may develop and restrict joint motion. In addition, there may be involvement of the esophagus, laryngeal, and pharyngeal muscles, causing potentially fatal dysphagia and aspiration pneumonia. These changes can be complicated by hypoventilation, particularly in a recumbent animal. In myopathies and botulism, the heart may be involved, causing yet another potentially fatal complication.

Assessment
Following the standard assessment, specific points that must be assessed in a patient with generalized lower motor neuron disease include the following:

- The severity and distribution of lower motor neuron signs should be recognized by making a distinction between an ambulatory and nonambulatory status and between nonambulatory tetraparesis and tetraplegia.

- Respiratory function should be assessed for evidence of hypoventilation (arterial partial pressure of carbon dioxide by arterial blood gas measurement) or aspiration pneumonia.
- Esophageal, pharyngeal, and laryngeal function should be assessed by careful questioning of the owner about voice changes, coughing after eating or drinking, and regurgitation. Thoracic radiographs should be taken to identify megaesophagus.
- Cardiac function should be assessed. Ideally, echocardiography should be performed in the presence of generalized myopathies.
- The presence and severity of muscle atrophy and joint range of motion should be evaluated to establish a baseline.

Prognosis and Recovery

Although the prognosis and course of recovery are closely linked to the underlying disease, the following general statements can be made:

- Esophageal, pharyngeal, and laryngeal dysfunction worsen the prognosis, particularly if the animal has aspiration pneumonia. This potential complication needs to be remembered by the physical therapist when performing exercises with the animal.
- Hypoventilation to the extent that the animal needs to be mechanically ventilated significantly worsens the prognosis.
- The more severe the muscle atrophy, the more protracted the recovery. The development of muscle contractures can preclude a recovery even when the underlying disease has been resolved.
- If the underlying disease process cannot be cured (eg, X-linked muscular dystrophy, inherited neuropathy such as the laryngeal paralysis polyneuropathy complex), the role of the physical therapist is to palliate the animal's signs. It is very important not to precipitate a crisis by causing aspiration pneumonia or an episode of myonecrosis. Physical therapists can also recommend appropriate protective and assistive devices and prevention and positioning techniques and can provide caregiver instruction for home care and safe transfer techniques in the event of hospice situations.

Some guidelines are available for the expected course of recovery for some of the common self-limiting diseases. The recovery from botulism requires the production of new proteins to replace those bound by the botulinum toxin and usually takes approximately 3 weeks [34]. If the animal can be supported through this period successfully, it should recover. Most dogs with polyradiculoneuritis take 3 to 6 weeks to recover from this immune-mediated disease [35]. In both of these diseases, the animals require intensive physical therapy and supportive care during the recovery period to survive.

Rehabilitation

The goals of a rehabilitation program for generalized neuromuscular disease are determined by the particular disease pathophysiology and specific neurologic deficits. Because generalized weakness and lower motor neuron dysfunction are common clinical signs of most neuromuscular disorders, rehabilitation of these patients includes attention to housing, maintaining joint range of motion, preventing neurogenic muscular atrophy, and restoring neuromuscular function. These goals can be achieved through a rehabilitation program that incorporates exercise and therapeutic modalities.

Passive and Reflexive Exercises
These exercises are performed as described previously.

Active Exercises
Sit-to-stand exercises, assisted and resistive walking
Active exercises are used in dogs with neuromuscular diseases as described earlier. Walking in an underwater treadmill is particularly useful in patients with generalized neuromuscular disorders because the buoyancy will help compensate for their weakened state [16]. Owing to the muscle weakness and risk of drowning, it is important to maintain control of the patient's head at all times while in the water.

Swimming
When swimming a patient with generalized neurologic disease, it is important to support them at all times using manual assistance or a life preserver. As is true for underwater treadmill use, the therapist must maintain control of the patient's head at all times to prevent drowning or aspiration. These patients fatigue easily; therefore, swimming should be limited to 1 to 3 minutes every 2 to 3 days.

Therapeutic Modalities
Neuromuscular stimulation
The application of NMES in patients with generalized neuromuscular dysfunction may be beneficial to increase tissue perfusion and minimize the onset of neurogenic muscle atrophy. NMES should be applied to muscle groups of affected limbs once a day for 15 minutes each.

SUMMARY
The rehabilitation of dogs with neurologic disease involves a combination of active and passive exercise, functional activities, and therapeutic modalities. The key to maximizing the patient's functional recovery is cooperation and participation of the patient, the owner, and the therapist.

References
[1] Olby NJ. Current concepts in the management of acute spinal cord injury. J Vet Int Med 1999;13:399–407.

[2] Jeffery ND, Blakemore WF. Spinal cord injury in small animals. 1. Mechanisms of spontaneous recovery. Vet Rec 1999;144:407–13.

[3] Summers BA, Cummings JF, De Lahunta A. Injuries to the central nervous system. In: Veterinary neuropathology. St. Louis: Mosby-Year Book; 1995. p. 189–207.

[4] Shi R, Blight AR. Compression injury of mammalian spinal cord in vitro and the dynamics of action potential conduction failure. J Neurophysiol 1996;76:1572.

[5] Griffiths IR. Some aspects of the pathology and pathogenesis of the myelopathy caused by disc protrusion. J Neurol Neurosurg Psychiatry 1972;35:403–13.

[6] Griffiths IR. Spinal disease in the dog. In Pract 1982;4:44–52.

[7] Olby NJ, DeRisio L, Muñana K, et al. Development of a functional scoring system in dogs with acute spinal cord injuries. Am J Vet Res 2001;62:1624–8.

[8] Olby NJ, Harris T, Burr J, et al. Recovery of pelvic limb function in dogs following acute intervertebral disc herniations. J Neurotrauma 2004;21:49–59.

[9] Olby NJ, Harris T, Muñana K, et al. Long-term functional outcome of dogs with severe thoracolumbar spinal cord injuries. J Am Vet Med Assoc 2003;222:762–9.

[10] Field-Fote EC. Combined use of body weight support, functional electric stimulation, and treadmill training to improve walking ability in individuals with chronic incomplete spinal cord injury. Arch Phys Med Rehabil 2001;82(6):818–24.

[11] Millis DL, Levine D, Taylor R. Canine rehabilitation and physical therapy. Philadelphia: WB Saunders; 2004.

[12] Brody LT. Mobility impairment. In: Hall CM, Brody LT, editors. Therapeutic exercise: moving toward function. 1st edition. Philadelphia: Williams and Wilkins; 1999.

[13] Jacobs PL, Nash MS, Rusinowski JW. Circuit training provides cardiorespiratory and strength benefits in persons with paraplegia. Med Sci Sports Exerc 2001;33(5):711–7.

[14] Sumida M, Fujimoto M, Tokuhiro A, et al. Early rehabilitation effect for traumatic spinal cord injury. Arch Phys Med Rehabil 2001;82(3):391–5.

[15] Harris-Love ML, Forrester LW, Macko RF, et al. Hemiparetic gait parameters in overground versus treadmill walking. Neurorehabil Neural Repair 2001;15(2):105–12.

[16] Levine D, Tragauer V, Millis DL. Percentage of normal weight-bearing during partial immersion at various depths in dogs. Presented at the Second International Symposium on Rehabilitation and Physical Therapy in Veterinary Medicine, Knoxville, TN, 2002.

[17] Marsolais GS, McLean S, Derrick T, et al. Kinematic analysis of the hind limb during swimming and walking in healthy dogs and dogs with surgically corrected cranial cruciate ligament rupture. J Am Vet Med Assoc 2003;222(6):739–43.

[18] Kesiktas N, Paker N, Erdogan N, et al. The use of hydrotherapy for the management of spasticity. Neurorehabil Neural Repair 2004;18(4):268–73.

[19] Hubbard TJ, Denegar CR. Does cryotherapy improve outcomes with soft tissue injury? J Athl Train 2004;39(3):278–9.

[20] Chae J, Bethoux F, Bohine T, et al. Neuromuscular stimulation for upper extremity motor and functional recovery in acute hemiplegia. Stroke 1998;29(5):975–9.

[21] Scremin AM, Kurta L, Gentili A, et al. Increasing muscle mass in spinal cord injured persons with a functional electrical stimulation exercise program. Arch Phys Med Rehabil 1999;80(12):1531–6.

[22] Fish CJ, Blakemore WF. A model of chronic spinal cord compression in the cat. Neuropathol Appl Neurobiol 1983;9:109.

[23] Yovich JV, et al. Ultrastructural alterations in the spinal cord of horses with chronic cervical compressive myelopathy. Prog Vet Neurol 1992;3:13.

[24] Uchida Y, Sugimara M, Onaga T, et al. Regeneration of crushed and transected sciatic nerves in young dogs. Journal of the Japanese Veterinary Medical Association 1993;46:775.

[25] Añor S. Monoparesis. In: BSAVA manual of canine and feline neurology. London: BSAVA Press; 2004.

[26] Evans HE, editor. The spinal nerves. In: Miller's anatomy of the dog. Philadelphia: WB Saunders; 1993. p. 829–93.

[27] Bailey CS. Patterns of cutaneous anesthesia associated with brachial plexus avulsions in the dog. J Am Vet Med Assoc 1984;185:889–99.

[28] Bailey CS, Kitchell RL. Cutaneous sensory testing in the dog. J Vet Intern Med 1987;1:128–35.

[29] Griffiths IR, Duncan ID. The use of electromyography and nerve conduction studies in the evaluation of lower motor neuron disease or injury. J Small Anim Pract 1978;19:329–40.
[30] Griffiths IR, Duncan ID, Lawson DD. Avulsion of the brachial plexus. 2. Clinical aspects. J Small Anim Pract 1974;15:177–83.
[31] Faissler D, Cizinauskas S, Jaggy A. Prognostic factors for functional recovery in dogs with suspected brachial plexus avulsion. J Vet Intern Med 2002;16:370.
[32] Kern H, Salmons S, Mayr W, et al. Recovery of long-term denervated human muscles induced by electrical stimulation. Muscle Nerve 2005;31(1):98–101.
[33] Johnson J, Levine D. Electrical stimulation. In: Millis DL, Levine D, Taylor RA, editors. Canine rehabilitation and physical therapy. Philadelphia: WB Saunders; 2004. p. 289–302.
[34] van Nes JJ, van der Most van Spijk D. Electrophysiological evidence of peripheral nerve dysfunction in six dogs with botulism type C. Res Vet Sci 1986;40:372–6.
[35] Cuddon PA. Electrophysiologic assessment of acute polyradiculoneuropathy in dogs: comparison with Guillain-Barre syndrome in people. J Vet Intern Med 1998;12:294–303.

Vet Clin Small Anim 35 (2005) 1411–1426

VETERINARY CLINICS
SMALL ANIMAL PRACTICE

Rehabilitation of Medical and Acute Care Patients

Dianne Dunning, MS, DVM[a],*, Krista B. Halling, DVM[b],
Nicole Ehrhart, VMD, MS[c]

[a]College of Veterinary Medicine, University of Illinois at Urbana-Champaign,
1008 West Hazelwood Drive, Urbana, IL 61802, USA
[b]Department of Clinical Studies, Ontario Veterinary College, University of Guelph,
Guelph, Ontario, Canada N1G 2W1
[c]Animal Cancer Center, Department of Clinical Sciences, Colorado State University,
300 West Drake Street, Fort Collins, CO 80523, USA

The primary goals of a clinical rehabilitation program in the intensive care or oncologic setting are to improve the animal's quality of life and reduce the complications associated with prolonged hospitalization or immunosuppressive therapy. Cancer and serious systemic illness result in several physiologic changes that involve multiple body systems. While the primary conditions are addressed with traditional modalities of medicine, the side effects, secondary changes, and complications can be ameliorated or even prevented with rehabilitation and supportive care. By applying the basic therapeutic modalities of massage, passive and active range of motion, postural drainage, low-intensity therapeutic exercise, electrical stimulation, and good general nursing care, one can improve the function of and decrease the animal's risk for complications associated with an intensive care admission or chemo- or radiotherapy. This article reviews problems facing the oncologic and critically ill animal, discusses basic techniques in the management of these animals, and highlights the essential role of rehabilitation in obtaining maximal functional capacity in the critically ill patient.

GENERAL APPLICATIONS OF REHABILITATION IN THE MEDICAL PATIENT

In the past, rehabilitation in companion animal medicine was limited to postoperative orthopedic and neurologic conditions. Although it is efficacious in both of these areas, the practice of rehabilitation can easily be modified and applied to many other animals, including those exhibiting clinical signs related to

---

*Corresponding author. North Carolina State University College of Veterinary Medicine, 4700 Hillsborough Street, Raleigh, NC 27606, USA. *E-mail address*: dianne_dunning@ncsu.edu (D. Dunning).

0195-5616/05/$ – see front matter
doi:10.1016/j.cvsm.2005.08.008

cardiopulmonary dysfunction, systemic disease, neuromuscular weakness, generalized weakness, trauma, and cancer. In humans, the role of rehabilitation is well established for a variety of diseases, with inpatient and outpatient physical therapy being available and covered by medical insurance for a variety of conditions including (but not limited to) the following [1]:

- Orthopedic conditions of the back, neck, shoulder, hip, knee and ankle
- Postsurgical conditions
- Amputations
- Fractures
- Joints and soft-tissue injuries
- Neurologic conditions such as stroke, Parkinson's disease, and multiple sclerosis
- Arthritis
- Cardiopulmonary and circulatory conditions
- Systemic diseases such as cancer, AIDS/HIV, and fibromyalgia
- Connective tissue conditions
- Functional capacity evaluations and work conditioning
- Workplace injuries
- Sports injuries

All rehabilitation regimens should be authorized by the primary care clinician before their initiation. In addition, the rehabilitation practitioner or therapist should fully review the animal's medical history and perform and record independent physical and rehabilitation examinations. From this review and discussion of the case with the primary care clinician, a problem list should be completed to guide the therapy and provide a baseline assessment from which one can fully evaluate the success or failure of the therapy. Depending on the patient's status, periodic reassessment should be performed as often as daily to modify the regimen and identify additional problems. Components of the rehabilitation evaluation commonly include, but are not limited to, limb girth measurement for estimation of muscle mass, edema and bruising scoring, goniometry, disability assessment with timed standing or walking, subjective mentation scoring, and pain assessment scoring.

Flexibility in the therapy regimen is essential for the critical care patient and in particular the radiation patient owing to the necessity for sedation and even anesthesia on the days of treatment. The rehabilitation regimen should not disrupt chemotherapy, antimicrobial, or fluid administration. Planning of various treatment regimens must be clear and strategic between services and clinicians to avoid compromise of the patient and the therapy. Animals with invasive monitoring, diarrhea, or urinary tract infection are limited in their ability to participate in an intensive rehabilitation program (ie, swimming or exercising in an underwater treadmill) but may still benefit from the therapeutic modalities of massage, mobilization, and limited therapeutic exercise. In addition, intravenous, epidural, and urinary catheters, telemetry pads, rectal probes, thoracostomy and feeding tubes, and oxygen supplementation are issues that must be taken into account when creating a therapeutic plan.

METABOLIC AND TISSUE CHANGES ASSOCIATED WITH SYSTEMIC ILLNESS

Although the physiologic changes associated with inactivity have been observed in veterinary medicine, most research and clinical reports in this area have involved humans [2–21]. Reduced physical activity that accompanies an admission to an intensive care unit (ICU) or oncology ward represents a significant stress to the body. In humans, decreased physical activity results in significant losses in functional capacity of the musculoskeletal and cardiovascular systems [3,5,6,8,15,17,18].

Patients in the ICU who are confined to bed rest for more than 1 week experience a rapid reduction of muscle mass and exercise intolerance [5]. Muscle atrophy caused by hospitalization and bed rest in humans is characterized by loss of myonuclei, decreased myocyte cytoplasm, myosin filament defects, and an increase in several proteolytic enzymes [2,10,21]. Some of these changes create inflammation within the inactive muscles, leading to production of reactive oxygen species (ROS) [20,21]. Molecular ROS factors, in turn, lead to contractile dysfunction, which is manifested as a reduced force of contraction without evidence of structural muscle damage or loss [20,21]. Inflammation contributes to acute and chronic myocyte damage and cell death through metabolic derangements in musculature, increased proteolysis, and disturbed regeneration of muscle fibers [13,22]. Elevated levels of proinflammatory factors have been implicated in reduced contractile force even in the absence of muscle damage [22]. In addition, inflammation is a normal consequence of injury or infection and a common phenomenon in the ICU. Cytokines initiate inflammation and contribute to muscle dysfunction [21]. Appendicular skeletal muscles are not alone in these changes. Similar alterations in muscle strength and endurance are seen in the diaphragm and intercostal muscles, which directly affect ventilation and decrease the cardiopulmonary response to exercise [5].

Inactivity in critically ill adults has been associated with an increased risk of decubital ulcers, pulmonary complications, deep vein thrombosis, and prolonged ICU and hospital stays [4,6,15,18,21]. Furthermore, cancer and systemic illness result in critical changes in metabolism and basal metabolic requirements and nutritional needs. The changes discussed herein most likely occur in dogs as well as humans and can be improved with a rehabilitation program. Any rehabilitation therapy regimen must be approached with caution and close monitoring. The heart rate and rhythm, the respiratory rate, and the animal's overall demeanor and response to therapy must be evaluated to detect stress or decompensation associated with the increased activity or intervention.

GENERAL NURSING CARE

Good general nursing care is an important component of any rehabilitation regimen. All therapies should take place in an area free from clutter and debris. Weak debilitated animals also benefit from textured flooring to provide firm footing during assisted standing or walking. Bedding should be checked and changed on a regular basis to prevent complications associated with decubital ulceration, urine scald, and soiling. Placing recumbent and nonambulatory animals on elevated racks facilitates air circulation and minimizes urine and fecal contamination. Disposable absorbable pads are also available to place under the animal's hind end.

The prevention of decubital ulceration and urine scald is significantly easier and more cost effective than the treatment of these complications [23]. Factors associated with pressure ulcers in humans in acute care hospitals include older age, male gender, sensory perception deficits, moisture, impaired mobility, nutrition, and friction or shear when transferring the patient from one surface to another with sheets or bedding [24]. Typical pressures over bony prominences when sitting or lying have been measured at 100 to 200 mm Hg [2,25,26]. Pressures greater than approximately 32 mm Hg exceed capillary filling pressure and result in potential tissue ischemia [2,25,26]. The standard recommendations of a 2-hour turning cycle for the immobile patient are based on animal models [2,25,26]. The location of pressure sores correlates well with pressure maps based on the anatomy of bony prominences and positioning.

Pressure sores are found in 3% to 10% of hospitalized human patients [2,25,26]. The prevalence correlates with advanced age and dependent mobility status [2,25,26]. More than 30% of hip fractures are complicated by pressure sores. Individuals with spinal cord injury have a lifetime risk ranging from 25% to 85% [2,25,26]. Specific risk factors for decubital ulcers in humans include the following [2,25,26]:

- Limitations in mobility (eg, paralysis, fracture, weakness, bed rest)
- Altered sensory feedback (sensory loss from spinal cord injury, peripheral neuropathy)
- Altered mental status (eg, pain medication, stupor, dementia, senility)
- Altered body mechanics (increased pressure over bony prominences secondary to spasticity, contractures, scoliosis, kyphosis)
- Malnutrition (weight loss, hypoalbuminemia)

Although individual risk factors in animals have not yet been identified, the skin of a recumbent animal should be inspected frequently to detect early signs of pressure sores [2,25,26]. Blanchable erythema is one of the first clinical signs of inflammation and pressure necrosis and is important in early detection of pressure-sensitive sites and the monitoring of current preventive strategies. Preventive strategies for patients at risk for decubital ulcers include turning the patient every 2 hours, soft bedding or an air mattress or water bed, and the use of doughnuts fashioned from cotton and tape and placed so that the open hole of the donut is over the pressure point to help minimize the pressure and distribute it over a greater surface area.

SPECIFIC TREATMENT TECHNIQUES
Positioning
Positioning in this context describes the use of body position as a specific treatment technique (Fig. 1) [19,27,28]. Positioning for animals in the ICU can be

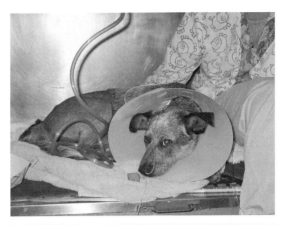

Fig. 1. Positioning of a dog in sternal recumbency with severe pulmonary contusions and pelvic fractures.

used to optimize oxygen transport through its effects of improving ventilation/perfusion, preventing atelectasis, increasing lung volumes by minimizing abdominal compression, reducing the work of breathing, and enhancing mucociliary clearance [19,27,28]. Positioning can also improve dependent limb edema, help prevent decubital ulcer formation, and improve patient comfort. The most common forms of positioning in recumbent animals are alternating between right and left lateral recumbency every 2 to 4 hours and positioning the animal in sternal recumbency with foam wedges, blankets, or pillows. For animals with unilateral lung disease, depending on its etiology, lying the animal with the affected side up or down can maximize remaining lung capacity and help resolve complicating atelectasis and edema from the dependent lung. In a patient with severe respiratory compromise, supplemental oxygen and close monitoring are necessary to ensure patient safety [27,28]. Attention should be paid to the animal's heart and respiratory rate, oxygen saturation, and demeanor, with periodic blood gas monitoring to detect respiratory decompensation [27,28].

Thoracic Postural Drainage Techniques

Thoracic postural drainage techniques use the position of the animal's body to promote removal of tracheobronchial secretions in animals with pulmonary disease (Fig. 2). Indications for thoracic postural drainage include pneumonia, lung lobe abscess, pulmonary contusions, and atelectasis from prolonged recumbency, mechanical ventilation, generalized weakness, or neurologic impairment. Thoracic radiographs or CT are imperative to guide postural drainage. The animal must be positioned so that the segmental bronchi are vertical to the affected lung to allow drainage of secretions into the larger airways [19,27,29]. By placing the animal's thoracic cavity in an inclined or declined position, the secretions can more easily reach the mainstem bronchi and trachea. Thoracic postural drainage sessions last 5 to 10 minutes performed two to four times

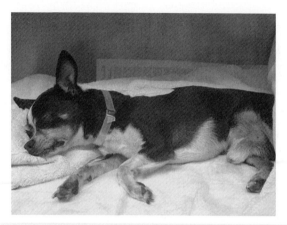

Fig. 2. Thoracic postural drainage. Note the elevated head position to improve left lung lobe drainage.

a day and are dictated by the comfort and tolerance level of the animal [27,28]. Coughing, percussion, and vibration may further enhance the flow up the mucociliary elevator [27,28]. A cough reflex may be elicited via digital pressure on the larynx and proximal portion of the trachea. All animals should be closely monitored for dyspnea and aspiration throughout the procedure, and supplemental oxygen should be available in case of hypoxemia.

Thoracic Percussion and Vibration

Thoracic percussion (coupage) and vibration are manual and mechanical techniques that are intended to promote clearance of airway secretions by the transmission of an energy wave through the chest wall [19,30]. Thoracic percussion is most commonly performed manually by clapping cupped hands on the chest wall over the affected area of the lung (Fig. 3) [19,27,29,31]. Correct technique and positioning over the affected lung segment are more important than the amount of force used, and only the affected lung lobe should be treated, because percussion causes atelectasis even when properly performed [27,29,31]. In an experimental study evaluating the effects of manual and mechanical thoracic percussion in a group of anesthetized, paralyzed, and ventilated dogs, both forms of percussion caused atelectasis based on postmortem and histopathologic evaluation. Despite the presence of atelectasis, gas exchange improved toward the end of percussion based on arterial blood gas analysis [31].

Vibration is also usually applied manually or mechanically by vibrating or pulsating the chest wall during expiration [19,30]. Manual expiratory vibration is performed with the animal in lateral recumbency and involves rapidly rattling the thoracic cavity with locked hands and arms [27]. Clinical studies in humans have shown manual percussion and vibration to be equal or superior to mechanical methods in the removal of proteinaceous material found in the alveoli of patients with pulmonary alveolar protein deposits while undergoing

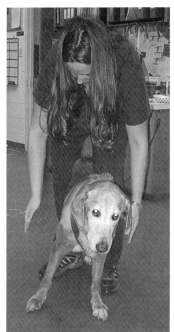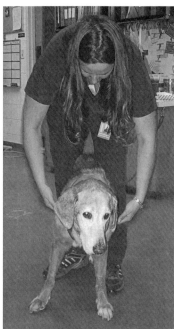

Fig. 3. Coupage is being performed on a Golden Retriever recovering from aspiration pneumonia. The therapist is standing above the patient with her hands cupped. She is gently and rhythmically tapping the chest of the patient.

whole-lung bronchopulmonary lavage [32]. Each thoracic percussion is usually 3 to 4 minutes in duration followed by vibration on the four to six subsequent expirations [27]. Three to four thoracic percussion/vibration therapy cycles are recommended following each postural drainage session [27]. Contraindications to thoracic percussion and vibration include hemodynamic instability, traumatic myocarditis, a flail chest, rib fractures, pleural space disease (chylo-, pyo-, hemo-, and pneumothorax), thrombocytopenia (<30,000 platelets/μL), open wounds, pain, and pulmonary or thoracic tumors [27].

Suction

The decision to ventilate a patient via endotracheal intubation or a tracheostomy is usually made by the attending clinician [33,34]. Advantages of tracheostomy ventilation in humans are that general anesthesia or heavy sedation is usually not required and the patient can participate in a more active rehabilitation regimen. Suction via an endotracheal tube or tracheostomy is used with the aim of removing secretions from the central airways and stimulating a cough [19,33,34]. Tracheal irritation from protracted intubation, ventilation, and a lack of oronasal mucosa air conditioning leads to increased volume and viscosity of respiratory secretions that will obstruct the trachea and lead to difficult breathing. The full care of mechanically ventilated patients is outside of the scope of this article but should be considered as a part of good general nursing care to maintain pulmonary function.

Mobilization

In general, activity in the ICU and oncologic setting can be divided into therapeutic and nontherapeutic movement [21]. Nontherapeutic movement consists of agitated nonpurposeful behaviors that are random and that have the potential to harm the animal or create an unsafe environment [21]. In these situations, sedation and pain management may be indicated for clinician and animal safety. Therapeutic movement is purposeful and does not injure the animal or create an unsafe condition (such as catheter line dislodgement) [21]. Mobilization is a subset of therapeutic movement that promotes function, prevents disability, and slows the onset of degenerative processes [19,21, 28,35,36]. Mobilization includes range of motion (active and passive), assisted standing, and facilitated walking.

Range of motion

One of the most common low-intensity forms of movement employed in the ICU and oncologic veterinary patient is range of motion. Nevertheless, little is known about the physiologic effects of stretching or range of motion on the muscle in these animals [21]. Generally, range of motion consists of therapeutic movement about a joint to maintain the integrity of the tendon, ligament, articular cartilage, and muscle, and may be passive, active assistive, active restrictive, or active in nature [27,28]. Range of motion is often combined with stretching to lengthen shortened tissue and to decrease muscle stiffness. Chronic effects of stretching include adding sarcomeres to muscle mass in deconditioned muscles [8,9,21,28,37].

In the controlled experimental setting in humans, range of motion does not seem to affect adversely cardiopulmonary parameters. In patients who are critically and systemically ill, limb movements performed passively by a physiotherapist have been shown to result in statistically significant increases in oxygen consumption, heart rate, and blood pressure over baseline values [19,38,39]. Despite these elevated physical parameters, passive range of motion (PROM) activity has been used safely, even in persons with intracranial disease, as long as Valsalva-like maneuvers are avoided [40,41]. In two separate clinical studies evaluating the effects of PROM on human patients with increased or normal intracranial pressure in neurosurgical ICUs, limb movement and PROM did not increase intracranial or cerebral perfusion pressures and in some cases was associated with suppression of abnormal intracranial pressure waves and improved consciousness [40,41].

In recumbent or debilitated animals, PROM should ideally be initiated early in the course of hospitalization. All joints of the appendicular skeleton should be placed through a multiple series of gentle, slow, pain-free cycles of flexion and extension. The length of each session is variable depending on the size of the animal and the level of disability; however, a standard PROM session for the ICU patient usually consists of each joint being flexed and extended

10 to 15 times with the animal fully relaxed and laterally recumbent [28,42]. If a joint is found to be developing a contracture, PROM is performed more frequently on that joint. If the animal can ambulate normally and has a near-normal level of activity, range of motion may not necessary, because normal ambulation with weight bearing is a more intensive form of activity [43]. Because these exercises do not involve any contribution of effort from the animal, PROM will not prevent muscle atrophy or increase muscle strength or endurance, and it has limited effects on peripheral circulation [28,42].

Facilitated standing and assisted walking
Experimental investigations in humans indicate that activity can affect serum levels of selected pro- and anti-inflammatory cytokines [21,44]. Intense prolonged activity that causes epithelial and myocyte stretch and changes in myocyte conformation clearly stimulates cytokine synthesis of tumor necrosis factor alpha (TNF-α), interleukin-1 (IL-1), IL-6, and IL-10 in healthy human athletes [21,44]. Exhaustive or prolonged exercise in humans produces significant increases in levels of TNF-α, IL-6, and IL-10 [21,45,46]. Low-to-moderate levels of exercise have very different effects in the critically ill and can improve blood flow to muscles and joints, inhibiting changes seen with disuse atrophy without concomitant increases in proinflammatory or anti-inflammatory cytokines [11,21,47,48]. Mild therapeutic activity in people improves circulation to myocytes and prevents macrophage infiltration into inactive muscles, consequently reducing the local load of potentially destructive cytokines [7,21]. It has been hypothesized that low levels of activity in the critically ill may prevent ischemia/reperfusion injury with subsequent inflammation, minimizing the risk of multiple organ dysfunction and acute respiratory distress syndrome [21,49].

In the nonambulatory and recumbent animal, facilitated standing and walking with a sling, cart, or therapy ball are important components of rehabilitation. Both movements work to improve circulation and lymphatic drainage. The physical act of standing and ambulation improves and in some cases retains an animal's mobility, functional capacity, and postural balance. The simple act of standing is a complicated activity in compromised patients that involves neuromuscular coordination to maintain normal postural balance and limb position (Fig. 4). Initial exercises are restricted to multiple facilitated stands with a sling or ball for a 1- to 2-minute duration that may be extended to assisted walks with a cart or sling or sessions in an underwater treadmill, with the animal's weight supported by the buoyancy of water or floatation devices.

Hydrotherapy in combination with massage is an excellent method to remove lymphedema and swelling from the distal extremities while relaxing and cleansing the patient. Postoperatively, hydrotherapy may be employed as soon as the surgical incision has established a fibrin seal, generally within 48 to 72 hours from surgery. Whirlpools, swimming pools, or underwater treadmill systems provide a reduced gravity environment that is ideal for performing nonconcussive active assisted exercise. The natural properties of water provide buoyancy and resistance to improve limb mobility and joint range of

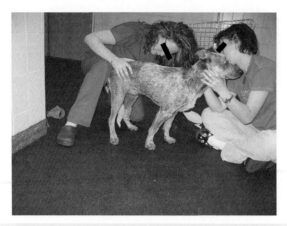

Fig. 4. Assisted standing for a dog with a femoral fracture. Note that the animal is supported at either end to prevent falling, and the limb position is adjusted to a normal weight-bearing position.

motion [50]. Caution should be used with any water exercise, particularly with the critically ill, because some dogs dislike water or resist swimming and may become distressed unless acclimatized to the regimen [28,51]. The authors recommend that the therapist accompany the pet in midchest deep water to provide assistance and assurance to the animal until it is accustomed to the activity. At no time should an animal be left unattended during a hydrotherapy regimen, because water aspiration and drowning are real risks.

Massage

Busy effective ICUs can be highly stressful environments. Sick animals in the ICU are often further stressed by prolonged separation from their owners and are subject to continuous high-intensity noise and bright light. In addition to disrupted sleep cycles, the constant and necessary nature of monitoring is often invasive and uncomfortable. Reducing stress for an animal is important to improve patient comfort. One of the most effective means of relaxing an animal and providing a positive stimulus is massage (Fig. 5). In humans, massage seems to decrease stress and provide tactile stimulation. It has been recommended as an intervention to promote growth and the development of preterm and low birth weight infants [52]. In another study in hospice patients, slow-stroke back massage was associated with modest clinical but statistically significant decreases in systolic blood pressure, diastolic blood pressure, and heart rate with an increase in skin temperature [53]. In animals, the effects of massage are undocumented to date, but massage still has a role as a clinical treatment tool because it is benign, noninvasive, and inexpensive to employ [51,54].

In general, massage is the therapeutic manipulation of soft tissues and muscle by rubbing, kneading, or tapping. Benefits of massage include increased local circulation, nerve sedation, reduced muscle spasm, attenuation of edema,

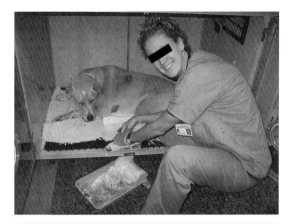

Fig. 5. Massage therapy provides relaxation and socialization for the critically ill and recumbent animal in a hectic and stressful ICU environment.

and break down of irregular scar tissue formation. The physiologic properties of massage stem from reflex and mechanical effects. Reflex effects are based on peripheral receptor stimulation producing central effects of relaxation while peripherally producing muscle relaxation and arteriolar dilation. Mechanical effects include increased lymphatic and venous drainage, removal of edema and metabolic waste, increased arterial circulation enhancing tissue oxygenation and wound healing, and manipulation of restrictive connective tissue, enhancing range of motion and limb mobility.

The most common techniques of massage used in veterinary medicine are effleurage, pétrissage, cross fiber, and tapotement. Effleurage (from the Latin *effluere* meaning to flow out) is a form of superficial or light stroking massage and is generally used in the beginning of all massage sessions to relax and acclimatize the animal. Pétrissage (from the French *pétrir* meaning to knead) is characterized by deep kneading and squeezing of muscle and surrounding soft tissues. Cross-fiber massage is also a deep massage that is concentrated along lines of restrictive scar tissue and is designed to promote normal range of motion [51,55] Tapotement involves percussive manipulation of the soft tissues with a cupped hand or instrument and is often used to enhance postural drainage for respiratory conditions. Contraindications to massage are unstable or infected fractures and the presence of a malignancy; however, in most patients, massage is an indispensable alternate for mobility in the critically ill animal with restricted mobility [56].

Electrical Stimulation

Electrical stimulation is a commonly used modality in rehabilitation and physical therapy. The two most common forms used in the critically ill animal are neuromuscular stimulation for improving range of motion activity, increasing muscle strength, and muscle re-education, and transcutaneous electrical nerve stimulation for modifying pain. Neuromuscular stimulation is indicated in any animal that is exposed to prolonged recumbency owing to systemic illness or neurologic impairment. Neuromuscular stimulation helps prevent disuse atrophy and improves limb performance by recruiting contracting fibers and increasing maximum contractible force of affected muscles (Fig. 6) [51,57]. The electrical stimulation device consists of a pulse generator and electrodes that are placed over selected weakened or paralyzed muscle groups to create an artificial contraction [51,57]. The pulse amplitude, rate, and cycle length may be varied to suit the comfort of the patient [51,57]. Reduction of muscle pain and edema owing to improved blood flow also occurs [51,57]. Combining neuromuscular stimulation with PROM exercises improves joint range of motion and prevents muscle contracture and is particularly indicated when dealing with muscle contracture and limb dysfunction originating from loss of range of motion [51,57]. Furthermore, neuromuscular stimulation is effective in promoting muscle re-education after prolonged disuse. A full discussion of electrical stimulation is outside the scope of this article, and the reader is referred to other texts for a more complete discussion of this modality in veterinary medicine [57].

Adjunct Pain Management

Assessing pain in the veterinary patient is challenging, especially when dealing with the critically ill animal that may be physically unable to display the common behavioral signs indicative of pain (vocalization, postural changes, trembling, restlessness, depression, disrupted sleep cycles, inappetence, aggression, and agitation) [58–61]. Furthermore, the physiologic parameters associated with pain (tachypnea, tachycardia, hypertension, dilated pupils, and ptyalism) may be masked or conversely exacerbated by the primary disease or its therapy [58–61]. Most systemic diseases and oncologic conditions present

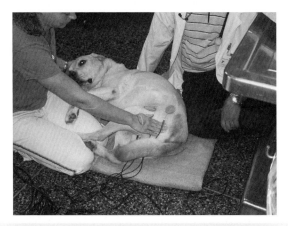

Fig. 6. Neuromuscular stimulation in a dog with muscular atrophy owing to a fibrocartilaginous embolus. Note that the electrode has been placed on the rehabilitationist's hand to facilitate pad positioning and to direct the electrical impulse.

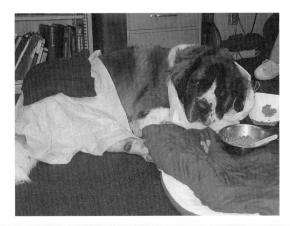

Fig. 7. Multimodal pain management in a postoperative hind limb amputee owing to osteo-sarcoma. Massage, icepacks, assisted standing, facilitated walking, and pharmaceutical intervention were employed in this patient to reduce postoperative pain, manage depression, and regain ambulatory function.

with a series of clinical signs that are arguably related to pain or at least malaise, and such patients would benefit from carefully planned multimodal pain management, in which rehabilitation has a supportive but important role (Fig. 7). Effective multimodal pain management reduces anxiety, decreases stress and its associated hormonal and metabolic derangements, and allows the animal to rest more comfortably.

In human patients, chronic noncancer pain is a common problem that is often accompanied by serious psychiatric comorbidity and disability [62]. Clinical studies in a variety of conditions of chronic pain have highlighted the effectiveness of physical therapy in a multidisciplinary pain management program to improve pain, depression, and disability scores [62,63]. Similarly, veterinary and human oncologists believe that the relief of cancer-related symptoms is essential in the supportive and palliative care of patients [64]. Complementary therapies such as acupuncture, mind-body techniques, and massage therapy can help when conventional treatment does not bring satisfactory relief or causes undesirable side effects [64]. Massage is increasingly applied to relieve pain and nausea symptoms in patients with cancer [65]. This practice is supported by evidence from several small randomized trials and a recent large study performed at Sloan-Kettering. The latter study involved 1290 patients and evaluated the effects of pre- and post-massage therapy on pain, fatigue, stress/anxiety, nausea, and depression using a 0 to 10 rating scale [65]. Symptom scores were dramatically reduced by approximately 50% even for patients reporting high baseline scores [65]. Outpatients improved about 10% more than inpatients. Furthermore, the benefits of massage therapy persisted, with outpatients experiencing no return toward baseline scores throughout the duration of a 48-hour follow-up period [65]. These data indicate that rehabilitation, even in its simplest form of massage therapy, is associated with substantial improvement in the symptom scores of cancer patients [65].

SUMMARY
Rehabilitation should begin as soon as the critically ill animal is stable, before the onset of complications associated with prolonged hospitalization. A proactive approach to rehabilitation in the medical, oncologic, and acute care animal will require less effort and reap greater rewards than one that is in response to a developing crisis. The nature of the treatment is influenced by factors such as the status of the animal, the etiology and extent of the disease, and the facilities, equipment, and trained personnel [66]. Most patients will experience improved recoveries with even simple fundamental techniques such as massage, cold-packing, PROM, and controlled exercise regimens that involve primarily an investment of time and training on the therapist's part.

References
[1] American Physical Therapy Association. Physical therapy and your insurance: a patient's guide to getting the best coverage. Available at: http://www.apta.org. Accessed October 2005.
[2] Allen C, Glasziou P, Del Mar C. Bed rest: a potentially harmful treatment needing more careful evaluation. Lancet 1999;354:1229–33.
[3] Anzueto A. Muscle dysfunction in the intensive care unit. Clin Chest Med 1999;20:1–25.
[4] Chulay M. Should we get patients out of bed who have a pulmonary artery catheter and introducer in place? Crit Care Nurse 1995;15:93–4.
[5] Cirio S, Piaggi G, De Mattia E, et al. Muscle retraining in ICU patients. Monaldi Arch Chest Dis 2003;59:300–3.
[6] Cook D, Attia J, Weaver B, et al. Venous thromboembolic disease: an observational study in medical-surgical intensive care unit patients. J Crit Care 2000;15:127–32.
[7] DeLetter M. Critical illness polyneuropathy and myopathy (CIPNM): evidence for local immune activation by cytokine-expression in the muscle tissue. J Neuroimmunol 2000;106:202–13.
[8] Gamrin L, Essen P, Forsberg A, et al. A descriptive study of skeletal muscle metabolism in critically ill patients: free amino acids, energy-rich phosphates, protein, nucleic acids, fats, and electrolytes. Crit Care Med 1996;24:575–83.
[9] Griffiths R, Palmer T, Helliwell T, et al. Effect of passive stretching on the wasting muscle in the critically ill. Nutrition 1995;11:428–32.
[10] Helliwell T, Wilkinson A, Griffiths R, et al. Muscle atrophy in critically ill patients is associated with the loss of myosin filaments and the presence of lysosomal enzymes and ubiquitin. Neuropathol Appl Neurobiol 1998;24:507–17.
[11] Hund E. Myopathy in critically ill patients. Crit Care Med 1999;27:2544–7.
[12] Lacomis D, Guiliani M, Cott A. Acute myopathy of intensive care: clinical electromyographic and pathologic aspects. Ann Neurol 1996;40:645–54.
[13] Marinelli W, Leatherman J. Neuromuscular disorders in the intensive care unit. Crit Care Clin 2002;18:915–29.
[14] Nevins M, Epstein S. Prolonged critical illness management of long term acute care. Clin Chest Med 2001;22:1–28.
[15] Nickerson N, Murphy S, Davila-Roman V, et al. Obstacles to early discharge after cardiac surgery. Am J Manage Care 1999;5:29–34.

[16] Norton L, Conforti C. The effects of body position on oxygenation. Heart Lung 1985;14: 45–52.
[17] Polkey M, Moxham J. Clinical aspects of respiratory muscle dysfunction in the critically ill. Chest 2001;119:1–23.
[18] Roebuck A, Jessop S, Turner R, et al. The safety of two-hour versus four-hour bed rest after elective 6-French femoral cardiac catheterization. Coron Health Care 2000;4:169–73.
[19] Stiller K. Physiotherapy in intensive care: toward an evidence-based practice. Chest 2000;118:1801–13.
[20] Tisdale M. Loss of skeletal muscle in cancer: biochemical mechanisms. Front Biosci 2001;6: D164–74.
[21] Winkelman C. Inactivity and inflammation: selected cytokines as biologic mediators in muscle dysfunction during critical illness. AACN Clinical Issues. Advanced Practice in Acute Critical Care 2004;15:74–82.
[22] Lundberg I, Dastmalchi M. Possible pathogenic mechanisms in inflammatory myopathies. Rheum Dis Clin North Am 2002;28:799–822.
[23] Maugham L, Cox R, Amsters D, et al. Reducing inpatient hospital usage for management of pressure sores after spinal cord lesions. Int J Rehabil Res 2004;27:311–5.
[24] Fisher A, Wells G, Harrison M. Factors associated with pressure ulcers in adults in acute care hospitals. Holist Nurs Pract 2004;18:242–53.
[25] Allman R. Pressure ulcers among hospitalized patients. Ann Intern Med 1986;105: 337–42.
[26] Barbenel J, Jordan M, Nicol S. Incidence of pressure-sores in the Greater Glasgow Health Board area. Lancet 1977;ii:548–50.
[27] Manning AM. Physical rehabilitation for the critically injured veterinary patient. In: Millis D, Levine D, Taylor R, editors. Canine rehabilitation and physical therapy. Philadelphia: Saunders; 2004. p. 404–10.
[28] Manning AM, Ellis DR, Rush J. Physical therapy for the critically ill veterinary patient. Part II. The musculoskeletal system. Comp Cont Educ Pract Vet 1997;19:803–7.
[29] Manning AM, Ellis DR, Rush J. Physical therapy for critically ill veterinary patients. Part I. Chest physical therapy. Comp Cont Educ Pract Vet19 1997;675–89.
[30] Pryor J. Mucociliary clearance. In: Ellis E, Alison J, editors. Key issues in cardiorespiratory physiotherapy. Oxford (UK): Butterworth-Heinemann; 1992. p. 105–30.
[31] Zidulka A, Chrome J, Wight D, et al. Clapping or percussion causes atelectasis in dogs and influences gas exchange. J Appl Physiol 1989;66:2833–8.
[32] Hammon W, McCaffree D, Cucchiara A. A comparison of manual to mechanical chest percussion for clearance of alveolar material in patients with pulmonary alveolar proteinosis (phospholipidosis). Chest 1993;103:1409–12.
[33] King LG, Hendricks JC. Use of positive-pressure ventilation in dogs and cats: 41 cases (1990–1992). J Am Vet Med Assoc 1994;204:1045–52.
[34] Campbell V, King LG. Pulmonary function, ventilator management, and outcome of dogs with thoracic trauma and pulmonary contusions: 10 cases (1994–1998). J Am Vet Med Assoc 2000;217:1505–9.
[35] Szaflarski N. Immobility phenomena in critically ill adults. In: Clochesy J, Breu C, Cardin S, et al, editors. Critical care nursing. 2nd edition. Philadelphia: Saunders; 1996. p. 1313–34.
[36] Hoffman K, Shanley JM, Oakley DA, et al. Care and management of the critically ill recumbent animal. Comp Cont Educ Pract Vet 1986;7:110–4.
[37] Hall C, Body L. Therapeutic exercise: moving toward function. Philadelphia: Lippincott; 1999.
[38] Norrenberg M, De Backer D, Moraine J, et al. Oxygen consumption can increase during passive leg mobilization. [abstract]. Intensive Care Med 1995;21:S177.
[39] Weissman C, Kemper M, Damask M, et al. Effect of routine intensive care interactions on metabolic rate. Chest 1984;86:815–8.
[40] Brimioulle S, Moraine J, Norrenberg D, et al. Effects of positioning and exercise on intracranial pressure in a neurosurgical intensive care unit. Phys Ther 1997;77:1682–9.

[41] Koch S, Fogarty S, Signorino C. Effect of passive range of motion on intracranial pressure in neurosurgical patients. J Crit Care 1996;11:176–9.

[42] Coby LA. Range of motion. In: Kisner C, Colby LA, editors. Therapeutic exercise: foundations and techniques. 4th edition. Philadelphia: FA Davis; 2002. p. 24–55.

[43] Bruce W, Frame K, Burbidge H, et al. A comparison of the effects of joint immobilization, twice-daily passive motion, and voluntary motion on articular cartilage healing in sheep. Vet Comp Orthop Trauma 2002;15:23–9.

[44] Pedersen B, Steensberg A, Fischer C, et al. Exercise and cytokines with particular focus on muscle-derived IL-6. Exerc Immunol Rev 2001;7:18–31.

[45] Nieman D. Exercise effects on systemic immunity. Immunol Cell Biol 2000;78:496–501.

[46] Pedersen B. Exercise and cytokines. Immunol Cell Biol 2000;78:532–5.

[47] Sargeant A, Davies C, Edwards R. Functional and structural changes after disuse of human muscle. Clin Sci (Colch) 1977;52:337–42.

[48] Neviere R, Mathiew D, Chagnon J. Skeletal muscle microvascular blood flow and oxygen transport in patients with severe sepsis. Am J Respir Crit Care Med 1996;153:191–5.

[49] Payen D, Faivre V, Lkaszewicz C, et al. Assessment of immunological status in the critically ill. Minerva Anesthesiol 2000;66:757–63.

[50] Payne J. General management considerations for the trauma patient. Vet Clin North Am Sm Anim Pract 1995;25:1015–29.

[51] Taylor R. Postsurgical physical therapy: the missing link. Comp Cont Educ Pract Vet 1992;12:1583–94.

[52] Vickers A, Ohlsson A, Lacy J, et al. Massage for promoting growth and development of preterm and/or low birth-weight infants. Cochrane Database Syst Rev 2004;(2). CD000390.

[53] Meek S. Effects of slow stroke back massage on relaxation in hospice clients. Image J Nurs Sch 1993;25:17–21.

[54] Ogilvie G, Robinson N. Complementary/alternative cancer therapy—fact or fiction? In: Ettinger S, Feldman E, editors. Textbook of veterinary internal medicine: diseases of the dog and cat. 5th edition. Philadelphia: Saunders; 2000. p. 374–9.

[55] Taylor R, Lester M. Physical therapy in canine sporting breeds. In: Bloomberg M, editor. Canine sports medicine and surgery. Philadelphia: WB Saunders; 1998. p. 265–75.

[56] Langer G. Physical therapy in small animal patients: basic principles and application. Comp Contin Educ Pract Vet 1984;6:933–6.

[57] Johnson J, Levine D. Electrical stimulation. In: Millis D, Levine D, Taylor R, editors. Canine rehabilitation and physical therapy. Philadelphia: Saunders; 2004. p. 289–302.

[58] Paddleford R. Analgesia and pain management. In: Manual of small animal anesthesia. 2nd edition. Philadelphia: WB Saunders; 1999. p. 227–46.

[59] Hendrix P, Hansen B, Bonagura J. Acute pain management. In: Kirk's current veterinary therapy XIII: small animal practice. Philadelphia: WB Saunders; 2000. p. 57–61.

[60] Hansen B, Mathews KA. Management of pain. Vet Clin North Am Sm Anim Pract 2000;30: 899–916.

[61] Lamont L. Feline perioperative pain management. Vet Clin North Am Sm Anim Pract 2002;32:747–63.

[62] Chelminski P, Ives T, Felix K, et al. A primary care, multi-disciplinary disease management program for opioid-treated patients with chronic non-cancer pain and a high burden of psychiatric comorbidity. BMC Health Serv Res 2005;13:3.

[63] Goldenberg D, Burckhardt C, Crofford L. Management of fibromyalgia syndrome. JAMA 2004;295:2388–95.

[64] Deng G, Cassileth B, Yeung K. Complementary therapies for cancer-related symptoms. J Support Oncol 2004;2:419–26.

[65] Cassileth B, Vickers A. Massage therapy for symptom control: outcome study at a major cancer center. J Pain Symptom Manage 2004;28:244–9.

[66] Downer A, Spear V. Physical therapy in the management of long bone fractures in small animals. Vet Clin North Am Sm Anim Pract 1975;5:157–64.

ELSEVIER
SAUNDERS

Vet Clin Small Anim 35 (2005) 1427–1439

VETERINARY CLINICS
SMALL ANIMAL PRACTICE

Rehabilitation and Conditioning of Sporting Dogs

Denis J. Marcellin-Little, DEDV, CCRP[a],*,
David Levine, PT, PhD, CCRP[a,b,c],
Robert Taylor, MS, DVM, CCRP[d]

[a]Department of Clinical Sciences, North Carolina State University College of Veterinary Medicine, 4700 Hillsborough Street, Raleigh, NC 27606, USA
[b]Department of Physical Therapy, University of Tennessee at Chattanooga, 615 McCallie Avenue, Chattanooga, TN 37403–2598, USA
[c]Department of Small Animal Clinical Sciences, University of Tennessee College of Veterinary Medicine, 2407 River Drive, Knoxville, TN 37996, USA
[d]Alameda East Veterinary Hospital, 9770 East Alameda Avenue, Denver, CO 80247, USA

Although dogs have been used extensively as a research model for human studies in the field of exercise physiology, little research has been conducted to determine the optimal amount of exercise needed for dogs in terms of the frequency, intensity, and duration of exercise that can help to optimize their health, fitness level, and recovery from orthopedic injuries. Studies to help determine this optimal level of exercise have been performed in human beings [1–4]. Sporting dogs are dogs that perform a variety of physical activities, including racing short and long distances with or without a lure, field trials, herding, tracking, agility, flyball, and Frisbee catching (disk dogs). The purpose of this article is to review the principles and applications of fitness training, rehabilitation, and reconditioning applying to sporting dogs.

FITNESS TRAINING AND CONDITIONING

Fitness is a general term used to describe the ability to perform physical work. It requires cardiorespiratory function, muscle strength, endurance, and flexibility. Fitness is a lifelong adaptation of the cardiovascular and musculoskeletal systems to exercise. Conditioning is the performance of specific physical exercises to prepare mentally and physically for the performance strenuous activity. A fit and conditioned athlete requires an owner, trainer, or handler's conscientious commitment to a well-rounded conditioning program. Training of the musculoskeletal and cardiopulmonary systems is a fundamental part of conditioning.

Corresponding author. E-mail address: Denis_Marcellin@ncsu.edu (D.J. Marcellin-Little).

0195-5616/05/$ – see front matter
doi:10.1016/j.cvsm.2005.08.002

Training is used to teach sporting dogs the specifics of sporting activities. Training also influences the dog's behavior.

Conditioning starts early in life. Strenuous exercise is not recommended before closure of the growth plates of long bones so as to avoid fractures or trauma to these growth plates. Physeal closure occurs at approximately 10 months of age in large dog breeds, a few months earlier in small dog breeds, and a few months later in giant dog breeds [5]. Before physeal closure, the conditioning of sporting dogs involves play with siblings and self-motivated activities (eg, walks, runs). It is important to make efforts to rule out developmental orthopedic diseases (DODs) in dogs chosen as future sporting dogs. This may be done by assessing the sire and dam, by performing an orthopedic examination at approximately 4 months of age, and by making radiographs of hip and elbow joints. Many physical attributes important to sporting dogs are inherited. These include size, speed, strength, endurance, and agility. The relative importance of these attributes varies greatly between sports (Table 1). Conditioning may be effective around puberty, when a surge in androgen hormones occurs in male dogs. This surge in androgens may help to promote muscle development [6]. Despite differences in muscle mass and size between male and female sporting dogs, there are no clear differences in performance between male and female dogs, including racing Greyhounds. The response to aerobic training increases after puberty in human beings [4]. Similarly, sexual maturity likely has an impact on the response to training in dogs.

Complete and balanced nutrition is critical to the conditioning and maintenance of sporting dogs. Nutrition is particularly important during growth, because excessive energy and calcium may increase the expression of faulty genes in dogs genetically predisposed to DODs [7]. Nutrition has to be adapted to the metabolic needs of working dogs during training and during the competitive period. These requirements may be dramatically increased during competitive periods (ie, a sled dog running 12 hours per day). Sled dogs have unique nutritional requirements resulting from their exercise profile. One study reported that sled dogs fed an extreme diet with no carbohydrate (39% protein and 61%

Table 1
Physical skills in canine sporting activities

Sport	Physical skills required[a]
Racing	
Greyhounds	Speed, strength
Sled dogs	Muscle and cardiorespiratory endurance
Field trial	Speed, strength, agility
Hunting	Muscle endurance
Herding	Speed, muscle endurance
Agility	Speed, balance, agility
Search and rescue	Endurance, balance
Flyball/disk	Speed, strength, agility, balance

[a]See text for full description.

fat on an energy basis) fared better than dogs receiving diets rich in carbohydrate (23% and 38% carbohydrate) [8]. Feeding of sporting dogs should not occur during periods of strenuous exercise. Gastric emptying was delayed by exercise lasting more than 1 hour in untrained dogs [9]. Hydration is also critical to sporting dogs, particularly when exercising in hot conditions.

Conditioning involves a physical effort placed on the cardiopulmonary system. Exercise increases heart rate and influences blood pressure in dogs. Over time, exercise also increases red blood cell counts [8]. Conditioning lowered the thyroid hormone concentration (T4 and free T4) in sled dogs in one study [10]. Heart rate monitoring during exercise has been used in dogs [11,12]. Exercise more than doubled the incidence of cardiac arrhythmias in Greyhounds in one study [11]. Heart rate during exercise is higher in overweight dogs than in lean dogs [12]. Training leads to an adaptation of the cardiovascular system over time. Although little is known about the specific changes occurring in heart rate at rest, during, and after exercise in sporting dogs, training leads to a lower resting heart rate and a lower resting blood pressure in people [13]. This is particularly true for endurance training [2], but it also occurs in response to strength training [14]. Training also boosts aerobic fitness in children and adolescents [15]. Although little is known about the relation between fitness and body fat in dogs, people with lower body fat tend to be fitter than people with higher body fat [16]. Exercise leads to a decrease in body fat in people [17,18]. The parameters evaluated when assessing a dog that is destined to be a working dog include its size, conformation, gait during general and specific activities, past and current orthopedic health, body condition score, fitness level, and behavior (eg, level of socialization, drive to perform, extraverted or introverted nature). Fitness and endurance may be evaluated in dogs by running on a treadmill, doing a 6-minute walk test, or by assessing performance during outdoor activities [19,20]. In one report, control dogs walked 573 ± 85.5 m in 6 minutes [20]. Physiologic (eg, heart rate, rectal temperature) and hematologic (eg, plasma creatine kinase, plasma lactate) factors are evaluated during fitness tests [21]. Endurance is adversely affected by restricted activity. Endurance decreased by 41% in 10 dogs whose activity was restricted for 8 weeks [19]. These changes were reversible in 8 weeks of retraining.

When designing a training program, frequency, intensity, and duration of exercises are chosen. The frequency is the number of exercise bouts per time period (per session, day, or week). The intensity is the load applied (eg, speed of trotting or galloping, weight used). The duration is the number of repetitions (in range of motion [ROM], jumping, or catching) or the length of time of exercise. Excessive frequency, intensity, or duration may have a negative impact on training, irritate an existing condition, or cause an injury because of insufficient rest, excessive muscle or cardiovascular fatigue, or excessive stress placed on tissues during activity. To our knowledge, there is no scientific information describing the optimal training amount for conditioning and maintenance of sporting dogs. In people, recommendations for maintenance of fitness include 30 minutes of moderate-intensity activity per day [22].

Strengthening

Strength can be defined as the ability of a muscle or muscle group to produce tension and a resulting force. Strength is required in sporting dogs that need speed (Fig. 1). These dogs have a higher muscle mass–to–body weight ratio than other dogs [23]. Strength is closely linked to speed, for example, in racing Greyhounds, which are extremely strong and may run faster than 70 km/h (45 mph). Growth hormone increases muscle mass in dogs [24].

Strengthening exercises follow a number of basic principles, including the principle of specificity and the overload principle. The principle of specificity refers to the need to train emphasizing the body systems that are used during the sport, and to train them in a manner consistent with how they are used during the sporting activity. In terms of strengthening exercises, the specific muscle groups whose strength is required to perform the desired activities need to be trained. These muscles also need to be strengthened in a way similar to how they are used during the activity (eg, aerobic versus anaerobic, duration of exercise). As an example, a dog involved in flyball needs to accelerate as quickly as possible in a straight line for just a few seconds and then jump four times, decelerate rapidly, turn, accelerate as quickly as possible, and jump over the hurdles again. In designing a strengthening program, there is a need to focus on strengthening pelvic limbs for acceleration and jumping and on strengthening the forelimbs for braking and turning. Specificity also should be present in the exercising environment (ie, surfaces, temperature, humidity, surroundings).

The overload principle is arguably the most critical factor in training. It states that to increase strength (or endurance), a load that exceeds the metabolic capacity of the muscle system or cardiopulmonary system must be achieved during exercise. The systems must also be exercised to fatigue to promote improvement. The principles of specificity and overload apply to conditioning sled dogs, in which pulling is an important specific exercise to illustrate the overload principle. A conditioned sled dog does not improve its fitness level by running on a treadmill or outside at 3 mph for 1 hour five times per week. This level of exercise does not increase its cardiopulmonary endurance

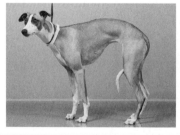 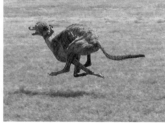

Fig. 1. The musculoskeletal tissues of sighthounds are specialized for speed. This Whippet (*left*) has large muscles in the pelvic limbs, back, and forelimbs. At a gallop (*right*), the bones, joints, muscles, and tendons of this Greyhound undergo high loads that may predispose them to mechanical failure.

or strength for competition, because it does not stress these systems enough to cause adaptation. If improving fitness is the goal, these dogs should exercise while pulling a sled at reasonably high intensities (race speed) for reasonably long periods. If time available during training is an issue and the dog has only 3 hours per training session, the speed could be increased 10% over normal race speeds to stress these systems adequately. Swimming, although a good endurance exercise, does not work the musculoskeletal system of a sled dog in the same manner as the sport. The stresses and subsequent adaptations on the bones, ligaments, and cartilage that occur with weight-bearing exercises are not provided to the same degree with swimming or underwater treadmills.

Strengthening exercises include trotting, trotting uphill, pulling weight or a cart, swimming, galloping, controlled ball playing, retrieving, dancing, and wheelbarrowing. Speed exercises include rapid acceleration and deceleration on level uphill and downhill terrain, ball playing, and playing and racing with other dogs.

Endurance

Endurance is critically important to sporting dogs that perform prolonged efforts, for example, long-distance races (ie, sled dogs) and herding. Aerobic endurance exercises usually target large muscle groups for a prolonged period (more than 15 minutes). They are performed several times per week. Long-term changes occurring in muscle undergoing aerobic training include increased vascularization, which increases the amount of oxygen brought to muscle. In conditioned endurance athletes, several other important changes occur. These changes include decreased resting heart rate and increased stroke volume because of increased vagal tone, which allows greater time for ventricular filling; decreased resting blood pressure, thought to be attributable to a decrease in circulating catecholamines in the bloodstream [25]; an increase in enzymes involved in the oxidative pathways so that ATP can be generated more rapidly; and increased capillary density within the muscle to allow for more efficient delivery of oxygen and greater oxygen uptake, resulting in improved performance. Training also positively affects the strength and stiffness of all musculoskeletal tissues. It makes cartilage and ligaments stiffer, and bones, muscle, and tendons are stronger [26–30]. Exercise does not seem to increase the likelihood of osteoarthritis in dogs free of predisposing factors (ie, obesity, limb malalignment) [31]. Endurance exercises are performed for sustained periods of 15 minutes or more. They include trotting, swimming, land or water treadmill activity, and sled pulling. Monitoring of variables, such as heart rate, during exercise is commonly performed in people but rarely done in dogs. Recommendations of percentage of maximum heart rate that dogs should train at for optimal conditioning are unknown but may help to determine more efficient training regimens.

Balance and Proprioception

Exercise enhances balance and proprioception [32]. Balance is the ability to adjust equilibrium at a stance or during locomotion to adjust to a change in direction or ground surfaces. Proprioception is the unconscious perception of movement and spatial orientation originating from the body. Sporting dogs need to have well-developed balance and proprioception to adjust to the specific challenges of their activities. Proprioception decreases with age in people [33]. Proprioceptive training includes activities that may be performed at low or high speed and require an awareness of limb position in space. They include walking in circles or a figure-of-eight and walking across obstacles of various shape, height, and spacing. Balance exercises are exercises requiring rapid responses to changes in slopes, such as walking on a trampoline, balance or wobble board, and swimming. Other balance and agility exercises include cavaletti rails, exercise balls, rapid changes of direction while trotting and galloping, ball playing, tug-of-war, dancing, and wheelbarrowing.

Adequate rest is important during conditioning to prevent muscle fatigue and lower the likelihood of overuse injuries. Conditioning, however, decreases rest requirements in dogs. Conditioning also minimizes the circulating lactic acid after intense muscular activity [34]. It decreases the likelihood of rhabdomyolysis, a syndrome resulting from hydrogen ion accumulation in muscles during exercise; muscle swelling and ischemia; erythrocyte death in muscles; myoglobinuria; and potential renal failure [35]. Rhabdomyolysis is primarily seen after intense exercise in poorly conditioned dogs. Sporting dogs often exercise all year long, with periodic higher intensity times corresponding to their competition season.

SPORTS INJURIES

Sporting dogs may experience a variety of orthopedic injuries and problems affecting their bones, joints, ligaments, muscles, and tendons (Table 2) [36–49], resulting from the increased physical demands placed on them. Overall, specific sports injuries are unusual in most sporting dogs [50]. Injuries in sporting dogs result from (1) trauma induced by the activity (ie, a disk dog rupturing a lateral collateral ligament while landing after a jump) or trauma induced by an accident occurring during activity (ie, a racing Greyhound catching the lure at high speed during a race, leading to a pile-up of the racers within that race), (2) chronic overload injuries (ie, fatigue fracture of a central tarsal bone fracture in a racing Greyhound or contracture of the tendon of insertion of the infraspinatus muscle in a hunting dog), and (3) preexisting orthopedic diseases (ie, a field trial dog with hip dysplasia showing signs of the disease after a field event). Overall, few surveys have reported the relative incidence of injuries and problems caused by trauma, overuse, and preexisting diseases in sporting dogs [51,52]. Traumatic injuries seem to be relatively unusual in sporting dogs, with the exception of dogs performing extremely intense activities (ie, racing Greyhounds). Stress fractures are also relatively unusual in sporting dogs, with the exception of racing Greyhounds, which have stress fractures of the acetabulum, metacarpal, radius, central tarsal bone, and possibly other bones [36,53,54]. Most orthopedic problems encountered in sporting dogs seem to result from classic DODs (ie, hip dysplasia, elbow dysplasia, patellar luxation, osteochondritis dissecans). These diseases often remain undiagnosed for months

Table 2
Common orthopedic injuries and problems linked to sporting activities in dogs

Structure	Injury	Dog affected	Treatment
Bone	Tarsal and carpal fractures [41–43]	Racing Greyhounds	Sx, bone screws
	Acetabular fractures [39]	Racing Greyhounds	Sx, bone plate
Joint	Interphalangeal luxations [44]	Racing Greyhounds	Sx (when severe)
Carpus	Accessory carpal bone fracture [42,43]	Racing Greyhounds	Sx, bone screws
Elbow	Traumatic FMCP [45]	Racing Greyhounds	Sx, excision
Shoulder	Medial glenohumeral ligament sprain [46]	Agility, hunting dogs	No Sx
Hock	Distal tibial fracture	Racing Greyhound	Sx, bone plate
	Central tarsal bone fracture [41,47]	Racing Greyhound	Sx, bone screw(s)
Stifle	Traumatic cruciate ligament avulsions [48,49]	All sporting dogs	Sx, stabilization
Hip	Craniodorsal luxation [50]	All sporting dogs	Sx, stabilization
Ligaments	Cranial cruciate ligament injuries [48,49]	Flyball dogs, Disk dogs	Sx, stabilization
Muscle	Tear: gracillis mm., tensor fascia lata mm [44]	Racing Greyhounds	Sx, repair
	Tear, long head of triceps mm	Racing Greyhounds	No Sx
	Contracture: infraspinatus mm [51,52]	Hunting dogs	Sx, release
Tendon	(Partial) common calcanean tendon tear [53]	Hunting dogs	Sx (when severe)
	Superficial digital flexor tendon [54]	Agility, herding	Sx, stabilization

Abbreviations: FMCP, fragmentation of the medial coronoid process; mm, muscle; Sx, surgical treatment.

to years until intense activity promotes the development of clinical signs. In most instances, changes, such as osteoarthritis, are present in the affected joints when the problem is diagnosed, confirming the chronicity of the problem. It is important to avoid overtraining high-performance dogs so as to avoid traumatic injuries resulting from high-impact activities performed while dogs are fatigued and to lower the likelihood of stress fractures. Sports requiring strength and speed require shorter training sessions than endurance sports. Overall, overtraining is difficult to define and is specific to each individual within each sport. The most effective protection against overtraining is to screen training dogs routinely for signs of lameness, pain, or tenderness while palpating joints and limbs or for exercise intolerance occurring during training and high-performance activities and to provide rest in fatigued dogs.

REHABILITATION OF SPORTING DOGS

Owners and trainers of dogs engaged in competitive activities often expect rapid and complete recovery after orthopedic injuries. Although the same general principles of rehabilitation are followed, the protocols may, at times, be accelerated in sporting dogs. One of the reasons for this acceleration is owner demand, which may be financial if the animal is racing and producing revenue or may be motivated solely by the desire to return to a hobby with the pet. The overall physical condition of a sporting dog is usually much greater than that of a house pet and may allow for this acceleration because of an increase in protective muscle mass, cardiorespiratory health, and motivation. The protocol followed must be developed in close communication with the surgeon and referring veterinarian. The following outlines the major phases of rehabilitation for the sporting dog and guidelines for the acute, subacute, and reconditioning rehabilitation phases.

Acute Rehabilitation

The acute phase of rehabilitation occurs after an injury or surgery. For patients being rehabilitated after surgery, one should first take into consideration the specifics of the patient (age, size, and behavior), the surgery (purpose, strength, and stability of repair), and what activities to avoid to prevent surgical complications. For example, a dog recovering from a tibial fracture stabilized with a bone plate has a low risk of mechanical failure compared with a dog recovering from an avulsion of the common calcanean tendon reattached using suture material. One should also consider contraindications to particular motions (eg, external rotation of the hip after craniodorsal coxofemoral joint luxation repair) and contractions of particular muscles (eg, active contraction of the gastrocnemius muscle after common calcanean tendon repair; Fig. 2). For example, no rotation or torque should be placed on the hock joint of an agility dog recovering from surgical repair of a luxated superficial digital flexor tendon for at least 6 weeks. Premorbid and comorbid conditions also greatly influence rehabilitation and need to be factored into the prognosis.

One should consider the anticipated rate and duration of tissue healing for the tissue involved. For skin healing, collagen has approximately 20% strength at 21 days and 70% strength at 1 year [55]. Muscle healing requires more than 6 weeks for adequate strength [55]. Tendon healing leads to 56% tensile strength at 6 weeks and 79% tensile strength at 1 year [55]. Ligament healing leads to 50% to 70% tensile strength at 1 year [55]. The median bone healing rate as judged by removal of external skeletal fixation frames ranged from 5 to 15 weeks in 12 studies [56]. Healing and recovery rates, however, vary with the patient's age, the severity of injury, and the specific tissue damage. Anemic patients should exercise cautiously. For example, exercise is not recommended in people with a hematocrit lower than 25%, and only light exercise is allowed in patients with a hematocrit lower than 30% [57].

Rehabilitation must also include consideration of how to enhance the patient's recovery. The acute rehabilitation of a sporting dog differs from the acute rehabilitation of a nonsporting dog in several ways. A dog that is highly conditioned before an injury typically recovers much more rapidly than a poorly

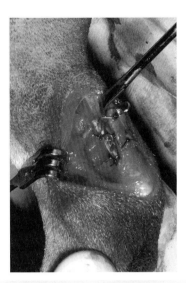

Fig. 2. This Dachshund ruptured his common calcanean and superficial digital flexor tendons. The tendons were repaired with monofilament nonabsorbable sutures. The rehabilitation after this injury takes into account the relative fragility of the repair, the high drive of the patient, and the need to apply progressively larger loads to the healing tissues.

conditioned dog, in part, because the increased muscle strength of conditioned dogs helps to support injured joints, resulting in less stress placed on these injured joints during their recovery. For example, a fit dog that has strong epaxial muscles undergoing a hemilaminectomy is likely to function better after surgery and to recover fully more rapidly than a deconditioned dog because of the strong musculature protecting his back. Also, the musculoskeletal tissues of well-conditioned dogs are stronger than the tissues of poorly conditioned dogs. Therefore, loss of strength and stiffness of musculoskeletal tissues after injury and surgery have a relatively lower impact on well-conditioned dogs. Limb disuse may be less likely in well-conditioned dogs because of potential behavioral factors (eg, eagerness to exercise, changes in pain threshold associated with past exercise experiences).

Sporting dogs may be required to recover from an injury as rapidly as possible to return to their activity because owners, trainers, or handlers generally want to keep the duration of their inactive period to a minimum. Their rehabilitation may be accelerated just as in human medicine, where athletes accelerate their rehabilitation as much as possible to return to sport as soon as they safely can. The average house pet that has undergone a tibial plateau leveling osteotomy may be rested for 3 weeks before beginning any rehabilitation. A dog actively competing in field trials may spend these same 3 weeks beginning cryotherapy and controlled exercises, such as ROM, short leash walks, and underwater treadmill walking, to prevent muscular and cardiovascular deconditioning and to accelerate the rehabilitation process.

Subacute Rehabilitation

The subacute phase can be thought of as the time immediately after the acute inflammatory phase during which some evidence of inflammation still exists but to a milder degree. It may last only 1 or 2 days or may persist for weeks. The initiation of the repair process signals the end of the subacute phase. During that phase, protection is still important but exercise is steadily increased concomitant with the patient's capacity. Ice is typically used in this phase, but heat may be used before exercise if it does not seem to increase inflammation.

It is beneficial to perform activities that are similar to those required during competition but to protect the injured tissues by training with less intensity. For example, a racing Greyhound recovering from an acetabular stress fracture places a significantly lower load on its pelvis when walking on an underwater treadmill compared with a land treadmill [53]. During this phase, the emphasis is on regaining ROM; increasing strength and endurance; and forming the foundation for the reconditioning phase of rehabilitation, where more aggressive activities, such as cutting, are performed. Protection of the injured area is still paramount in this phase, because tissues are healing and rehabilitation is helping them to remodel in the strongest and most anatomically normal way. An example is that performing ROM exercise of a stifle joint after extracapsular imbrication three times per day helps to increase ROM by aligning collagen in the skin, fascia, and muscle along the normal lines of stress (flexion/extension). This leads to a stronger scar, a more normal and anatomically correct stifle, and, potentially, a more functional joint. During this phase, other limbs also need to be exercised to maintain conditioning and the cardiorespiratory systems should be exercised as much as possible to prevent deconditioning.

Reconditioning

The reconditioning phase of rehabilitation is undertaken after the injury has healed to the point where the dog is ready to begin training to re-enter the sporting event. For example, reconditioning may be initiated in a dog that is walking and trotting without lameness after a cranial cruciate ligament injury or in a dog with a fracture that has a mature bridging callus. The emphasis now shifts from protection of the injured area to loading the area aggressively in preparation for return to activity. The entire body must be considered in rehabilitation and prepared for the sport and not just the injured joint or body part.

Reconditioning is similar to exercise in the first two phases of rehabilitation in its basic principles, but because there is no longer any injured tissue to protect, the limiting factor to the duration and intensity of exercise may be the overall cardiovascular fitness or other physical limitations. Common sense dictates that a fit and conditioned athlete requires an owner's conscientious commitment to a well-rounded conditioning program. Proper conditioning is paramount to the training of dogs for any event. Competitive exercise places strenuous demands on the body, particularly the cardiovascular and musculoskeletal systems. A conditioned dog is able to perform its particular sport or task more effectively and is less likely to suffer serious injury than a poorly conditioned dog.

Reconditioning should involve the training of the muscular system and the cardiovascular system and should be sport specific. For example, a racing Greyhound that performs in the southern United States in high heat and humidity must have high-impact exercise reintroduced under similar conditions. Exercising indoors on an underwater treadmill, although beneficial in many ways, does not reproduce the conditions in which that athlete must perform. Likewise, the high intensity and short duration of the races (commonly 5/16 of a mile or 503 m) requires training close to maximal oxygen consumption in comparison to a sled dog, which performs up to 14 hours per day at submaximal oxygen consumption levels.

SUMMARY

Although the field of conditioning and rehabilitation in sporting dogs continues to evolve and to become more popular, much is to be learned about how to exercise dogs most effectively and monitor their progression during exercise regimens. Research needs to be conducted to determine the optimal amount of exercise needed for normal and sporting dogs in terms of the frequency, intensity, and duration of exercise that helps to optimize their health, fitness level, and recovery from orthopedic injuries.

References

[1] Smith DJ. A framework for understanding the training process leading to elite performance. Sports Med 2003;33:1103–26.
[2] Jones AM, Carter H. The effect of endurance training on parameters of aerobic fitness. Sports Med 2000;29:373–86.
[3] Banister EW, Carter JB, Zarkadas PC. Training theory and taper: validation in triathlon athletes. Eur J Appl Physiol Occup Physiol 1999;79:182–91.
[4] Borms J. The child and exercise: an overview. J Sports Sci 1986;4:3–20.
[5] Ticer JW. General principles. In: Radiographic technique in small animal practice. Philadelphia: WB Saunders; 1975. p. 97–102.
[6] Lamb DR. Androgens and exercise. Med Sci Sports 1975;7:1–5.
[7] Dammrich K. Relationship between nutrition and bone growth in large and giant dogs. J Nutr 1991;121(Suppl):S114–21.
[8] Kronfeld DS, Hammel EP, Ramberg CF Jr, et al. Hematological and metabolic responses to training in racing sled dogs fed diets containing medium, low, or zero carbohydrate. Am J Clin Nutr 1977;30:419–30.
[9] Kondo T, Naruse S, Hayakawa T, et al. Effect of exercise on gastroduodenal functions in untrained dogs. Int J Sports Med 1994;15:186–91.
[10] Evason MD, Carr AP, Taylor SM, et al. Alterations in thyroid hormone concentrations in healthy sled dogs before and after athletic conditioning. Am J Vet Res 2004;65:333–7.
[11] Ponce Vazquez J, Pascual Gomez F, Alvarez Badillo A, et al. Cardiac arrhythmias induced by short-time maximal dynamic exercise (sprint): a study in greyhounds. Rev Esp Cardiol 1998;51:559–65.
[12] Kuruvilla A, Frankel TL. Heart rate of pet dogs: effects of overweight and exercise. Asia Pac J Clin Nutr 2003;12(Suppl):S51.

[13] Dickhuth HH, Rocker K, Mayer F, et al. Endurance training and cardial adaptation (athlete's heart). Herz 2004;29:373–80.

[14] Stone MH, Fleck SJ, Triplett NT, et al. Health- and performance-related potential of resistance training. Sports Med 1991;11:210–31.

[15] Baquet G, van Praagh E, Berthoin S. Endurance training and aerobic fitness in young people. Sports Med 2003;33:1127–43.

[16] Chen KY, Acra SA, Donahue CL, et al. Efficiency of walking and stepping: relationship to body fatness. Obes Res 2004;12:982–9.

[17] Nemet D, Barkan S, Epstein Y, et al. Short- and long-term beneficial effects of a combined dietary-behavioral-physical activity intervention for the treatment of childhood obesity. Pediatrics 2005;115(Suppl):e443–9.

[18] Ara I, Vicente-Rodriguez G, Jimenez-Ramirez J, et al. Regular participation in sports is associated with enhanced physical fitness and lower fat mass in prepubertal boys. Int J Obes Relat Metab Disord 2004;28:1585–93.

[19] Nazar K, Greenleaf JE, Pohoska E, et al. Exercise performance, core temperature, and metabolism after prolonged restricted activity and retraining in dogs. Aviat Space Environ Med 1992;63:684–8.

[20] Boddy KN, Roche BM, Schwartz DS, et al. Evaluation of the six-minute walk test in dogs. Am J Vet Res 2004;65:311–3.

[21] Sneddon JC, Minnaar PP, Grosskopf JF, et al. Physiological and blood biochemical responses to submaximal treadmill exercise in Canaan dogs before, during and after training. J S Afr Vet Assoc 1989;60:87–91.

[22] Blair SN, LaMonte MJ, Nichaman MZ. The evolution of physical activity recommendations: how much is enough? Am J Clin Nutr 2004;79:913S–20S.

[23] Gunn HM. The proportions of muscle, bone and fat in two different types of dog. Res Vet Sci 1978;24:277–82.

[24] Molon-Noblot S, Laroque P, Prahalada S, et al. Effect of chronic growth hormone administration on skeletal muscle in dogs. Toxicol Pathol 1998;26:207–12.

[25] Appel LJ, Champagne CM, Harsha DW, et al. Effects of comprehensive lifestyle modification on blood pressure control: main results of the PREMIER clinical trial. JAMA 2003;289:2083–93.

[26] Tipton CM, James SL, Mergner W, et al. Influence of exercise on strength of medial collateral knee ligaments of dogs. Am J Physiol 1970;218:894–902.

[27] Johnson KA, Skinner GA, Muir P. Site-specific adaptive remodeling of Greyhound metacarpal cortical bone subjected to asymmetrical cyclic loading. Am J Vet Res 2001;62:787–93.

[28] Cherdchutham W, Meershoek LS, van Weeren PR, et al. Effects of exercise on biomechanical properties of the superficial digital flexor tendon in foals. Am J Vet Res 2001;62:1859–64.

[29] Luthi JM, Howald H, Claassen H, et al. Structural changes in skeletal muscle tissue with heavy-resistance exercise. Int J Sports Med 1986;7:123–7.

[30] Newton PM, Mow VC, Gardner TR, et al. The effect of lifelong exercise on canine articular cartilage. Am J Sports Med 1997;25:282–7.

[31] Levine D, Prall E, Hanks J, et al. Running and the development of osteoarthritis. Part I, animal studies. Athletic Therapy Today 2003;8:6–11.

[32] Waddington GS, Adams RD. The effect of a 5-week wobble-board exercise intervention on ability to discriminate different degrees of ankle inversion, barefoot and wearing shoes: a study in healthy elderly. J Am Geriatr Soc 2004;52:573–6.

[33] Pai YC, Rymer WZ, Chang RW, et al. Effect of age and osteoarthritis on knee proprioception. Arthritis Rheum 1997;40:2260–5.

[34] Amberger C. Relapsing rhabdomyolysis in a greyhound. Description of a case. Schweiz Arch Tierheilkd 1995;137:180–3.

[35] Davis PE, Paris R. Azoturia in a Greyhound: clinical pathology aids to diagnosis. J Small Anim Pract 1974;15:43–54.

[36] Boudrieau RJ, Dee JF, Dee LG. Central tarsal bone fractures in the racing Greyhound: a review of 114 cases. J Am Vet Med Assoc 1984;184:1486–91.

[37] Johnson KA, Dee JF, Piermattei DL. Screw fixation of accessory carpal bone fractures in racing Greyhounds: 12 cases (1981–1986). J Am Vet Med Assoc 1989;194: 1618–25.

[38] Johnson KA. Accessory carpal bone fractures in the racing greyhound. Classification and pathology. Vet Surg 1987;16:60–4.

[39] Davis PE. Toe and muscle injuries of the racing greyhound. NZ Vet J 1973;21: 133–46.

[40] Görtz K, Van Ryssen B, Taeymans O, et al. Traumatic fracture of the medial coronoid process in a dog. Radiographic, computed tomographic, arthroscopic, and histological findings. Vet Comp Orthop Traumatol 2004;17:159–62.

[41] O'Neill T, Innes JF. Treatment of shoulder instability caused by medial glenohumeral ligament rupture with thermal capsulorrhaphy. J Small Anim Pract 2004;45:521–4.

[42] Boudrieau RJ, Dee JF, Dee LG. Treatment of central tarsal bone fractures in the racing Greyhound. J Am Vet Med Assoc 1984;184:1492–500.

[43] Hayashi K, Manley PA, Muir P. Cranial cruciate ligament pathophysiology in dogs with cruciate disease: a review. J Am Anim Hosp Assoc 2004;40:385–90.

[44] Harari J. Caudal cruciate ligament injury. Vet Clin North Am Small Anim Pract 1993;23: 821–9.

[45] Evers P, Johnston GR, Wallace LJ, et al. Long-term results of treatment of traumatic coxofemoral joint dislocation in dogs: 64 cases (1973–1992). J Am Vet Med Assoc 1997;210: 59–64.

[46] Steiss JE. Muscle disorders and rehabilitation in canine athletes. Vet Clin North Am Small Anim Pract 2002;32:267–85.

[47] Dillon EA, Anderson LJ, Jones BR. Infraspinatus muscle contracture in a working dog. NZ Vet J 1989;37:32–4.

[48] Worth AJ, Danielsson F, Bray JP, et al. Ability to work and owner satisfaction following surgical repair of common calcanean tendon injuries in working dogs in New Zealand. NZ Vet J 2004;52:109–16.

[49] Mauterer JV Jr, Prata RG, Carberry CA, et al. Displacement of the tendon of the superficial digital flexor muscle in dogs: 10 cases (1983–1991). J Am Vet Med Assoc 1993;203: 1162–5.

[50] Johnson JA, Austin C, Breur GJ. Incidence of canine appendicular musculoskeletal disorders in 16 veterinary teaching hospitals from 1980 to 1989. Vet Comp Orthop Traumatol 1994;7:56–69.

[51] Prole JH. A survey of racing injuries in the Greyhound. J Small Anim Pract 1976;17: 207–18.

[52] Sicard GK, Short K, Manley PA. A survey of injuries at five greyhound racing tracks. J Small Anim Pract 1999;40:428–32.

[53] Wendelburg K, Dee J, Kaderly R, et al. Stress fractures of the acetabulum in 26 racing Greyhounds. Vet Surg 1988;17:128–34.

[54] Muir P, Johnson KA, Ruaux-Mason CP. In vivo matrix microdamage in a naturally occurring canine fatigue fracture. Bone 1999;25:571–6.

[55] Williams N. Wound healing: tendons, ligaments, bone, muscles, and cartilage. In: Taylor R, editor. Canine rehabilitation and physical therapy. St. Louis, MO: WB Saunders; 2004. p. 100–12.

[56] Marcellin-Little DJ. External skeletal fixation. In: Slatter DH, editor. Textbook of small animal surgery. 3rd edition. Philadelphia: WB Saunders; 2003. p. 1818–34.

[57] Goodman CC, Fuller KS, Boissonnault WG. Appendix B. Pathology: implications for the physical therapist. 2nd edition. Philadelphia: WB Saunders; 2003. p. 1178–9.

Vet Clin Small Anim 35 (2005) 1441–1451

VETERINARY CLINICS
SMALL ANIMAL PRACTICE

ELSEVIER
SAUNDERS

Assistive Devices, Orthotics, and Prosthetics

Caroline Adamson, MSPT, CCRP[a],*, Martin Kaufmann, AT[b],
David Levine, PT, PhD, CCRP[c,d,e],
Darryl L. Millis, MS, DVM, CCRP[d],
Denis J. Marcellin-Little, DEDV, CCRP[e]

[a]Alameda East Veterinary Hospital, 9770 East Alameda Avenue, Denver, CO 80247, USA
[b]Orthopets, 11314 Jersey Way, Thornton, CO 80233, USA
[c]Department of Physical Therapy, University of Tennessee at Chattanooga, 615 McCallie Avenue, Chattanooga, TN 37403-2598, USA
[d]Department of Small Animal Clinical Sciences, College of Veterinary Medicine, The University of Tennessee, 2407 River Drive, Knoxville, TN 37966, USA
[e]Department of Clinical Sciences, North Carolina State University College of Veterinary Medicine, 4700 Hillsborough Street, Raleigh, NC 27606, USA

Assistive devices can have an important role in the overall well-being and functional abilities of an animal with neurologic or orthopedic impairments (Fig. 1). In addition to providing increased independence for the pet, these devices can provide additional autonomy for the owner. They give support to a weak or nonfunctioning body part and may assist with rehabilitation [1–3]. They can help to prevent decubital ulcers, increase an animal's mobility, and prevent complications in recumbent patients. These devices are available in a variety of forms, including boots, slings, two-wheeled and four-wheeled carts, and prosthetics [1–3].

BOOTS

Boots or "booties" are an excellent way to protect the feet when an animal with neurologic deficits is knuckling or turning its feet over and walking on the dorsum of the foot when ambulating. Animals that have poor proprioception are not aware of the placement of their paws and tend to walk on the dorsum of their paws or drag the nails when walking. Boots act as socklike coverings and are securely fastened by Velcro straps at the top. Most have a rubber sole to prevent slipping and are machine washable. Boots are also commonly worn by active dogs on long hikes to protect them from jagged rocks and other dangerous elements. Boots may be used for working dogs to protect their feet

*Corresponding author. E-mail address: cadamson@aevh.com (C. Adamson).

0195-5616/05/$ – see front matter
doi:10.1016/j.cvsm.2005.08.009

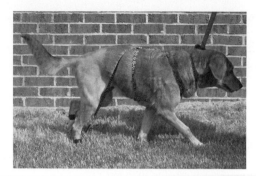

Fig. 1. A Labrador Retriever is walking with the assistance of elastic bands designed to provide traction on her hind feet at the beginning of the swing phase of her gait. These bands may be used to help patients with decreased proprioception or weakness of the pelvic limbs.

from glass and other sharp debris, and for sled dogs to protect against cold-induced injuries and trauma from the repetitive nature of the sport.

The boots should be removed periodically (several times daily) to assess the skin condition, especially in neurologically impaired patients, and if possible when performing therapeutic exercise to increase weight bearing and proprioception through the bottom of the pads. If not fitted properly, boots can interrupt circulation, become cumbersome, impede gait patterns or strides, and potentially cause more problems if the animal stumbles and falls. A proper fit is essential, and appropriate education instructions for skin care and rehabilitative exercises must be communicated to the owner.

Boots can be ordered through a variety of veterinary or specialty rehabilitation companies with products designed specifically for dogs. Outdoor adventure stores, pet stores, and online businesses may also sell supplies for dogs. When choosing the boots, one should ensure that they are machine washable, waterproof or water resistant, made of a durable material so they do not wear down quickly, and have a nonskid bottom to prevent slipping. Old socks may also be used to help provide padding; however, caution should be taken if the top is secured with tape to avoid cutting off circulation.

SLINGS

Slings come in a variety of shapes and sizes. Some products may be strapped around the belly or fitted for the forelimbs, hindlimbs, or both. They should have long hand-held straps attached to allow proper body mechanics to avoid personal injury to the handler when supporting the pet. Slings aid in transitioning a recumbent animal to a standing position, especially larger dogs. They can also assist with ambulation and prevent falls on slippery floors, especially after surgery, to avoid further injury to the animal. Support slings are also available for forelimb assistance and patients with amputations.

Slings are available in a variety of sizes to provide the best fit. It is important to select a properly sized sling for safety and comfort of the patient. A sling used for the forelimbs should not obstruct respiration, and urine flow should not be compromised with hindlimb slings in male dogs. Slings should have a soft lining against the animal's skin to avoid irritation and sores, and they should be washable. Slings should not be too thin, especially around the groin and belly region, to avoid excessive pressure and sores. They can be conveniently designed for male and female patients.

Slings are useful during the rehabilitation phase and can be used for supported standing during therapeutic exercises, such as repeated sit to stands. With a sling supporting the caudal abdomen or hindlimbs, the hind end is assisted to a standing position, with the therapist making sure the feet are in a standing position. As the dog is allowed to sit back down, it is assisted to a standing position again, repeating the exercise. When documenting patient progress, the amount of assistance given through sling support can be rated as minimum, moderate, or maximal.

In dogs with degenerative myelopathy, crossing the hind limbs under the abdomen while walking is common. In an effort to assist ambulation and keep the legs properly positioned, a rolled towel may be taped to the middle of a sling to maintain the hindlimbs in a normal position or in slight abduction, improving independent ambulation. If the towel is too large, overabduction of the hindlimbs may occur and adversely affect gait.

CARTS

Sometimes a combination of forelimb and hindlimb devices may be necessary to provide total body support and prevent decubitus ulcers. Carts, or canine wheel chairs, are beneficial to provide support, allow independence for the owner and animal, and prevent the deleterious effects of recumbency. Carts can be designed with two or four wheels for dogs that are permanently disabled [4,5]. It is relatively easy for one person to place an animal into the lightweight frame, and the wheels are designed to traverse most terrains.

Carts should not be used in place of a rehabilitation program. If ordered early in the rehabilitation phase, the owners may become too dependent on the cart's support and use it as a replacement for exercise and rehabilitation. Carts also should not be used in place of therapeutic exercises that may help to improve function. The owners should be instructed to carry out the rehabilitation program before ordering a cart to encourage the patient to ambulate and achieve as complete a recovery as possible, including neurologic function and muscle strength.

As is true when introducing any new device, the transition into the cart should be a positive experience. To reduce unnecessary stress on the animal, one should be familiar with the cart and its parts before placing an animal in the device. Animals should be supervised at all times when in a cart so that they do not fall out, tumble down a flight of stairs, tip over, or become stuck on an object. Animals should be able to eat and drink while in their carts, although bowls may need to be elevated. A rest period out of the cart is necessary on frequent occasions, especially for larger dogs, because it is difficult for animals to rest comfortably while in a cart. Frequent skin assessment is important to ensure no areas of skin breakdown occur. Patients standing in a cart may be unable to tolerate for more than a short time period the cardiac, pulmonary, or neuromusculoskeletal stress of being in a cart. For animals such as those with wobbler's disease that are in a cart with all four limbs supported or that are completely non–weight bearing, 30 minutes at one time is sufficient. After this time, there is a potential for ischemic damage owing to vascular compression and compromised circulation.

ORTHOTICS AND PROSTHETICS

Orthotic and prosthetic intervention has been used for many years in human rehabilitation to achieve mechanical and rehabilitative goals [1,6]. An orthotic is defined as a device used to support or protect an injured limb (Figs. 2 and 3). A prosthetic device is designed to replace a missing limb or body part (Fig. 4). The use of prosthetic devices has been limited in the field of veterinary medicine, although published case reports have existed for over 40 years [7].

Functional Considerations for Orthotic Prescriptions

The goal of orthotic prescription may include one or any combination of the following: rest, immobilization, joint protection, control, assisting movement, preventing movement, and correction. These goals are achieved through the selected application of forces. If the desired goal is to assist movement of a part of the body, the orthotic device must be able to substitute for, or assist with, the action of the muscles. Alternatively, orthotic intervention may be indicated for immobilization to reduce pain or provide joint protection immediately following surgery or injury. In these cases, the orthosis substitutes for

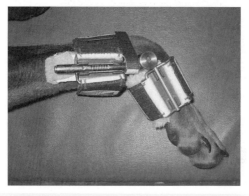

Fig. 2. A hinged brace has been fitted to the antebrachium of a Doberman Pinscher with a contracture of her antebrachial flexor muscles. The cause of the contracture was not known, although transient radial nerve palsy was suspected. The brace has two dynamic hinges that place an adjustable amount of torque to stretch the contracted antebrachial flexor muscles over a period of hours each day.

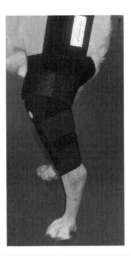

Fig. 3. A brace has been placed on the pelvic limb of a Labrador Retriever recovering from stabilization of a cranial cruciate deficient stifle joint. The brace is made of neoprene and is secured to the limb using three wide straps with hoop and loop fasteners and a strap connecting it to the opposite pelvic limb. A hinged metal bar is sewn into the brace laterally.

the lack of intrinsic stability normally achieved by the bony, ligamentous, or muscular components [8,9].

The orthotic prescription should take into account whether the purpose of the appliance is to control or to assist movement. A basic understanding of the injured anatomic structures that render certain movements unstable is

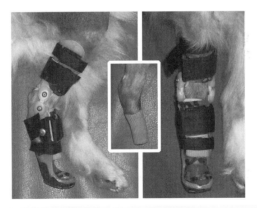

Fig. 4. A hinged prosthesis has been designed for a Shetland Sheepdog who lost his digits and metatarsal pad after an ischemic event that followed ligation of the femoral artery that was deemed necessary during excision of a soft tissue sarcoma of the thigh region. The prosthesis has two passive hinges, two lined plastic shells with hoop and loop fasteners, and a rubber sole with a non-skid textured surface. A silicon liner protects the skin within the prosthesis (*inset*).

necessary to incorporate the appropriate support and rigidity into the orthosis. An orthosis may provide correction, using the viscoelastic characteristics of the intervening soft tissues to cause a deformation over time; however, there is a potential for harm to the tissues if orthotic devices are used incorrectly.

Degrees-of-Freedom

Before selecting an orthotic device, the physical rehabilitation therapist should consider the kinematic characteristics of the region of interest, including an analysis of the degrees-of-freedom. This rationale entails an evaluation of the translation along, and the rotation about, each of the coordinate axes of the respective segments or joints to be braced. Although most treatment strategies typically address one or more potential degrees-of-freedom, an awareness of all inherent motions and coupled relationships between segments is important to maximize the effectiveness of the orthosis. The orthosis can attempt to control motion of one joint and consequently alter motion in another joint or plane. The attempt to control or to limit two or more degrees-of-freedom continues to present challenges to orthotic designers. The continual evolution of orthoses in the quest for the optimal appliance that controls translation and rotation without sacrificing functional performance is the ultimate goal.

Achieving Desired Outcomes Through Orthotic Devices

The desired outcomes of orthotic interventions are achieved through selected application and transmission of forces via the orthotic appliance. Indirect transmission of force through structures such as muscles, fascia, tendons, fat, viscera, and bone helps to achieve these outcomes. One important concept underlying many of the strategies in force application is the phenomenon known as creep. Creep is the deformation that follows the initial loading of a viscoelastic material and occurs over a period ranging from several seconds to several days. After this period, biologically mediated changes in the mechanical properties of the tissues occur owing to adaptation [10,11].

Additional Factors in the Consideration of Orthotic Appliances

In addition to the mechanical and rehabilitative goals of orthotic and prosthetic intervention, other prescriptive considerations are equally important for achieving a successful outcome. The sensitivity of the skin and underlying tissues must be considered, because these factors may limit the magnitude and direction of forces that may be applied to the skin. Orthotic prescription should take into account other biologic functions of the skin, including skin integrity and cleanliness. Attention must be given to adequate ventilation and the ease of cleaning the appliance, especially for long-term use.

Orthoses should be assessed for their effect on all levels of functional performance. This assessment should not be restricted to the impact of the orthosis on the ultimate performance of the patient. The effect of the orthosis on transitional functional tasks such as sit to stand, particularly for patients with neurologic or musculoskeletal deficits, is equally critical [9]. Likewise, an awareness of the patient's ability to tolerate the appliance is essential.

Ideally, the orthotic prescription should incorporate a predictive component or a "vision" for the future of the wearer. Reassessment of the objectives and timely orthotic modifications should accompany changes in the neurologic or musculoskeletal status of the patient. Cost will undoubtedly be a major concern that presents a challenge to providing effective orthotic and prosthetic management.

Prosthetics

Amputations in dogs and cats are most commonly due to trauma (65%) and neoplasia (35%) [12,13]. Chronic infections, such as with osteomyelitis, as well as denervation leading to a nonfunctional limb may also lead to amputation. In denervation, soft-tissue lesions as well as self-mutilation may necessitate the amputation. Prosthetics have not gained widespread use in veterinary medicine owing to the nature of quadrupeds adapting well to a three-legged gait. Two surveys in the veterinary literature have shown amputation to be overwhelmingly satisfactory when used [12,13]. In one of these surveys, it was found that owners were initially reluctant to consider amputation for their pets [13]. Forelimb amputations have been found to be more debilitating than pelvic limb amputations. Dogs and cats with multiple orthopedic or soft-tissue injuries are more likely to have difficulty using a prosthetic. One specific indication for prosthetics would be the animal with a bilateral amputation that has left it unable to ambulate. A prosthesis consists of several components, including the socket (which contacts the residual limb), the pylon or shank (which is the structural support), and the ground contact device (such as an artificial foot). Prosthetics are attached to the patient through suspension systems that typically involve suction (using air or skin contact with a material such as silicone or urethane) or a harness.

If a prosthetic will be considered postoperatively, this should be taken into account by the surgeon, because it may alter the level of the amputation to allow the residual limb to fit into a prosthetic. A human prosthetist will most likely be involved to mold the prosthetic from the limb and construct the device. Osseointegration (or osteointegration) is implanting a prosthetic device into a bone and allowing for ingrowth or outgrowth into or onto the prosthesis. It has been used in human medicine for cosmetic surgery, bone-anchored hearing aids, implant dentistry, and limb prosthetics, and has also been studied in rats, rabbits, and dogs [14]. This procedure has potential benefits for small animal patients with bilateral amputations and in situations when the skin condition would make a traditional prosthesis unsuitable. Prosthetics have historically been underused in veterinary medicine, but with the emergence of rehabilitation as a specialty field, their use is likely to increase. Much information remains to be learned about the optimal materials to be used, support systems, training, and eventual outcomes.

SUMMARY

Deciding on which supportive device, orthotic, or prosthetic is best suited for a given patient is a complex process involving many different factors. The ability to manage biomechanical abnormalities successfully can be enhanced by an understanding of the properties of the various materials that comprise these devices, their effect on functional performance, and other associated patient factors. Veterinary health care providers are faced with the challenge of effectively addressing the physiologic and fiscal needs of the patient in a rapidly changing patient care environment.

APPENDIX: CASE STUDIES

Case 1

Signalment

The patient, "Peabody," was a 12-year-old male Golden Retriever mix.

History

Peabody underwent a scapulectomy of approximately two-thirds of the right dorsal scapula owing to an osteosarcoma.

Clinical presentation

The patient presented to the Department of Sports Medicine & Rehabilitation at Alameda East Veterinary Hospital 5 weeks postsurgery non–weight bearing on the right forelimb. He would occasionally touch the right limb to the ground in standing, although he was severely abducted at the elbow. Chronic instability in the shoulder region produced a large seroma around the surgical site. After further investigation, the operative report revealed removal of the cranial, caudal, and dorsal majority of the scapula. With loss of approximately two thirds of the patient's scapula, the origination points for shoulder musculature were virtually eliminated, making it impossible for Peabody to regain a normal stride without assistance. Shoulder extensor origination points were removed, eliminating use of the supraspinatus, infraspinatus, subscapularis, and trapezius muscles. The teres major and spinal portion of the deltoid was eliminated, limiting shoulder flexion. In addition, origination points for the rhomboids and serratus ventralis musculature were removed. Triceps and biceps musculature remained intact; therefore, Peabody maintained the ability to support his weight against gravity on the right forelimb and to flex and extend the elbow. The free-floating scapular fragment continued to aggravate the seroma.

Treatment

A passive shoulder extension-assist brace was designed to support weight bearing and to encourage a normal gait pattern (Fig. 5). As Peabody shifted weight onto his left forelimb, the brace allowed passive shoulder extension through the right forelimb swing phase of gait. It also provided lateral stability at the shoulder during the stance phase of gait.

Re-evaluation

After 3 weeks of gait training and adjusting the speed of passive extension of the shoulder brace, Peabody was partial-to-full weight bearing with a mild limp on 100% of strides on the right forelimb while donning the brace. A large

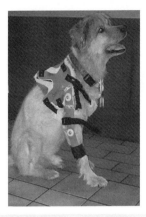

Fig. 5. Passive shoulder extension-assist brace.

decrease in the size of the shoulder seroma and increased lateral stability of the shoulder were also observed.

Case 2

Signalment

The patient, "Bronte Fuzzbucket," was a 14-week-old female Golden Retriever.

History

Bronte was the runt of a litter of five pups as a result of a "backyard" breeding. Her mother was 8 months old at the time and died of birthing complications. Bronte was born with a missing right paw. All of the other pups in the litter had no apparent or known deformities. Bronte was able to ambulate on her own but unable to jump into a car or on and off a bed. She taught herself how to navigate stairs and was awkwardly able to ascend and descend independently. The referring veterinarian recommended amputation of the residual limb. Bronte's owners adopted her from the local Golden Retriever rescue organization and decided to investigate other options.

Clinical presentation

Bronte presented to the Department of Sports Medicine & Rehabilitation at Alameda East Veterinary Hospital with severe muscle atrophy in the right forelimb, especially in the shoulder flexors and extensors and triceps musculature. At 7 cm above the olecranon, the right forelimb muscle mass measured 14.5 cm; the left measured 17.5 cm. Full elbow range of motion was present, and elbow flexion was measured at 55 degrees. She was able to touch occasionally the right residual limb to the floor and to use it for balance by dropping her head and flexing the left elbow to lower her front. The entire metacarpal pad remained at the distal portion of the residual limb.

A radiograph was taken to determine the stability and anatomy of the remaining limb (Fig. 6). The radiograph revealed agenesis of the limb distal to

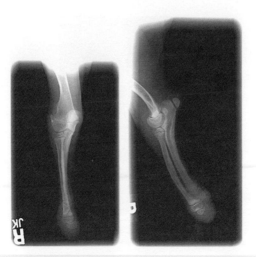

Fig. 6. Radiograph of Bronte's residual right forelimb.

the antebrachium with one carpal bone, the radiocarpal bone, present. The ulnar shaft showed twice than normal thickening, and cranial bowing of the radius was observed.

Treatment

It was determined that Bronte had enough of her residual limb to fabricate a prosthetic device to support the malformed limb. The leg was casted, and a prosthetic was constructed (Fig. 7).

Re-evaluation

After a few minor adjustments, Bronte has advanced to wearing the prosthesis 4 hours per day. She shows some exaggeration of elbow flexion through the

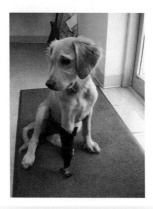

Fig. 7. Bronte donning her new forelimb prosthesis.

swing phase of gait but is weight bearing on 100% of strides. Minor skin break down has impeded full-time wear of the brace. The time spent wearing the prosthesis will slowly be increased and adjustments in size made as she continues to grow. A radiograph will be taken each month to observe any weight-bearing changes the brace may have on bony formation of the forelimb.

References

[1] Hamilton S. Orthotics, slings, and carts. In: Proceedings of the 2nd International Symposium on Rehabilitation and Physical Therapy in Veterinary Medicine. Knoxville (TN): University of Tennessee; 2002. p. 242–7.

[2] Marcellin-Little DJ. Assistive ambulation devices. In: Proceedings of the 3rd International Symposium on Rehabilitation and Physical Therapy in Veterinary Medicine. Raleigh (NC): North Carolina State University; 2004. p. 275–8.

[3] Clark GN. Orthotics, prosthetics, and ambulatory carts: use of supportive devices in canine patients. In: Proceedings of the First International Symposium on Rehabilitation & Physical Therapy in Veterinary Medicine, Corvallis, OR. 1999. p. 141.

[4] Leighton RL. A cart for small dogs with posterior paralysis. Vet Med Small Anim Clin 1966;61:554–6.

[5] Balasubramananian S, Thilagar S. Use of a cart to aid ambulation in a cat following posterior paralysis. Vet Rec 1991;128:335.

[6] Levine JM, Fitch RB. Use of an ankle-foot-orthosis in a dog with traumatic sciatic neuropathy. J Small Anim Pract 2003;44:236–8.

[7] Howard DM. Artificial legs for a dog. J Am Vet Med Assoc 1961;139:564.

[8] Smith EM, Juvinall RC. Mechanics of orthotics. In: Redford JB, editor. Orthotics etcetera. 3rd edition. Baltimore: Williams & Wilkins; 1986. p. 26–32.

[9] Fuerbach JW, Grabiner MD, Hoh TJ, et al. Effect of an ankle orthosis and ankle ligament anesthesia on ankle joint proprioception. Am J Sports Med 1994;22:223–9.

[10] Byars EF, Snyder RD, Plants HL. Engineering mechanics of deformable bodies. 4th edition. New York: Harper and Row Publishers; 1983. p. 224–37.

[11] Burstein AH, Wright TM. Fundamentals of orthopaedic biomechanics. Baltimore: Williams & Wilkins; 1994. p. 137–40.

[12] Carberry CA, Harvey HJ. Owner satisfaction with limb amputation in dogs and cats. J Am Anim Hosp Assoc 1987;23:227–32.

[13] Withrow SJ, Hirsch VM. Owner response to amputation of a pet's leg. Vet Med Small Anim Clin 1979;74(3):332–4.

[14] Brånemark R. A biomechanical study of osseointegration: in vivo measurements in rat, rabbit, dog and man [dissertation]. Gothenburg, Sweden; 1996.

Vet Clin Small Anim 35 (2005) 1453–1471

VETERINARY CLINICS
SMALL ANIMAL PRACTICE

ELSEVIER
SAUNDERS

Wound Healing in the Veterinary Rehabilitation Patient

June Hanks, PhD, PT[a],*, Gary Spodnick, DVM[b]

[a]Department of Physical Therapy, University of Tennessee at Chattanooga,
615 McCallie Avenue, Chattanooga, TN 37403-2598, USA
[b]Veterinary Specialty Hospital of the Carolinas, 6405-100 Tryon Road, Cary, NC 27511, USA

W ound healing is a biologically complex cascade of predictable overlapping events and is a natural restorative response to tissue injury. The continuum of interrelated processes is classically divided into the inflammatory, proliferative, epithelialization, and remodeling phases. Each phase is regulated by biochemical mediators such as cytokines, growth factors, and other cellular components that stimulate or inhibit the cellular responses that facilitate healing (Table 1). The biologic process for wound healing is the same for all wounds, although the specific mechanisms may vary. Superficial and partial-thickness wounds complete healing principally through epithelialization and progress through the repair process more quickly than full-thickness wounds that rely primarily on contraction. Unlike acute wounds, chronic wounds may lack an orderly progression through wound healing phases, allowing for prolonged inflammation, repeated injury, and infection. This article reviews the wound healing process, discussing factors that may delay normal healing progression and potential modalities and treatments to aid healing.

REVIEW OF WOUND HEALING PHYSIOLOGY
Inflammatory Phase
Two important events occur during the inflammatory phase of wound healing that commences at the time of wounding or injury and typically lasts for 3 to 7 days. The first event involves cessation of bleeding and culminates with the formation of a primary platelet plug and blood clot. Within minutes of wounding, blood vessels constrict, reducing hemorrhage, aiding platelet aggregation, and containing healing factors to the wound environment. Platelets adhere to exposed vascular collagen and to each other via adhesive glycoproteins such as fibrinogen, fibronectin, and von Willebrand's factor, resulting in the primary platelet plug. Activated platelets release growth factors such as platelet-derived growth factor (PDGF), transforming growth factor beta (TGF-β), and

---

*Corresponding author. E-mail address: june-hanks@utc.edu (J. Hanks).

0195-5616/05/$ – see front matter
doi:10.1016/j.cvsm.2005.08.005

Table 1
Various cytokines and growth factors important in wound healing

Cytokine	Cell of origin	Function
PDGF	Platelets, macrophages, endothelial cells	Cell chemotaxis
		Mitogenic for fibroblasts
		Stimulates angiogenesis
		Stimulates wound contraction
TGF-α	Macrophages, T-lymphocytes, keratinocytes	Mitogenic for keratinocytes and fibroblasts
		Stimulates keratinocyte migration
TGF-β	Platelets, T-lymphocytes, macrophages, endothelial cells, keratinocytes	Cell chemotaxis
		Stimulates fibroplasia
		Stimulates angiogenesis
EGF	Platelets, macrophages	Mitogenic for keratinocytes
		Stimulates keratinocyte migration
Fibroblast growth factor	Macrophages, mast cells, T-lymphocytes, endothelial cells	Chemotactic for fibroblasts
		Mitogenic for fibroblasts
		Stimulates angiogenesis
TNF	Macrophages, mast cells, T- lymphocytes	Activates macrophages
		Mitogenic for fibroblasts
		Stimulates angiogenesis
KGF	Keratinocytes	Stimulates epithelialization
VEGF	Endothelial cells	Stimulates angiogenesis
Interleukins	Macrophages, mast cells, lymphocytes	Induces fever
		Activates neutrophils, macrophages, T-cells
		Induces ACTH release

Abbreviations: EGF, epidermal growth factor; KGF, keratinocyte growth factor; TGF, transforming growth factor; TNF, tumor necrosis factor; VEGF, vascular endothelial growth factor.

epidermal growth factor (EGF), as well as proteases and the vasoactive amines serotonin and histamine [1–3]. The growth factors facilitate cellular mitogenesis, chemotaxis of leukocytes, and collagen synthesis. The initial vasoconstriction period is followed by a more persistent period of local vasodilation that facilitates blood flow to the area and migration of the necessary inflammatory cells and factors into the wound environment. Polymorphonuclear neutrophils (PMNs) migrate to the wound space within the first 24 hours of wounding and are important in the phagocytosis of bacteria and necrotic debris and in breaking down the extracellular matrix through the release of elastase and collagenase [4]. Although they are larger and slower than PMNs, macrophages invade the wound site to assist in phagocytosis and to direct the repair process through chemotaxis of other inflammatory cells and secretion of cytokines and growth factors, including tumor necrosis factor alpha (TNF-α), interleukin-1 (IL-1), basic fibroblast growth factor (bFGF), PDGF, TGF-α, TGF-β, and EGF [1,5].

Proliferative Phase

The proliferative phase of healing begins as early as 48 to 72 hours after injury and may last as long as 14 to 21 days [6]. Crucial events of the proliferative phase include angiogenesis, granulation tissue formation, epithelialization, and wound contraction. Local ischemia, growth factors, and chemical mediators stimulate angioblasts adjacent to the injury site to grow into the affected area and form endothelial buds that eventually form a functioning capillary bed. Under the influence of TNF-α and IL-1, fibroblasts that infiltrate the wound site during the inflammatory phase are stimulated to synthesize and deposit an extracellular matrix containing the fibrous elements of collagen, elastin, and reticulin, and a nonfibrous ground substance composed of water, salts, and glysosaminoglycans. In a process called fibroplasia, collagen production begins as soon as 3 days after wounding and continues until the wound bed is filled, which may take 2 to 4 weeks. Intermolecular bonds form between collagen fibers, rendering the collagen matrix resistant to destruction. The endothelial cells migrate along and within the scaffolding created by fibroblastic activity to yield a well-vascularized granulation tissue bed. As the defect is filled with granulation tissue, keratinocytes multiply and migrate from the wound edges across the wound surface to re-epithelialize the wound. Current research indicates that epithelial cells may interact with the underlying matrix of fibronectin, fibrin, and collagen, which provides signals for epithelial cell proliferation and migration [7]. The water content of the wound bed appears to facilitate epithelial migration, because wounds with adequate tissue humidity heal more quickly than desiccated wounds [8,9]. Once epithelialization is complete, the keratinocyte resumes its normal form and establishes new linkages to other epidermal cells and the basement membrane. The final component of proliferation is wound contraction, the centripetal movement of wound edges resulting in a diminution of the wound size. Wound contraction is mediated by the myofibroblast, a specialized type of fibroblast containing actin. Wound contraction should be distinguished from a pathologic process known as wound contracture. In contracture, wound contraction is excessive, resulting in limited motion of the underlying tissues. This event can be a particular problem in the limbs where it can limit joint mobility as well as acting as a natural tourniquet, causing impairment of venous drainage from the distal limb and edema (Fig. 1).

Remodeling Phase

The final phase of wound healing is the remodeling phase that begins with granulation tissue formation during the proliferative phase and continues for 6 months to years, depending on the size and severity of the wound [6,10]. Collagen synthesis and degradation are regulated by growth factors such as FGF,

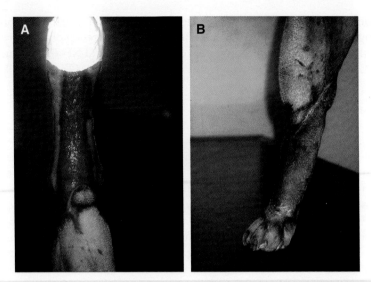

Fig. 1. (A) Full-thickness skin loss affecting the distal limb of a Shar Pei dog. The wound encompassed approximately 180 degrees of the circumference of the dorsum of the paw and surrounded the talocrural joint. The paw is edematous, and flexion in the joint is limited owing to wound contracture. (B) 14-day postoperative appearance of the limb after removal of scar tissue and reconstruction of the defect using a skin flap. A skin expander was implanted in the medial crus, and the flap was developed from the expanded skin.

TGF-β, and PDGF, and by collagenases called matrix metalloproteinases (MMPs). Tissue inhibitors of MMPs maintain the equilibrium between continued collagen degradation and synthesis of the extracellular matrix components [2,11]. During remodeling, collagen becomes more organized, type III collagen is replaced by type I collagen, collagen cross-linking occurs, and wound strength increases. Peak tensile wound strength returns to about 80% of prewounding levels during the process of scar maturation. The transition of the scar from a rosy pink to pale color reflects the regression of blood vessels during the remodeling process [12].

SPECIFIC CAUSES FOR NONHEALING WOUNDS
Some wounds fail to progress in an orderly and timely manner through the biologic sequences comprising the phases of healing, resulting in a nonhealing or poorly healing wound. Before healing can occur, causative factors must be identified and addressed. Wound healing may be disrupted by underlying pathophysiologic intrinsic factors, by environmental influences, or by inappropriate management (iatrogenic factors). The location of a wound in a well-vascularized area allows delivery of oxygen and micronutrients critical to healing. A wound over a bony surface or joint may result in delayed healing owing to difficulty in maintaining approximation of wound edges. Local infection may delay collagen production and increase breakdown [13]. Aging

affects wound healing potential, with increasing age resulting in decreased collagen density, impaired vascularity of the dermis, atrophy of the dermis, a lower rate of epithelialization, and decreased tensile strength in remodeled tissue [14]. Neurologically impaired skin from central nervous system dysfunction, spinal cord injury, or lesions compressing nervous tissue may lead to pressure ulceration.

A myriad of causes may adversely affect wound healing through decreased oxygen tension, impaired leukocyte function, and delayed collagen synthesis. Ischemic ulcers resulting from vessel occlusion are susceptible to infection [15]. Immunocompromised patients may not be able to produce an effective inflammatory response. Nonhealing wounds may be associated with excessive bioburden from necrotic tissue or resistant infection, such as that caused by methicillin-resistant *Staphylococcus aureus, Actinocmyces*, and *Nocardia*. Fungal organisms such as *Pythium, Histoplasma,* and *Blastomyces* may delay healing. Tissue samples from such wounds should be obtained for bacteriologic and histologic evaluation, and the laboratory should be notified so that special techniques, media, and stains (acid-fast stains for *Mycobacteria* and silver stains for fungal organisms) can be employed to aid in the identification of such organisms. Treatment of these wounds may involve initial surgical debridement and medical therapy with an appropriate antibiotic or antifungal medication. Attempts at primary wound closure should be delayed until the underlying cause has been removed and adequately treated.

Malignant cutaneous wounds secondary to local invasion of a primary tumor or metastasis from another site may present initially as inflammation with induration, redness, heat, and tenderness with subsequent ulceration as the tumor infiltrates the skin. Biopsies of suspected neoplasms should be obtained as soon as possible to diagnose and determine an appropriate treatment regimen. The purpose of chemotherapy is to disrupt the cell cycle, and, as such, it may delay wound healing. Attention should be given to controlling bacterial colonization through debridement and cleansing, managing exudate through appropriate dressing application, and reducing pain through systemic and topical medications.

Identification of foreign bodies within a chronic wound can be difficult, but most often, these wounds are characterized by the presence of a draining tract. Plant or woody material, porcupine quills, nonabsorbable suture material or other surgical implants such as orthopedic implants, gauze sponges, or osteomyelitis and bony sequestra may act as foreign bodies. A surgical implant may be the source of infection and wound drainage. Although stable fractures will heal in the presence of infection, resolution of the infection typically necessitates removal of the implant; however, it may not be possible or desirable to remove the implant until the bone has healed. Most of the time, the infection can be controlled with appropriate antibiotic therapy and perhaps additional surgery, such as sequestrectomy.

Certain medications such as corticosteroids may impair all phases of wound healing by inhibiting prostaglandin production, leukocyte migration to the wounded area, and the rate of wound contraction [16,17]. Nutritional deficits, especially protein-calorie malnutrition, may result in reduced phagocytosis, collagen synthesis, and angiogenesis [18].

Inappropriate wound management may lead to impaired healing. Solutions such as povidone-iodine, sodium hypochlorite, and hydrogen peroxide may reduce bacterial counts in wounds, but evidence is lacking to suggest that prolonged use enhances wound healing. In fact, these solutions may be cytotoxic to living cells [19,20]. To combat toxicity, some have suggested diluting antiseptic solutions; however, even with significant dilution, cytotoxicity remains, and there is a reduced bactericidal effect [17]. Whirlpool treatment may be appropriate for wounds with necrotic tissue or thick exudates but should not be used for wounds demonstrating good granulation tissue, because the whirlpool increases edema, traumatizes the healing tissue, and retards epithelialization. The hydration status of the wound bed must be considered. Desiccation and eschar formation can inactivate growth factors and impede epithelial cell migration [21].

ULTRASOUND

In ultrasound therapy, ultrasonic beams are produced when alternating current is applied to a piezoelectric transducer. When the beams are delivered to the body, compression and separation occur of the biologic tissues that are exposed to the ultrasonic beam. For therapeutic ultrasound, the frequency of sound waves can vary between 1 and 3.3 MHz, with penetration into deeper tissues with lower frequencies (1 MHz). Physiologic effects of nonthermal ultrasound include stable cavitation and microstreaming. Stable cavitation refers to the formation and vibration of micron-sized bubbles within tissue fluids, whereas microstreaming refers to the movement of fluids in the area of the vibrating bubbles. These simultaneous events are presumed to enhance healing through increased permeability of cell membranes [22,23], increased synthesis of proteins, and increased release of growth factors [14], although conclusive evidence is lacking. [24] The delivery of therapeutic ultrasound requires the use of some type of coupling medium such as gel, a hydrogel sheet, or a transparent film dressing. Underwater application may also be used, preferably in a plastic or rubber basin or tub. The method of ultrasound application may be through direct contact with the wounded area or application to the wound periphery. Application during the acute inflammatory phase is recommended and may enhance entry into the proliferative phase [14]. Some evidence suggests that thermal ultrasound may induce the inflammatory response in chronic wounds [14], but pulsed nonthermal ultrasound is most commonly used [14]. Evidence of the efficacy of pulsed nonthermal ultrasound in influencing wound healing has been demonstrated in a few small studies [25], but systematic reviews comparing the use of ultrasound with sham treatment indicate no significant differences in healing rates of chronic pressure ulcers and venous ulcers in humans [26]. Studies of the effect of ultrasound on incisional wound healing indicate an acceleration of angiogenesis [27] and an increase in strength of healed tissue [28,29].

ELECTRICAL STIMULATION

The rationale for applying electrical current to enhance wound healing is based on several theories, including potential restoration of the body's "electrical current of injury" to trigger healing of chronic wounds. The normal electronegativity of the epidermis when compared with the dermis creates a bioelectrical current that may be disrupted by a break in the skin. Other mechanisms include the attraction and activation of the cellular components associated with all phases of healing, modifying the electrical potential of the wounded area, increasing circulation and enhancing oxygen tension, enhancing antibacterial properties and autolytic debridement capabilities of tissues, and reducing edema [17]. Recommended treatment parameters vary but generally include a stimulation frequency of 80 to 125 Hz at an intensity of 75 to 200 V to produce a comfortable paresthesia. If there is loss of sensation, the intensity of stimulation should be limited to a submotor level [30]. Studies have included the use of various current types, including a high-voltage pulsed current, a low-intensity direct current, and a microcurrent. Although more research is needed to validate the efficacy of polarity choices with continuous or monophasic pulsed current, consistent outcomes have been demonstrated with use of the cathode over the wound site at the initiation of treatment with a change in polarity as healing plateaus [31]. As an adjunctive therapy, electrical stimulation is indicated for clean, necrotic, or infected chronic wounds of various etiologies, including pressure ulcers [32–35], vascular wounds [36,37], and neuropathic ulcers [38]. The use of electrical stimulation is contraindicated in patients with osteomyelitis, malignancy, actively bleeding wounds, or in the presence of metal ions [30].

Extensive research supports the use of electrical stimulation for facilitation of wound healing [32–37,39]. Comparison among studies is difficult owing to variations in wound etiologies and treatment parameters; however, a meta-analysis of the effects of various types of electrical stimulation on chronic wound healing reported faster healing rates in chronic wounds [40]. Further research is needed to differentiate the characteristics of the most effective types and treatment parameters to facilitate maximal healing.

EMERGING MODALITIES

Negative Pressure Wound Therapy

Supportive evidence is increasing for the use of negative pressure wound therapy for chronic granulating wounds that fail to progress to closure. A piece of sterile open-cell foam is placed in a clean thoroughly debrided wound bed. Open-ended tubing is placed in the foam dressing within the wound bed. A thin film dressing is placed to provide an airtight seal, covering the entire wound area with overlap to normal peripheral tissue. The tubing is passed underneath or through a hole cut in the film dressing and then connected to a collection container and pump mechanism. The negative pressure pump is turned on to pull wound fluid into the collection canister. Pump pressure is adjustable between 50 and 200 mm Hg and is typically set at 125 mm Hg. The pump may run continuously or intermittently, and the dressing should be left in place for 48 to 72 hours. Dressings for infected wounds should be changed every 12 hours. The objective of negative pressure wound therapy is to enhance the formulation of granulation tissue by reducing wound edema, increasing blood flow, and removing infectious fluid [41,42]. The negative pressure changes the shape of cells, stimulates cellular proliferation, increases bacterial clearance, and draws cells toward the wound center to facilitate wound closure [43,44]. Animal studies indicate faster granulation of the wound bed, a reduction in bacterial colonization, and improved perfusion and oxygenation with negative pressure wound therapy [44]. Studies indicate enhanced healing of a variety of wound types, including pressure ulcers, vascular wounds, neuropathic ulcers, grafts, and flaps. Caution should be exercised with application to wounds with great potential for active bleeding or in patients on anticoagulation therapy. Contraindications include necrotic wounds, fistulas to body cavities or organs, exposed blood vessels, and osteomyelitis [17].

Monochromatic Near-infrared Photo Energy

A modality gaining recognition for treating a variety of wound types and sensory loss is monochromatic near-infrared photo energy, often referred to by its manufacturer's name, the Anodyne Therapy System (Anodyne Therapy, LLC, Tampa, Florida). In this therapy, photo energy is emitted from diodes in a flexible pad. The therapy has been shown to augment wound healing [45,46], increase microcirculation [47], improve neural function and pain [48,49], and improve sensation in human patients with diabetic peripheral neuropathy [47,50,51].

Growth Factors

The use of specific growth factors in the treatment of diabetic and pressure ulceration has yielded promising, although controversial, results. A recombinant PDGF product, becaplermin gel, is commercially available (Regranex gel, Johnson & Johnson, New Brunswick, New Jersey) and has been approved by the US Food and Drug Administration for the treatment of lower extremity diabetic neuropathic ulcers in humans [52]. PDGF is released from the alpha granules of platelets and is responsible for the stimulation of neutrophils and macrophages and for the production of TGF-β. It is a mitogen and chemotactic agent for fibroblasts and smooth muscle cells and stimulates angiogenesis, collagen synthesis, and collagenase [52,53]. When used in combination with other appropriate wound care measures such as wound debridement, pressure-relieving measures, infection control, and proper bandaging, PDGF stimulates and improves wound healing [52,53].

Nerve growth factor (NGF) has been used experimentally in humans as a topical treatment for severe noninfected pressure ulcers of the foot. NGF is a polypeptide in a family of neurotrophic factors exerting effects on developing peripheral sensory and sympathetic neurons. It can promote the regeneration of injured cells that express NGF receptors in the peripheral and central nervous systems [54]. NGF may also have an important role in wound healing in mouse skin [55]. Epithelial cells and fibroblasts are capable of producing NGF and are receptive to its effects. These observations have led to experimental studies in which daily topical application of a solution of NGF produced significantly accelerated rates of pressure ulcer healing when compared with standard therapy [54]. Although not yet commercially available, NGF and other growth factors currently undergoing investigation show promising results as an adjunctive treatment for nonhealing wounds in humans. Applications for the treatment of chronic wounds in veterinary patients warrant further study.

THE SPECIAL CASE OF PRESSURE SORES (DECUBITAL ULCERS)

The prevalence of pressure sores in people in the United States is reported to be between 1.3 to 3 million, and pressure sores are estimated to affect 5% to 10% of hospitalized patients [56,57]. Pressure sores are a source of numerous complications contributing to high rates of morbidity and mortality in humans. Treatment of pressure sores can result in huge costs to the health care system [57–59]. Although similar statistics are not available in veterinary medicine, pressure sores are similarly known to be a cause of increased patient morbidity and expense to the owner. Pressure sores are generally caused by prolonged pressure to the skin overlying a bony prominence, resulting in local or regional tissue ischemia. The progression of pressure sores is influenced by several other factors aside from direct pressure, including shear forces, friction, and moisture [59–61]. Underlying conditions, such as neurologic injuries (paralysis), vascular diseases causing impaired circulation, metabolic diseases (diabetes or hyperadrenocorticism), and malnutrition, can place animals at a much greater risk for the development of pressure sores. Most pressure sores observed in veterinary medicine occur in nonambulatory patients or in patients that cannot or are unwilling to change their body position. Obese patients and large breeds of dogs are at increased risk for pressure sores owing to body weight issues.

Common anatomic locations for pressure sores include the greater trochanter, tuber ischium, calcaneus, lateral malleolus of the tibia, and the lateral aspect of the fifth digit of the paw in the pelvic limbs and the acromion, olecranon, and lateral epicondyle of the humerus, and the lateral aspect of the fifth digit of the paw in the thoracic limbs. The most commonly affected site is the greater trochanter region. An exception to this occurs in small dogs with thoracolumbar spinal cord injuries resulting in pelvic limb paralysis. These dogs most commonly develop pressure sores over the tuber ischii owing to the upright seated posture they often assume (Fig. 2). Impaired cutaneous sensation in the perineal region may contribute to the formation of these ulcers. Pressure sores are also commonly seen under casts or other coaptation devices if the pressure points are not adequately protected. Decubital ulcer formation in cats is an unusual occurrence most likely owing to their small size.

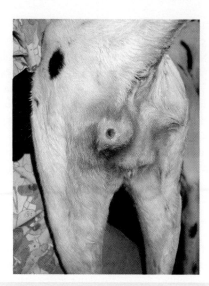

Fig. 2. Stage III pressure ulcer over the tuber ischium in a dog with a spinal injury causing caudal paralysis. Note the full-thickness necrosis of the overlying skin and the craterlike appearance of the lesion.

Prevention of pressure sores is certainly more cost effective than treating them; however, this is often easier said than done. Recognition of the at-risk patient is the first step toward preventing their development. Patients with limited mobility for whatever reason, especially large recumbent dogs, are at high risk for pressure sores. Providing the patient with special bedding is an effective way to minimize some of the risk. In humans, use of a low-pressure alternating air mattress system is effective in reducing the incidence of decubital ulcers. By alternating pressure and the sequence of chamber inflation in the mattress, the system provides regular periods of pressure relief and stimulation of blood flow to regions of the skin located over bony prominences [61]. This system has reduced the need for frequent repositioning of the recumbent patient. In veterinary medicine, such sophisticated mattress systems are not yet available, although standard air mattresses and waterbeds are available for animal use. A fine nylon mesh hammock suspended in an aluminum frame is available for animals (Fig. 3). Keeping the patient's skin clean and dry is critical for preventing pressure sores because moisture has a role in their development. Urine drains through the nylon mesh, keeping the patient drier, and the inherent elasticity of the nylon may help reduce the development of pressure points. Additionally, elevated coated metal racks or grates can be used to limit contact with urine and feces. Covering the grate with a synthetic fleece can provide additional padding for the patient. The fleece can be changed when it becomes soiled. For large recumbent or nonambulatory dogs, regular repositioning of the patient every 2 to 4 hours may still be necessary to prevent pressure sores.

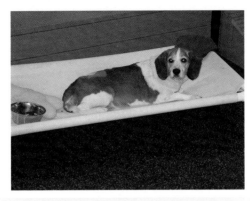

Fig. 3. Nonambulatory postoperative laminectomy patient on a nylon mesh hammock.

Suspended apparatuses or slings have been fabricated to assist the recumbent or paralyzed dog with standing. Although these devices are commercially available, they can be manufactured from PVC pipe, nylon mesh, and nylon strapping. Mechanical systems designed for movement of human patients can be adapted to veterinary medicine. These systems consist of a motorized hoist attached to an overhead track system to allow easy movement of the patient and to aid standing in the recumbent or infirmed patient (Fig. 4).

Regardless of these efforts, assessment of the skin, particularly in the previously mentioned at-risk locations, should be part of routine daily examination.

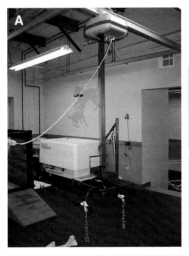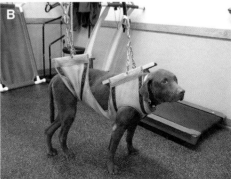

Fig. 4. (A) Hoist system mounted to overhead track system for moving patients. (B) Patient suspended in nylon mesh sling connected to the hoist. Such a system facilitates movement of patients in the clinic and allows patient "off-loading."

Early recognition and monitoring of these lesions generally results in more rapid healing of pressure sores. The presence of a dense hair coat may not only foster ulcer development owing to retention of moisture (urine and feces) but also may impair early recognition of impending pressure sores and delay initiation of preventive steps and treatment of the lesion. If detected early, lesions are not allowed to progress and can be managed in a more conservative manner (nonsurgical). The cost and patient morbidity can be minimized. Once a pressure sore is detected, the lesion should be staged and described. Taking measurements or even digital photographs of the lesion can be of value in documenting the wound's progress and can eliminate subjectivity and interobserver differences when making treatment decisions. Once classified, appropriate treatment (conservative versus surgical) of the wound can begin.

Classification and Treatment

Pressure sores are classified in humans according to the degree of tissue damage [56,60]. These classification schemes are used to determine treatment protocols for pressure sores and can similarly be applied to animals. Table 2 summarizes a commonly used classification scheme.

All nonviable tissue should be removed from the wound, regardless of its classification. Debridement accelerates wound healing by creating an environment that is free from necrotic and infected tissues, impediments to the normal wound healing process. In stage I and II lesions, debridement can generally be accomplished with local anesthesia and sedation. Stage I and II pressure sores are typically managed by second intention healing after the wound is debrided. Effective wound bed preparation involves establishing a moist wound-healing environment. Promotion of well-vascularized granulation tissue while facilitating wound drainage can be achieved effectively with wet-to-dry bandaging techniques. A variety of topical wound medications have been reported to

Table 2
Pressure sore classification

Stage	Description
Stage I	Nonblanchable erythema of intact skin and intact epidermis (pre-ulcer) are present. In pigmented skin, discoloration of skin, edema, and induration may be present.
Stage II	Superficial or partial-thickness skin loss involves epidermis, dermis, or both. Necrotic tissue or discharge may be present. The ulcer remains superficial and may appear as an abrasion, blister, or shallow crater.
Stage III	Full-thickness skin loss involves damage or necrosis of subcutis extending down to but not through deep fascia. Ulcer appears as deep crater, and there may be undermining of adjacent tissues.
Stage IV	Deep extension of the ulcer exists with necrosis or damage to muscle, bone, or supporting structures (tendon, joint capsule). Undermining and sinus tracts may be present.

promote wound healing, especially during the early inflammatory stages of wound repair. Acemannan (CaraSorb) and a D-glucose polysaccharide, maltodextrin (Intracell), are two such products. Acemannan promotes fibroblast proliferation, neovascularization, epidermal growth, and enhanced collagen deposition [62]. Maltodextrin is hydrophilic and reportedly causes chemotaxis of neutrophils and macrophages, which have a role in wound healing [63]. Porcine collagen (Vet BioSISt) is an acellular resorbable collagen matrix derived from swine intestinal submucosa. This product contains types I, III, and V collagen, fibronectin, hyaluronic acid, chondroitin sulfate, heparan sulfate, and TGF-β and FGF. Its use in one study resulted in an earlier appearance of granulation tissue over exposed bone in a comparison with control wounds treated with a conventional bandage only [64]. In the presence of healthy granulation tissue, contraction and epithelialization of the wound can occur. Use of nonadherent or semi-occlusive bandages is effective in promoting epithelialization. A polyethylene oxide occlusive dressing (BioDres) seems to promote earlier epithelialization by maintaining a moist wound environment [65]. A novel technique for promoting and facilitating wound healing is wet wound healing. A transparent, flexible, round chamber that is adhered to the skin surrounding the wound provides an in vivo tissue culture system. Analgesics, antibiotics, growth factors, growth media, and cells can be delivered into the chamber, facilitating wound healing and becoming a platform for tissue engineering. Although still experimental, the device holds promise as a mechanism for delivering gene therapy directly to the wound [66].

Stage III and IV pressure sores typically require reconstruction (Fig. 5). Although single-stage procedures have the advantage of saving time and money, the author(G.S.) prefers a two-stage approach because the potential for complications and graft or flap failure is greater with a single-staged procedure. Initial intervention consists of aggressive debridement and a period of open wound management followed by reconstruction of the wound after infection is well controlled. All grossly evident necrotic tissue, including bone, should be removed during the debridement phase [67]. Specimens for bacteriologic testing and biopsy, if necessary, should be obtained during this procedure. Open wound management with daily bandage changes (or more frequent changes depending on the amount of exudation present in the wound) should be performed. The author's preferred method of open wound management includes the use of a wet-to-dry bandaging technique. Empiric antibiotic therapy should be initiated pending the results of the bacterial culture and antibiotic sensitivity testing. Most patients requiring surgery typically have concurrent or comorbid diseases that may affect anesthesia and wound healing. Permanently paralyzed or debilitated dogs are prone to future or recurrent pressure sore development even after successful wound closure. Successful management of pressure sores depends on the patient becoming ambulatory. Dogs having a poor prospect for regaining the ability to ambulate have a guarded to poor prognosis for maintaining permanent healing of the ulcer. These factors should be considered when making a decision regarding surgical intervention.

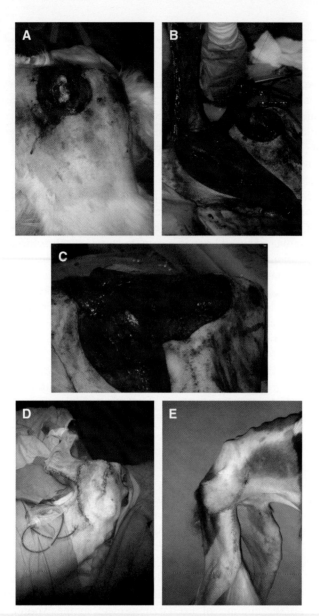

Fig. 5. Stage IV trochanteric decubital ulcer with osteomyelitis in a Borzoi. (*A*) Appearance of the wound after 5 days of open wound management using a wet-to-dry bandage technique. Note the exposed bone of the greater trochanter. (*B*) Intraoperative photograph showing developed cranial sartorius muscle flap and an axial pattern skin flap based on the ventral branch of the deep circumflex iliac vessels. (*C*) The muscle flap has been sutured in place over the greater trochanter. The muscle enhances blood supply to the area and provides robust padding over the prominent trochanter. (*D*) The skin flap has been transposed caudally to reconstruct the cutaneous defect, and the donor site along the cranial thigh has been closed primarily. A Jackson-Pratt closed suction drain has been used to provide drainage from the surgical wound. (*E*) Appearance of the healed wound 14 days after surgery at the time of suture removal. A nearly identical wound in the contralateral limb was successfully managed using the same reconstructive techniques.

Several options for wound closure are available to the surgeon, including direct closure, skin grafting, skin flaps, muscle flaps, and composite flaps (myocutaneous flaps). Although simple and tempting, direct closure techniques in which the skin edges are undermined, advanced, and sutured are subject to failure. Closure in this manner usually creates tension in the skin and places the incision line directly over the bony prominence, leading to dehiscence of the wound. Free skin grafting is a relatively simple procedure yielding good results for closure of noninfected, shallow, granulating wounds. In veterinary medicine, most free grafts are full-thickness meshed grafts. Free grafting procedures require immobilization for the first 10 to 14 days after surgery to prevent disruption of revascularization of the graft. The graft should be protected from mechanical loading and strain for the first 3 to 4 weeks after surgery. Nonhealing wounds in the distal extremities are probably best closed using free grafts. Skin flaps can be divided into local flaps that depend on the subdermal plexus for circulation and axial pattern flaps that have a well-defined arterial and venous vascular pedicle incorporated into their base. Axial pattern flaps have a much wider range of reconstructive capabilities with regard to flap size, versatility, and tissue constituents. Most skin flaps are robust, provide thicker tissue for resurfacing the wound, and do not require revascularization from the recipient site because they have an inherent blood supply. Muscle flaps are well suited for the reconstruction of deep wounds in which vascularity is impaired. Muscle flaps are highly vascular and can enhance the blood supply to otherwise marginally ischemic tissues. They provide ample padding over bony prominences, obliterate dead space, and provide a stable vascular bed for overlying skin grafts or flaps. Composite flaps typically consist of muscle and overlying skin. The most common composite flap used in veterinary reconstructive surgery is the latissimus dorsi composite flap. Stage IV decubital ulcers are probably best managed using a combination of muscle and skin flaps or a composite flap.

The location of the pressure sore dictates which techniques of wound resurfacing and closure can be employed. Deep pressure sores located over the greater trochanter are probably best closed using a cranial sartorius muscle flap and an axial pattern flap based on the ventral branch of the deep circumflex iliac vessels (Fig. 5). Ischial ulcers are well suited for reconstruction using a semitendinosus muscle flap and subdermal plexus skin flap. Wounds over the olecranon are well within the proximity of a thoracodorsal axial pattern flap or a latissimus dorsi myocutaneous flap [68]. Use of surgical drains is important to prevent fluid accumulation in the dead space under the muscle or skin flap. Although Penrose drains are adequate for this purpose, active closed suction drains allow for qualitative and quantitative evaluation of the fluid and provide the surgeon with greater latitude in drain placement. Penrose drains must exit in a gravity dependent location. These drains are usually kept in place for 5 to 7 days or when fluid production in the wound has fallen to about 1 mL/kg/day.

Regardless of whether a pressure sore is managed conservatively or requires surgical intervention, the wound should be "off-loaded." Protecting the healing wound from moisture, microorganisms, pressure, shearing forces, and friction is essential to a successful outcome [60,61]. Pressure relief can be achieved using bandaging techniques. Thick soft "donuts" can be constructed from rolled cotton or cast padding. The donut or ring encircles the lesion and prevents contact of the bony prominence with hard surfaces when the patient is laterally recumbent. Depending on the location, it can be difficult to maintain the donut in position. Securing the ring directly to the skin with adhesive spray followed by taping the donut to the skin can be effective, but the position of the bandage still needs to be checked regularly. An alternative to a ring is to make two rolls of cotton padding that are placed on the skin on either side of the wound in parallel fashion. These rolls are similarly taped to the skin of the patient. Other types of splints, such as Spica splints (for the forelimb), casts, and Robert Jones bandages can be effective ways of protecting a healing decubital ulcer. Care should be exercised when bandaging wounds reconstructed with skin flaps so that the base of the flap (vascular pedicle) is not compromised by the bandage.

SUMMARY

Management of wounds is an important part of physical therapy and rehabilitation in humans and animals. Patients that have sustained trauma often have wounds over the extremities that must be treated concurrently with other conditions. Proper wound care, along with some of the newer modalities, should be applied for successful treatment of open wounds. Many veterinary patients have orthopedic or neurologic conditions that result in prolonged recumbency, placing them at risk for decubital ulcers. Proper awareness for the prevention of pressure sores is best. When these wounds occur, appropriate treatment is critical to limit morbidity.

References

[1] Karukonda SPK, Flynn TC, Boh EE, et al. The effects of drugs on wound healing. Part I. Int J Dermatol 2000;39:250–7.

[2] Shultz GS, Mast BA. Molecular analysis of the environment of healing and chronic wounds: cytokines, proteases, and growth factors. Wounds 1998;10:1–9.

[3] Harding KG, Morris HL, Patel GK. Healing chronic wounds. BMJ 2002;324:160–3.

[4] Lawrence WT. Physiology of the acute wound. Clin Plast Surg 1998;25(3):321–40.

[5] Kerstein MD, Bensing KA, Brill LR, et al. The physiology of wound healing. Philadelphia: The Oxford Institute for Continuing Education and Allegheny University of Health Sciences; 1998.

[6] Porth CM. Pathophysiology: concepts of altered health states. 7th edition. Philadelphia: Lippincott Williams & Wilkins; 2005. p. 398–9.

[7] Singer AJ, Clark RA. Cutaneous wound healing. N Engl J Med 1999;341(10):738–46.

[8] Breuing K, Eriksson E, Liu P, et al. Healing of partial thickness porcine skin wounds in a liquid environment. J Surg Res 1992;52:50–8.

[9] Svensjo T, Pomahac B, Yao F, et al. Accelerated healing of full-thickness skin wounds in a wet environment. Plast Reconstr Surg 2000;106:602–14.

[10] Calvin M. Cutaneous wound repair. Wounds 1998;10(1):12–32.

[11] Tarnuzzer RW, Schultz GS. Biochemical analysis of acute and chronic wound environments. Wound Repair Regen 1996;4:321–5.

[12] Gogia PP. Clinical wound management. Thorofare (NJ): Slack; 1995.

[13] Rico RM, Ripamonti R, Burns AL, et al. The effect of sepsis on wound healing. J Surg Res 2002;102(2):193–7.

[14] Sussman C, Dyson M. Therapeutic and diagnostic ultrasound. In: Sussman C, Bates-Jensen BM, editors. Wound care: a collaborative practice manual for physical therapists and nurses. 2nd edition. Gaithersburg (MD): Aspen Publications; 2001.

[15] Norris S, Provo B, Stotts N. Physiology of wound healing and risk factors that impede the healing process. AACN Clin Issues 1990;1:545–52.

[16] Lampe KE. Methods of wound evaluation. In: Kloth LC, McCulloch JM, editors. Wound healing alternatives in management. 3rd edition. Philadelphia: FA Davis; 2002. p. 153–97.

[17] Myers BA. Wound management: principles and practice. Upper Saddle River (NJ): Prentice Hall; 2004.

[18] Stotts NA, Wipke-Tevis DD. Co-factors in impaired wound healing. In: Krasner DL, Rodeheaver GD, Sibbald RG, editors. Chronic wound care: a clinical source for healthcare professionals. 3rd edition. Wayne (PA): HNP Communications; 2001. p. 265–72.

[19] Lineaweaver W, Howard R, Soucy D, et al. Topical antimicrobial toxicity. Arch Surg 1985;120(3):267–70.

[20] Burks RI. Povidone-iodine solution in wound treatment. Phys Ther 1998;78(2):212–8.

[21] Ennis WJ, Meneses P. Factors impeding wound healing. In: Kloth LC, McCulloch JM, editors. Wound healing alternatives in management. 3rd edition. Philadelphia: FA Davis; 2002. p. 68–91.

[22] Cameron MH. Physical agents in rehabilitation: from research to practice. St. Louis (MO): Saunders; 2003.

[23] Belanger AY. Evidence-based guide to therapeutic physical agents. Philadelphia: Lippincott Williams & Wilkins; 2002.

[24] Baker KG, Robertson VJ, Duck FA. A review of therapeutic ultrasound: biophysical effects. Phys Ther 2001;81(7):1351–8.

[25] Peschen M, Weichenthal M, Schopf E, et al. Low-frequency ultrasound treatment of chronic venous leg ulcers in an outpatient therapy [abstract]. Acta Derm Venereol 1997;77(4):311–4.

[26] Baba-Akbari Sari A, Flemming K, Cullum NA, et al. Therapeutic ultrasound for pressure ulcers. Cochrane Database Syst Rev 2005;3.

[27] Young RS, Dyson M. Macrophage responsiveness to therapeutic ultrasound. Ultrasound Med Biol 1990;16(8):809–16.

[28] Byl NN, McKenzie AL, West JM, et al. Low dose ultrasound effects on wound healing: a controlled study with Yucatan pigs. Arch Phys Med Rehabil 1992;73:656–64.

[29] Byl NN, McKenzie AL, Wong T, et al. Incisional wound healing: a controlled study of low dose and high dose ultrasound. J Orthop Sport Phys Ther 1993;18(5):619–28.

[30] Sussman C, Byl NN. Electrical stimulation for wound healing. In: Sussman C, Bates-Jensen BM, editors. Wound care: a collaborative practice manual for physical therapists and nurses. 2nd edition. Gaithersburg (MD): Aspen Publications; 2001. p. 497–545.

[31] Kloth LC, Feedar JA. Acceleration of wound healing with high voltage, monophasic, pulsed current. Phys Ther 1988;68:503–8.

[32] Griffin JW, Tooms RE, Mendius RA, et al. Efficacy of high voltage pulsed current for healing of pressure ulcers in patients with spinal cord injury. Phys Ther 1991;71(6):433–44.

[33] Unger P, Eddy J, Sai R. A controlled study of the effects of high voltage pulsed current (HVPC) on wound healing. Phys Ther 1991;71(Suppl 6):S119.

[34] Unger P. A randomized controlled trial of the effect of HVPC on wound healing. Phys Ther 1991;71(Suppl 6):S118.

[35] Fitzgerald GK, Newsome D. Treatment of a large infected thoracic spine wound using high voltage pulsed monophasic current. Phys Ther 1993;73(6):355–60.

[36] Houghton PE, Kincaid CB, Lovell M, et al. Effect of electrical stimulation on chronic leg ulcer size and appearance. Phys Ther 2003;83(1):17–28.

[37] Goldman R, Rosen M, Brewley B, et al. Electrotherapy promotes healing and microcirculation of infrapopliteal ischemic wounds: a prospective pilot study. Adv Skin Wound Care 2004;17(6):284–94.

[38] Baker LL, Chambers R, DeMuth SK, et al. Effects of electrical stimulation on wound healing in patients with diabetic ulcers. Diabetes Care 1997;20(3):405–12.

[39] Gogia PP, Marquez RR, Minerbo GM. Effects of high voltage galvanic stimulation on wound healing. Ostomy Wound Manage 1992;38(1):29–35.

[40] Gardner SE, Frantz RA, Schmidt FL. Effect of electrical stimulation on wound healing: a meta-analysis. Wound Repair Regen 1999;7(6):495–503.

[41] Mendez-Eastman S. Negative pressure wound therapy. Plast Surg Nurs 1998;18(1):33–7.

[42] Morykwas M, Argenta L, Shelton-Brown E, et al. Vacuum-assisted closure: a new method for wound control and treatment. Animal studies and basic foundation. Ann Plast Surg 1997;38(5):553–61.

[43] Bates-Jensen BM, Edvalson J, Gary DE, et al. Management of the wound environment with advanced therapies. In: Sussman C, Bates-Jensen BM, editors. Wound care: a collaborative practice manual for physical therapists and nurses. 2nd edition. Gaithersburg (MD): Aspen Publications; 2001. p. 282–6.

[44] Kloth LC. Adjunctive interventions for wound healing. In: Kloth LC, McCulloch JM, editors. Wound healing alternatives in management. 3rd edition. Philadelphia: FA Davis; 2002. p. 316–81.

[45] Burke TJ. 5 Questions and answers about MIRE treatment. Adv Skin Wound Care 2003; 16(7):369–71.

[46] Horwitz LR, Burke TJ, Carnegie D. Augmentation of wound healing using monochromatic infrared energy. Adv Wound Care 1999;12:35–40.

[47] Powell MW, Carnegie DE, Burke TJ. Reversal of diabetic peripheral neuropathy and new wound incidence: the role of MIRE. Adv Skin Wound Care 2004;17:295–300.

[48] Noble JG, Lowe AS, Baxter GD. Monochromatic infrared irradiation (890 nm): effect of a multisource array on conduction in the human median nerve. J Clin Laser Med Surg 2001;19(6):291–5.

[49] Thomasson TL. Effects of skin-contract monochromatic infrared irradiation on tendonitis, capsulitis and myofascial pain. J Neurol Orthop Med Surg 1996;16:242–5.

[50] Leonard DR, Farooqi MH, Myers S. Restoration of sensation, reduced pain and improved balance in subjects with diabetic peripheral neuropathy. Diabetes Care 2004;27(1): 168–72.

[51] Kochman AB. Monochromatic infrared photo energy and physical therapy for peripheral neuropathy: influence on sensation, balance and falls. J Geriatric Phys Ther 2004;27(1): 16–9.

[52] Embil JM, Papp K, Sibbald G, et al. Recombinant human platelet-derived growth factor—BB (becaplermin) for healing chronic lower extremity diabetic ulcers: an open-label clinical evaluation of efficacy. Wound Repair Regen 2000;8:162–8.

[53] Bello YM, Phillis TJ. Recent advances in wound healing. JAMA 2000;283(6):716–8.

[54] Landi F, Luigi A, Russo A, et al. Topical treatment of pressure ulcers with nerve growth factor: a randomized clinical trial. Ann Intern Med 2003;139:635–41.

[55] Li AK, Koroly MJ, Schattenkerk ME, et al. Nerve growth factor: acceleration of the rate of wound healing in mice. Proc Natl Acad Sci USA 1980;77:4379–81.

[56] Lyder CH. Pressure ulcer prevention and management. JAMA 2003;289:223–6.

[57] Allman RM, Laprade CA, Noel LB, et al. Pressure sores among hospitalized patients. Ann Intern Med 1986;105:337–42.

[58] O'Brien SP, Gahtan V, Wind S, et al. What is the paradigm: hospital or home health care for pressure ulcers? Am Surg 1999;65:303–6.

[59] Sørensen JL, Jørgensen B, Gottrup F. Surgical treatment of pressure ulcers. Am J Surg 2004;188(1A Suppl):42–51.

[60] Brem H, Lyder C. Protocol for the successful treatment of pressure ulcers. Am J Surg 2004;188(1A Suppl):9–17.

[61] Edlich RF, Winters KL, Woodward CR, et al. Pressure ulcer prevention. J Long Term Eff Med Implants 2004;14(4):285–304.

[62] Tizard IR, Carpenter RH, McAnally BH, et al. The biological activities of mannans and related complex carbohydrates. Mol Biother 1989;1:290–6.

[63] Swaim SF, Gillette RL. An update on wound medications and dressings. Comp Contin Educ 1998;20:1133–44.

[64] Swaim SF, Gillette RL, Sartin EA, et al. Effects of a hydrolyzed collagen dressing on the healing of open wounds in dogs. Am J Vet Res 2001;61:1574–8.

[65] Swaim SF. Current concepts in open wound management. Proc Am Coll Vet Surg 2001;36: 394–7.

[66] Eriksson E, Vranckx J. Wet wound healing: from laboratory to patients to gene therapy. Am J Surg 2004;188(1A Suppl):36–41.

[67] Parsons B, Strauss E. Surgical management of chronic osteomyelitis. Am J Surg 2004; 188(1A Suppl):57–66.

[68] Pavletic MM. Atlas of small animal reconstructive surgery. 2nd edition. Philadelphia: WB Saunders; 1999. p. 338–9.

Vet Clin Small Anim 35 (2005) 1473–1484

VETERINARY CLINICS
SMALL ANIMAL PRACTICE

Logistics of Companion Animal Rehabilitation

Denis J. Marcellin-Little, DEDV, CCRP[a,b,*],
Kim Danoff, DVM, CCRP[c],
Robert Taylor, MS, DVM, CCRP[d],
Caroline Adamson, MSPT, CCRP[d]

[a]North Carolina State University College of Veterinary Medicine, 4700 Hillsborough Street, Raleigh, NC 27606, USA
[b]Animal Rehabilitation and Wellness Hospital, Suites 107, 108, 700 Blue Ridge Road, Raleigh, NC 27606, USA
[c]Veterinary Holistic and Rehabilitation Center, 360 Maple Avenue West, Suites A, B, Vienna, VA 22180, USA
[d]Alameda East Veterinary Hospital, 9770 East Alameda Avenue, Denver, CO 80247, USA

C ompanion animal rehabilitation is a segment of veterinary medicine aimed at identifying and addressing acute and chronic physical disorders in dogs, cats, and other companion animals. This segment of medicine has undergone rapid growth in recent years. Rehabilitation is based on the use of physical modalities (ie, heat, cold, electricity), manual therapy, therapeutic exercises, ambulation support, and environment modifications to assist with and promote improved function and recovery from an injury. The practice of companion animal rehabilitation relies on qualified professionals with specific knowledge, specialized equipment, and supplies. Rehabilitation is being taught at multiple veterinary schools and in other education programs [1]. Rehabilitation services may be available for outpatients or inpatients within general and specialty practices and at independent rehabilitation practices. Owner-implemented home exercise programs may also be designed for patients needing rehabilitation. The purpose of this article is to present and discuss the business issues specific to animal rehabilitation, including personnel, equipment, supplies, and facilities.

PERSONNEL

Clinicians and their support staff are the most important resource when providing physical rehabilitation. The specific medical knowledge fundamental to animal rehabilitation includes knowledge of anatomy and physiology, pathophysiology of orthopedic and neurologic diseases and injuries (Table 1),

*Corresponding author. E-mail address: denis_marcellin@ncsu.edu (D.J. Marcellin-Little).

0195-5616/05/$ – see front matter
doi:10.1016/j.cvsm.2005.09.001

Table 1
Classic medical problems treated in rehabilitation clinics

Problems	Common consequences	Occurrence
Orthopedic problems		
CCL injury	Loss of HL muscle mass, weight shift, OA	Common
Hip dysplasia	Pain in hip extension, loss of HL muscle mass	Common
Fracture patients	Loss of limb use, muscle mass	Relatively uncommon
Osteoarthritis	Loss of mobility, weight gain	Common
Traumatic sprain, luxations	Loss of joint motion	Relatively uncommon
Joint contractures	Loss of limb use	Uncommon
Neurologic problems		
TL disk herniation	Loss of motor function, urinary and/or fecal continence	Common
FCE	Loss of motor function, urinary and/or fecal continence	Uncommon
Degenerative myelopathy	Loss of proprioception, motor function	Relatively uncommon
Cd Cerv spondylomyelopathy	Loss of proprioception, motor function	Relatively uncommon
Other medical problems		
Obesity	Loss of mobility, OA	Common
Limb osteosarcoma	Amputation, loss of mobility	Uncommon

Abbreviations: CCL, cranial cruciate ligament; Cd Cerv, caudal cervical; FCE, fibrocartilaginous embolism; HL, hind limb; OA, osteoarthritis; TL, thoracolumbar.

gait and functional assessment, pain management, the healing and recovery process of musculoskeletal and neurologic tissues, wound healing, nursing care of nonambulatory and incontinent patients, nutrition and weight loss, use of rehabilitation modalities, therapeutic exercises, and exercise prescription. All personnel involved in rehabilitation need to be aware of the general health of rehabilitation patients and their physical limitations, including their ability to ambulate and likelihood of joint luxation or mechanical failures of fracture fixation (Table 2). Everyone should be familiar with indications, precautions, and contraindications of patient handling and treatments.

A veterinarian is fundamental to rehabilitation services (see Table 2). The veterinarian assesses the general health profile of patients. For example, the veterinarian is key to assessing for signs of peritonitis in a trauma patient recovering from orthopedic surgery or to assess for signs of hypoxemia in a tetraplegic patient with respiratory insufficiency. Veterinarians also assess patients with potential systemic or hormonal diseases that may have an impact on neuromuscular function. For example, peripheral neuropathy may be present in dogs with diabetes [2], dogs receiving corticosteroids may develop tendon ruptures [3], or dogs with hypothyroidism may develop myopathy or peripheral

Table 2		
Roles and responsibilities in a rehabilitation clinic		
Professionals	Knowledge and skills	Responsibilities
Veterinarian	Physical, orthopedic, and neurologic examinations	Disease diagnosis
	Functional assessment, pain assessment	Outcome assessment
	Knowledge of metabolic, orthopedic, neurologic diseases	
Physical therapist	Limb palpation, functional assessment	Design of rehabilitation program
	Therapeutic ultrasound, electrical stimulation	Specialized care delivery
	Therapeutic exercise prescription	Outcome assessment
		Owner education, discharge planning
Veterinary technician	Pain assessment, functional assessment	Care delivery
	Client and clinician communication	Performance assessment

neuropathy [4]. Veterinarians oversee the pain management protocols of rehabilitation patients. These protocols may include epidural, local, and bolus or continuous-rate infusion intravenous medications in severe and acute pain situations. With subacute and chronic pain, the pain management protocols include oral medications, cold, heat, massage, and exercises. In most states, the veterinarian is the gatekeeper for veterinary care, and if care is rendered by another health care professional, it is done on a prescriptive basis. In the final analysis, the veterinarian is legally responsible for the care provided to his or her patients. In situations in which physical therapists or other health care professionals operate in the veterinary facility under veterinary supervision or prescription, they are considered an extension of the veterinarian's care and liability.

Physical therapists (PTs) bring expertise to a rehabilitation clinic (see Table 2). PTs have a solid knowledge base in human orthopedic and neurologic diseases, tissue healing, goniometry, functional assessment, use of therapeutic modalities, protected weight-bearing strategies, development of outpatient and home exercise programs, ambulation assistive devices, and wound management. Their role is to outline specific functional impairments or disabilities in conjunction with the veterinarian; construct a problem list; set realistic and attainable goals specific to the patient; implement a treatment plan specific to the goals set; consistently assess response and tolerance to therapy; adjust intensity, mode, frequency, and duration of treatments as needed; recognize and address any problems that may arise (problem solving); provide clear and concise patient education; and discharge the patient in a timely and efficient manner when goals are attained. PTs may be board certified in one or more specialties, including orthopedic, neurologic, pediatric, sports, cardiovascular and pulmonary, clinical electrophysiologic, and geriatric board certifications. Some PTs also have specialized knowledge of joint manipulation (manual therapy), massage, orthoses, and prostheses as well as other focused clinical areas. PTs have a strong foundation in evidence-based medicine, because many of the protocols used in human physical therapy have been validated through controlled clinical studies [4]. It is logical to have the input of a physical therapist to help assess patients needing rehabilitation, to help design their rehabilitation program, and to conduct specific therapy. PTs may participate in therapy as consultants or practice employees based on practice arrangements and local veterinary and physical therapy practice acts [5]. PTs may increase their knowledge of companion animal rehabilitation through courses offered at meetings and through university-based programs. In some cases, a physical therapy assistant (PTA) can be a part of the team. PTAs are trained to administer therapy but do not perform assessments or develop treatment plans.

Initially, a clinician has to assess the patient thoroughly to develop an objective opinion of the extent of the animal's orthopedic or neurologic physical limitations; the severity and chronicity of these limitations; and the presence of complicating factors, including obesity, cardiovascular problems, chronic wasting diseases, or lack of physical fitness. That initial evaluation is key to the development of the initial rehabilitation program. As such, the initial assessment of the patient must be accurate, it must be sensitive (ie, all problems should be detected), and it must be specific (ie, all detected problems should be accurately judged). Also, this accurate assessment should be placed in proper perspective; the likelihood of success of therapy should be known based on the scientific literature and the clinician's clinical experience, and that information should be fairly presented to the owner. Making this objective assessment and discussing it objectively with the owner require solid scientific and clinical knowledge in orthopedics, neurology, and rehabilitation. This knowledge may come from a single clinician, a veterinarian trained in physical rehabilitation, or a team that includes a veterinarian and a PT.

Other medical professionals have medical knowledge related to rehabilitation, neurologic, and orthopedic problems. They include prosthetists, occupational therapists, hand therapists, chiropractors, doctors of osteopathy practicing osteopathic manipulative treatments, medically oriented massage therapists, and others. These professionals have clinical experience that is often beneficial to veterinarians working on animal rehabilitation.

Licensed veterinary technicians (LVTs) play a key role in animal rehabilitation (see Table 2). Hospitalized rehabilitation is labor-intensive. Patients require specialized nursing care, ambulation assistance, and rehabilitation care. LVTs play a key role in delivering that inpatient care. They assist with treatment, handling, and transfers, carrying out basic therapy procedures under the supervision and direction of a PT or veterinarian. LVTs collect functional feedback from owners admitting outpatients for therapy. LVTs assess pain status, changes in limb use, joint stability, overall performance during therapeutic exercises, and the general well-being of hospitalized rehabilitation patients. LVTs slightly modify therapy (ie, treadmill speed, pauses during therapeutic exercise sessions, duration of cold therapy) based on patient performance and tolerance. LVTs objectively communicate information regarding limb use and performance during therapy to veterinarians and PTs and to the owner. LVTs may increase their knowledge in companion animal rehabilitation through courses offered at meetings and through university-based programs.

FACILITIES

Overall, a rehabilitation service or clinic should be a quiet, safe, and easily accessible space where functionally impaired patients are treated as outpatients or inpatients. Rehabilitation clinics should have easy access because many patients have limited mobility. Urination and defecation areas should be placed near the entry. The number of steps at the entry point and throughout the clinic should be minimized. Entrance and exits should be carefully planned to minimize patient interactions and contact. A dock may be helpful to load and unload large dogs traveling in the rear of sports utility vehicles (Fig. 1). Plastic or aluminum ramps should be available to facilitate patient transfer. Flooring is particularly important in rehabilitation clinics because of the large number of patients with impaired mobility. Optimal flooring should provide excellent traction and be relatively easy to clean and maintain. The use of nonskid flooring should be a consideration for assessment, therapy, and housing areas. Flooring should be nonporous to avoid penetration of water and organic material. Roll- or tile-based nonskid rubber flooring has the advantage of providing excellent dry and wet traction and good shock absorption. It may be glued to a concrete slab. Rubber flooring is more difficult to clean and maintain than epoxy flooring and is significantly more costly than vinyl flooring. Seamless epoxy flooring with quartz aggregate has the advantage of providing good dry traction and

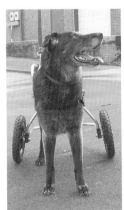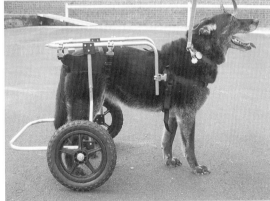

Fig. 1. Observation of gait and lameness may be performed outdoors on a smooth surface. This 14-year-old mixed-breed dog being fitted for an ambulation cart is walking outside a rehabilitation clinic in a large and quiet parking lot. A loading dock, visible behind the dog, may be used to assess the gait of other patients walking at the eye level of the observer.

durability and is relatively easy to maintain. Terrazzo and tile flooring is easy to maintain but provides low traction and shock absorption. Large thick rubber mats (ie, horse stall mats) may be used to cover slippery surfaces.

Patient housing is an important consideration in the design of a rehabilitation clinic. Large nonambulatory dogs, particularly dogs recovering from neurosurgery and trauma, are common rehabilitation inpatients (Fig. 2). Patients with limited mobility should rest on surfaces that minimize the likelihood of decubitus ulcers. These surfaces may include foam mats with impervious surfaces, mesh beds, or water beds. Urinary-incontinent dogs should be kept on porous or absorbing surfaces that decrease the likelihood of urine scalding. Dogs with mechanically weak surgical repair at risk of joint luxation or mechanical failure should be kept in a space that decreases the likelihood of stumbling or falling. Hosting rehabilitation inpatients in small separate rooms or kennels and using sound-absorbing materials help to minimize the tension and noise in patients that are often stressed by their ongoing neurologic or orthopedic problems. The size and behavior of the patient with regard to confinement influences housing choices (ie, jumping dog, restless dog, dog aggressive toward other dogs). Kennels with low-skid rubber mats decrease the risk of slipping compared with soft bedding on a stainless steel cage floor. In-house transportation between bedding, sleeping, urination and defecation, and assisted exercise areas is an important consideration. Quad-carts, transport tables with adjustable height, a hoist, or a ceiling rail system may greatly facilitate the transport of large nonambulatory patients. A safe and ergonomic bathing station is helpful to keep incontinent patients clean. A dryer or drying cage is useful to dry some patients after baths and aquatic exercises. Cages or kennels should be available to host day patients dropped off for therapy.

The assessment of rehabilitation patients may require a combination of indoor and outdoor space. The gait evaluation includes stance, walk, pace, trot, and sometimes gallop. Some high-performance dogs may be challenged

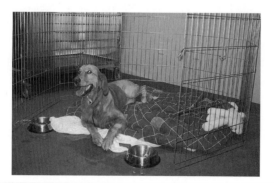

Fig. 2. A nonambulatory Golden Retriever is housed in an exercise pen (x-pen) at floor level on padded mats placed on the nonskid impervious rubber flooring. Food and water are readily accessible. The patient had septic osteomyelitis involving the ilium and sacrum.

by climbing or walking down slopes or steps, jumping up and down, or circling at various speeds. This should be done in a safe and quiet place, often outdoors (see Fig. 1). In geographic areas with a large amount of snow, extreme cold, or excessive heat, it may be beneficial to have indoor space available for these gait evaluations. This space can also be used to perform therapeutic exercises (Table 3; Fig. 3). One or more examination rooms should be available for the assessment of rehabilitation patients. This room should have nonskid flooring and be vast enough to allow the examination of large patients. A large floor mat (1.2 m × 1.8 m–1.5 m × 2.1 m [4 ft × 6 ft–5 ft × 7 ft]) is necessary to examine large nonambulatory patients.

As a general rule, rehabilitation therapy should be delivered in an environment as quiet and free of distraction as possible. A quiet treatment room may set up to deliver cold, heat, therapeutic ultrasound, electrical stimulation, massage, range-of-motion exercises, wound management, and slings and splints (Fig. 4). This room may be smaller than the examination room. Exercise areas are important in a rehabilitation clinic. Space is required to host a land treadmill, steps or stairs, cavaletti rails, large exercise balls, and other exercise equipment (see Table 3). Exercises that involve walking or trotting are done along the long part of rectangular areas (Fig. 5). Exercises requiring circling may be done in square areas. Facilities with underwater treadmills and swim tanks should have readily accessible floor drains, a nearby water source, and ground-fault interrupted electrical outlets and circuits in proximity (Fig. 6). Because of the moisture released from swim tanks, the surrounding paint and ceiling should be moisture resistant and the aquatic exercise room should be properly vented. Overall, rehabilitation clinics require a large amount of space if they intend to offer complete therapy options available regardless of weather conditions (see Table 3). In many cases, initial efforts to provide physical therapy and rehabilitation begin in an examination room or unoccupied space in the veterinary office. With success and demand comes the need for dedicated space. This may involve remodeling or creating new space. Construction costs are dictated by many things, including region, remodeling versus new construction, and the amount of special engineering needs. A recent dedicated physical

Table 3
Potential space requirements in companion animal physical rehabilitation

Equipment	Dimensions	Surface required
Gait evaluation area	3 m × 10 m/9 ft × 30 ft	30 m²/270 sq ft
Treatment mat or table	2 m × 2 m/6 ft × 6 ft	4 m²/36 sq ft
Land treadmill	2 m × 4 m/6 ft × 12 ft	8 m²/72 sq ft
Underwater treadmill	5 m × 10 m/15 ft × 30 ft	50 m²/450 sq ft
Cavaletti rails	2 m × 10 m/6 ft × 30 ft	20 m²/180 sq ft
Half and full steps[a]	2 m × 8 m/6 ft × 24 ft	16 m²/144 sq ft
Total		128 m²/1152 sq ft

Abbreviations: m, meters; m², square meters; sq ft, square feet.
  [a]Each half step is 7.5-cm high (3 inches high); each full step is 15-cm high (6 inches high).

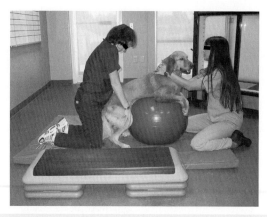

Fig. 3. The dog in Fig. 2 is exercising on a therapy mat measuring 1.2 m × 1.8 m (4 ft × 6 ft) and an exercise ball. The exercise is aimed a strengthening his pelvic limbs, stretching his hip region, and promoting a caudal weight shift.

therapy and rehabilitation complex cost $125 per square foot and an additional $100 per square foot for equipment and special engineering.

EQUIPMENT AND SUPPLIES

Rehabilitation services are made more effective with the use of specialized equipment. This equipment provides cold, heat, therapeutic ultrasound, and neuromuscular stimulation and enables dogs to perform safe and effective

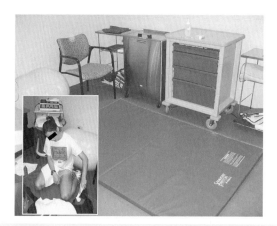

Fig. 4. A quiet treatment room measuring approximately 3.3 m × 3.3 m (10 ft × 10 ft) includes a therapy mat measuring 1.2 m × 1.8 m (4 ft × 6 ft), a dedicated cold pack freezer, a moist heat pack hydrocollator, a cart for wound management and splinting supplies, a Physio-Roll exercise ball (Sportime, Atlanta, Georgia) and a therapeutic ultrasound and electrical stimulation combination machine shown in the inset behind the therapist.

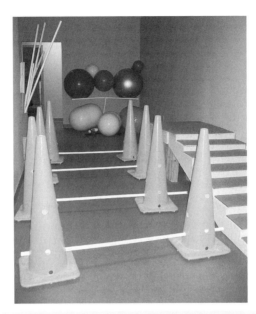

Fig. 5. An exercise area has nonskid rubber flooring. Cavaletti rails are set (*left*) and may be easily moved. Half steps and full steps are in place (*right*). Exercise balls are stored in the back. The PVC tubes seen on the left are used to create other cavaletti rail configurations.

therapeutic exercises (Table 4). The size and amount of specialized equipment should be adapted to the anticipated caseload; for example, a clinic with a low caseload can keep cold packs in the freezer compartment of a refrigerator, but a clinic with a higher caseload benefits from a dedicated cold pack freezer (see Fig. 3). Similarly, a clinic with a low caseload may use microwavable moist heat packs for heat therapy, but a clinic with a higher caseload benefits from a dedicated hydrocollator (see Table 4). Exercise equipment in rehabilitation clinics includes exercise balls, half and full steps, cavaletti rails, balance and wobble boards, land and underwater treadmills, and swim tanks (see Table 4). Additional equipment and supplies may include a sand box, trampoline, and soft mats also used to stimulate balance and proprioception. Strengthening exercise equipment is a key part of rehabilitation clinics. Underwater treadmills are popular because of the fact that they enable nonambulatory patients with good motor function and weakly ambulatory patients to walk while part of their weight is supported by warm water (see Fig. 6). They also enable injured patients and patients with relatively weak surgical repairs to exercise with the relative safety of the confined treadmill and water as a source of buoyancy and a shock absorber. Swim tanks may be present in rehabilitation clinics. They enable patients to perform low- or high-intensity non–weight-bearing exercises. Swim tanks in rehabilitation clinics range from 2 m × 3 m × 1.5 m (7 ft × 10 ft × 5 ft) to indoor or outdoor swimming pools. Clinics owning a swim tank may place a submersible underwater treadmill within the tank.

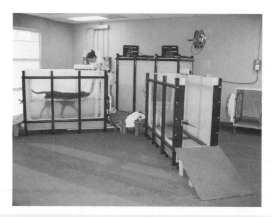

Fig. 6. Two underwater treadmills are placed above ground in a rehabilitation clinic. The treadmills are placed at an angle to each other to facilitate patient observation during therapy and to have a centralized operating location. A third tank holds water used to operate the two therapy tanks. Water is available on the wall behind the tanks to fill and wash the tanks. The room has three floor drains (not shown). Nonskid rubber flooring covers a concrete slab and covers the ramps used to access the treadmills.

Rehabilitation clinics use a variety of ambulation assistive device to support nonambulatory and weakly ambulatory patients during sessions of assisted stance or assisted ambulation. These devices include quad aluminum or polyvinyl chloride (PVC) carts with mesh or neoprene slings and a hoist [6]. Large carts and hoists may be larger than some doorways, so it is important to check their width and the width of door frames before purchase.

Supplies are needed to wrap or splint weak or injured limbs during or after rehabilitation sessions. These supplies include contact material (ie, gauze, petroleum jelly–impregnated gauze, gel dressing), cast padding, rolled gauze, self-adhesive elastic tape, and a variety of splinting materials (ie, aluminum, fiberglass, thermoplastic). Other equipment and supplies used in rehabilitation clinics include slings, chest harnesses, personal floatation vests, elastic exercise bands, and sport-specific exercise equipment (ie, agility tunnels). Rehabilitation clinics may use diagnostic equipment of various sizes and sophistication. Force plates or platforms and kinematic analysis systems may be set up in the assessment or exercise area.

FEE STRUCTURE

The fee structure for rehabilitation services should separate conventional veterinary medical care, housing and nursing care, and rehabilitation. Housing and nursing care charges should be adapted to the ease and intensiveness of patient care. Larger dogs that are nonambulatory and fecally incontinent, with compromised urination, long hair, and skin irritation from recumbency or urine scalding and that may be fear biters are quite challenging and labor-intensive.

Table 4
Specialized equipment and supplies used in companion animal rehabilitation

Equipment	Role	Potential candidates
Cold pack freezer	Rapid cooling and storage of cold packs	Trauma and postoperative patients
		OA patients with flare-ups
Hydrocollator	Rapid heating and storage of hot packs	Patients with contractures
		OA patients with loss of ROM
Therapeutic ultrasound	Heating deep tissues, pain relief	Patients with contractures
Electrical stimulation	Strengthen muscles (NMES)	Patients with chronic limb disuse
	Pain relief (TENS)	Acute and chronic pain
Land treadmill	Diagnose lameness	Exercise weak ambulatory patients
	Provide controlled exercise	
Underwater treadmill	Provide controlled and supported exercise	Exercise weak ambulatory patients
		Exercise patients with weak repairs
Swim tanks	Provide controlled and supported exercise	Exercise weak ambulatory patients
Cavaletti rail	Stimulate active ROM and stretch	Neurologic patients
		Patients with chronic limb disuse
Half-step and full-step stairways[a]	Functional strengthening	Trauma patients
Balance and wobble boards	Stimulate balance and proprioception	Neurologic patients
		Patients with chronic limb disuse
Swiss balls, Physio-Rolls	Support dogs, stretch joint, shift weight	Weak ambulatory patients
		Patients with chronic limb disuse
Trampoline, sand box	Stimulate balance and proprioception	Neurologic patients
		Patients with chronic limb disuse
Slings and harnesses	Facilitate ambulation	Neurologic and orthopedic patients
Ambulation carts	Provide assisted ambulation	Nonambulatory patients
Protective footwear	Protect limbs	Neurologic patients, denervation
Orthoses	Provide joint support	Patients with denervation or luxations
Prostheses	Provide limb support	Patients with partial amputations
Large padded floor mats	Allow comfortable lateral recumbency	Patients being evaluated and treated

Abbreviations: NMES, neuromuscular stimulation; OA, osteoarthritis; ROM, range of motion; TENS, transcutaneous electrical nerve stimulation.

[a] Each half step is 7.5-cm high (3 inches high); each full step is 15-cm high (6 inches high).

A smaller nonambulatory patient with short hair is significantly less labor-intensive. Day patients may be charged for daycare expenses. The initial rehabilitation assessment is charged based on its complexity and duration. Rehabilitation services may be charged based on the time spent with medical care providers or based on the modalities used. Packages may be offered at a slight discount to encourage sustained regular rehabilitation visits. Weight loss programs, conditioning, and wellness programs may be offered at a price lower than rehabilitation services requiring more intense supervision and adjustments.

In the final analysis, physical therapy and rehabilitation services must perform economically. The cost of the equipment, manpower, and amount of time needed to perform the service can be used to develop a fee structure. The classic gross income and salary for veterinarians dictate that their gross income should cover all the overhead costs and their salary should be 15% to 30% of their gross income.

BUSINESS COMMUNICATIONS

Rehabilitation services are most often provided as a part of a veterinary practice to ensure the constant supervision of patients undergoing rehabilitation. This is particularly true when patients are hospitalized. The rehabilitation center may function as a sole dedicated rehabilitation practice, as part of a general practice, or as part of a specialty practice. That structure influences the referral base and marketing plan of the rehabilitation center. A dedicated rehabilitation practice may be a resource for all practices in its close geographic area. A rehabilitation center attached to a practice tends to support the compromised patients treated within that practice but may also be providing services to the local veterinary community. In most cases, the facility cannot survive without outside referrals, and every effort should be made to involve the local referral community to visit, participate, and refer patients.

References

[1] Boyle K, Marcellin-Little DJ, Levine D. An interdisciplinary animal physical rehabilitation course for physical therapy and veterinary students. J Vet Med Educ 2002;29:183–5.
[2] Johnson CA, Kittleson MD, Indrieri RJ. Peripheral neuropathy and hypotension in a diabetic dog. J Am Vet Med Assoc 1983;183:1007–9, 1965.
[3] Rewerts JM, Grooters AM, Payne JT, et al. Atraumatic rupture of the gastrocnemius muscle after corticosteroid administration in a dog. J Am Vet Med Assoc 1997;210:655–7.
[4] Rothstein JM. On the second edition of the Guide to Physical Therapist Practice. Phys Ther 2001;81:6–8.
[5] Model Veterinary Practice Act. AVMA membership directory and resource manual. Schaumburg, IL: American Veterinary Medical Association; 2001. p. 319.
[6] Vaughan RW, Short SJ, Kirkland KD. Construction of a cart and sling for rehabilitation of immobile dogs. Vet Med Small Anim Clin 1983;78:191–4.

Vet Clin Small Anim 35 (2005) 1485–1517

VETERINARY CLINICS
SMALL ANIMAL PRACTICE

CUMULATIVE INDEX 2005

A

Abdomen
  acute. See *Acute abdomen.*
  examination of, in emergency patients, 299–300
  feline infectious peritonitis effects on, 48–49
  neuroanatomy of, 375–376

Abdominal fluid, in acute abdomen, 385–387
  biochemical analysis and culture of, 388–390
  cytologic analysis of, 387–388

Abdominal pain, perception of, 375–376

Abductor pollicis longus tenosynovitis, canine lameness due to, 1241–1243

Absolute anchorage, in control of tooth movement in small animal orthodontics, 874

Acepromazine, for trauma patients, 487

Achilles rupture, rehabilitation for, 1384–1385

Acid(s), urine bile, in feline hepatic lipidosis, 236

Acromegaly, feline, 181–187
  clinical signs of, 181–185
  diagnosis of, 185–186
  pathogenesis of, 181
  prognosis of, 187
  treatment of, 186–187

Active exercises
  in acute spinal cord injury rehabilitation, 1396–1398
  in chronic spinal cord injury rehabilitation, 1401–1402
  in peripheral nerve injury rehabilitation, 1404–1405

Acute abdomen
  abdominal fluid accumulations in, detection and retrieval of, 385–387
  approach to, **375–396**
  biochemical abdominal fluid analysis and culture for, 388–390
  causes of, 379, 380–383
  clinical signs of, 376–379
  cytologic abdominal fluid analysis for, 387–388
  defined, 299
  diagnosis of, 385
  history of, 376–379
  imaging of, 390–394
  initial stabilization of, 379, 383–385
  management of, 379, 383–385
  physical examination of, 376–379
  surgical evaluation of, 394–395
  trauma-associated, causes of, 379, 384

Acute care patients
  general nursing care for, 1413–1414
  rehabilitation in, **1411–1426**. See also *Rehabilitation, in acute care patients.*
  systemic illness in, metabolic and tissue changes associated with, 1413

Acute hematogenous osteomyelitis, 1096–1097

Acute renal failure, 366–371
  clinical signs of, 368
  described, 366–367
  pathophysiology of, 367–368
  treatment of, 368–371
    new directions in, 371

Acute spinal cord injury, 1390–1399
  assessment of, 1391–1393
    deep pain perception, 1392–1393
    gait, 1392
    respiratory function, 1393
  pathophysiology of, 1390–1391
  prognosis of, 1393–1395
  recovery from, 1393–1395
  rehabilitation for, 1394–1399
    active exercises, 1396–1398
    cold-packing, 1398–1399
    flexor reflex stimulation, 1396
    goals of, 1394–1395
    neuromuscular stimulation, 1399
    passive range of motion, 1395–1396
    patellar reflex stimulation, 1396
    therapeutic modalities, 1398–1399
    therapeutic ultrasound, 1399

α-Adrenoceptor agonists, for pain in feline patients, 140

Note: Page numbers of article titles are in **boldface** type.

0195-5616/05/$ – see front matter
doi:10.1016/S0195-5616(05)00141-5

β-Adrenoceptor blocking agents, for feline hyperthyroidism, 176

Aggression
analgesia and chemical restraint for, 484–489
to humans, by geriatric pets, 682–683

Aging
effects on brain, 689–692
immunologic effects of, 745–746
in dogs and cats, nutrition for, **713–741.**
See also *Geriatric pets, nutrition for.*
metabolic effects of, 745–746
pharmacologic effects of, 746
physical effects of, 745–746
physiologic effects of, 745–746

α-Agonist(s), for trauma patients, 486

α-₂-Agonists, for oral and dental procedures, 1053

Airway(s)
assessment of, in emergency patients, 287
lower, respiratory distress of, 312–313
upper, respiratory distress of, 310–312

Airway obstruction, upper, analgesia and chemical restraint for, 491–492

Albuminuria
implications of, 593–594
in dogs and cats, 590–594

Alveolar bone, functions of, 821

Ambulation activities, in acute spinal cord injury rehabilitation, 1397

Ameloblastoma, clinical presentation of, 1014

American Veterinary Dental College
approved case-log abbreviations, in tooth identification, **1059–1063**

Amino acid(s), in feline hepatic lipidosis, 254–255

Amitriptyline, for interstitial/idiopathic cystitis, 158–159

Ammonia testing, in feline hepatic lipidosis, 237

Amputation, for joint disorders, 1368–1369

β-Amyloid, in cognitive decline, 690

Analgesia/analgesics
for infants, 506–507
for neonates, 506–507
for nursing mothers, 505–506
for oral and dental procedures, **1041–1058.** See also *Dental procedures, regional anesthesia and analgesia for.*
for pain in feline patients, 131–137
for pediatric patients, 506–507
for pregnant dogs and cats, 510

for weanlings, 506–507
in emergency patients, **481–515**
adjuvant drugs, 510–512
for aggression, 484–489
for arrhythmias, 500–501
for cardiovascular compromise, 494–498
for chest trauma, 493
for dehydration, 500
for diaphragmatic hernia, 493
for dilation volvulus, 501–503
for gastric volvulus, 501–503
for gastrointestinal pain, 501
for intravenous catheter placement, 504
for lower respiratory injury, 492–493
for neurologic compromise, 489
for pancreatitis, 503–504
for peritonitis, 503–504
for respiratory compromise, 489–491
for shock, 498–500
for upper airway obstruction, 491–492
for urinary catheter placement, 504
for visceral pain, 501
in intra-arterial catheter placement, 504
NSAIDs, 510
nursing care–related, 512
LLLT in, 1341–1342
multimodal, for oral and dental procedures, rationale for, 1041–1042

Anchorage
absolute, in control of tooth movement in small animal orthodontics, 874
in control of tooth movement in small animal orthodontics, 873
friction and, 874–876
reinforced, in control of tooth movement in small animal orthodontics, 873

Anconeal process, ununited, rehabilitation for, 1375–1376

Anesthesia/anesthetics
for emergencies, **435–453**
anticholinergics, 441
case studies, 444–451
etomidate, 440
general anesthesia, 436–441
in monitoring, 442–444
in pain management, 441–442
ketamine, 440
propofol, 438–439
sedation, 436

thiopental, 439–440
for esophagostomy/endoscopic
    gastrostomy tube placement, in
    feline hepatic lipidosis, 246
for geriatric patients, **571–580**
    barbiturates in, 576–577
    dissociative anesthetic agents, 577
    etomidate, 577
    halothane, 578
    inhalants, 577
    isoflurane, 578
    maintenance of, 578–579
    monitoring and support of, 579
    propofol, 577–578
    sevoflurane, 579
in gold standard of veterinary oral
    health care, 782–783
in oral tumor management, 1017
local
    for oral and dental procedures,
        1044
    for pain in feline patients, 139–140
regional, for oral and dental procedures,
    1041–1058. See also *Dental
    procedures, regional anesthesia and
    analgesia for.*

Angular impulse, 1262

Angular kinetics, 1261–1262

Anodyne Therapy System, 1460

Anterior uveitis, 456–458
    prognosis of, 458
    treatment of, 458

Antibiotic(s)
    for gingivostomatitis, 902–904
    prophylactic, in fracture patients, 1145

Antibody(ies)
    in blood, in feline infectious peritonitis
        diagnosis, 56–57
    in CSF, in feline infectious peritonitis
        diagnosis, 58
    in effusion, in feline infectious peritonitis
        diagnosis, 57–58
    in feline infectious peritonitis diagnosis,
        55–58

Antibody antigen complex detection, in feline
    infectious peritonitis diagnosis, 59

Anticholinergic agents
    for emergencies, 441
    in preanesthetic sedation of geriatric
        patients, 574–575

Antidepressant(s), tricyclic
    for oral and dental procedures, 1057
    for pain in feline patients, 141

Antigen(s)
    detection of, in feline infectious
        peritonitis, 59–61

in tissue, in feline infectious peritonitis,
    60–61

Anti-inflammatory drugs
    for gingivostomatitis, 904–905
    nonsteroidal (NSAIDs)
        for oral and dental procedures,
            1053–1054
        for osteoarthritic pain in geriatric
            dogs and cats, 658–660
        for pain in feline patients,
            137–139
        in emergency patients, 510

Antithyroid therapy, trial course of, in feline
    hyperthyroidism, 175

Antiviral chemotherapy, for feline infectious
    peritonitis, 63–65

Anxiety, separation, in geriatric pets, 683–684

Appendicular osteosarcoma, in dogs,
    1159–1161

Appendicular skeleton
    long bones of, tumors of, 1159–1162
    traumatic luxations of, **1173–1199**
        initial assessment of, 1173–1174
        management of, 1175–1196
            carpal luxation, 1178–1180
            digital luxation, 1175–1178,
                1196
            elbow luxation, 1180–1183
            hip luxation, 1184–1188
            hock luxation, 1193–1196
            metacarpal luxation,
                1178–1180
            metatarsal luxation, 1196
            patellar luxation, 1188–1189
            shoulder luxation,
                1183–1184
            stifle luxation, 1189–1193

Appetite stimulants, for feline hepatic
    lipidosis, 249–250
    avoidance of, 260

Applicable mechanical theory, in
    biomechanics of rehabilitation,
    1255–1263
    angular kinetics, 1261–1262
    energy, 1263
    linear kinetics, 1259–1261
    moments and levers, 1255–1259
    power, 1263
    work, 1262–1263

Aquatic biomechanics, 1281–1282

Aquatic exercises, biomechanics of,
    1281–1282

Arch bars, in small animal orthodontics, 881

Arch expansion devices, in small animal
    orthodontics, 882

Arrhythmia(s), analgesia and chemical restraint for, 500–501

Arterial blood pressure, monitoring of, for perfusion abnormalities in emergency patients, 325–326

Arthritis, **1073–1091**
   described, 1073
   diagnosis of, 1081
   management of, 1082–1086
   pathophysiology of, 1073–1080
   rheumatoid, 1086–1088
   septic, 1102–1105. See also *Septic arthritis.*

Arthrodesis, for joint disorders, 1368

Arthroplasty, excision, for joint disorders, 1367–1368

Articular fractures, rehabilitation for, 1358–1359

Assisted walking
   for medical and acute care patients, 1419–1420
   in acute spinal cord injury rehabilitation, 1397

Assistive devices, **1441–1450**
   boots, 1441–1442
   carts, 1443
   case studies using, 1446–1449
   orthotics, 1443–1446
   prosthetics, 1445–1446

Auscultation, in heart diseases in aging dogs, 605–607

Avulsion of tendon of long digital extensor muscle, rehabilitation for, 1383–1384

Axial osteosarcoma, in dogs, 1162–1163

Axial skeleton, tumors of, 1162–1166

Azathioprine, for gingivostomatitis, 905

B

Bacteria, zoonoses due to, control of, 12–14

Balance, in conditioning of sporting dogs, 1430–1431

Balance exercises, in acute spinal cord injury rehabilitation, 1398

Barbiturate(s), for geriatric patients, 576–577

Behavior problems, in geriatric pets, **675–698**
   aggression to humans, 682–683
   causes of, 677–680
   cognitive dysfunction syndrome, 685–695
   compulsive disorders, 685
   diagnosis of, 680–681
   distribution of, 675–677
   excessive vocalization, 684–685
   fear, 683–684
   house soiling, 683
      medical conditions and, 678–679
      nocturnal restlessness, 684–685
      phobias, 683–684
      primary problems, 680
      repetitive disorders, 685
      separation anxiety, 683–684
      treatment of, 681–685

Biceps tendon lesions, classification of, 1203

Biceps tenosynovitis, rehabilitation for, 1382

Bicipital tenosynovitis, 1203–1206
   diagnosis of, 1204–1205
   management of, 1206

Bilateral mandibular fracture, repair of, 994–1006

Bilateral pelvic fractures, rehabilitation for, 1365

Bilateral rostral mandibulectomy, 1021–1023

Bilateral rostral maxillectomy, 1027–1029

Bile acids, urine, in feline hepatic lipidosis, 236

Biochemical testing, of geriatric patients, **537–556**

Biomechanics
   aquatic, 1281–1282
   defined, 1255
   of dancing, 1280–1281
   of exercise modification, 1274–1277
   of joint motion, 1270–1271
   of rehabilitation, **1255–1285**. See also *Rehabilitation, biomechanics of.*
   of skeletal muscle, 1271–1274
   of therapeutic exercises, 1277–1282
   of treadmill walking, 1277–1278
   of wheelbarrowing, 1278–1280
   terminology and formulas in, 1256–1257

Bird tongue, 790–791

Bleeding
   active, in assessment of emergency patients, 292
   in assessment of emergency patients, 292

Blindness, sudden, 476

Blood
   antibodies in, in feline infectious peritonitis diagnosis, 56–57
   polymerase chain reaction in, in feline infectious peritonitis diagnosis, 58–59

Blood chemistry, in heart diseases in aging dogs, 613–614

Blood pressure, arterial, monitoring of, for perfusion abnormalities in emergency patients, 325–326

Blood substitutes, in biochemical testing of geriatric patients, 543

Blood tests, in feline hepatic lipidosis, 236–239

Body temperature, in assessment of emergency patients, 290

Bone(s)
    alveolar, functions of, 821
    LLLT effects on, 1340–1341
    multilobular tumor of, 1163–1164
    of cranium, in dogs and cats, 763–769

Bone grafts, in fracture repair, 1153–1155
    in geriatric dogs and cats, 665

Bone healing, after fracture repair, 1147–1148

Bone tumors, metastatic, 1165–1166

Boots, 1441–1442

Borna disease virus, 109–113
    clinical signs of, 110–111
    diagnosis of, 111–113
    epizootiology of, 109–110
    pathogenesis of, 110
    treatment of, 113
    zoonotic risk of, 113

Brain, aging effects on, 689–692

Brain stem, examination of, in emergency patients, 304

Breath sounds
    bronchial, in heart diseases in aging dogs, 607
    examination of, in emergency patients, 293–296

Breathing, examination of, in emergency patients, 287, 293–296

Bronchial breath sounds, in heart diseases in aging dogs, 607

Buprenorphine
    for oral and dental procedures, 1052
    for pain in feline patients, 135–136

Butorphanol
    for oral and dental procedures, 1052
    for pain in feline patients, 133–134
    for trauma patients, 486, 487

C

Calcium, for feline hyperthyroidism, 176–177

Cancer
    in cats, 632
    in dogs, 628–629
    oral, 711

Canine elbow dysplasia (CED), 1126–1130
    causes of, 1126
    clinical signs of, 1126–1127
    described, 1126

diagnosis of, 1127–1128
    elbow incongruity, 1130
    fragmented medial coronoid process, 1128
    osteochondrosis dissecans, 1129–1130
    pathogenesis of, 1126
    prognosis of, 1128
    signalment of, 1126
    treatment of, 1128
    ununited anconeal process, 1129

Canine hypothyroidism, 641–649
    clinical features of, 643–645
    described, 641–642
    diagnosis of, 645–647
    primary, 642–643
    prognosis of, 648–649
    secondary, 643
    treatment of, 647–648

Canine lameness, causes of, **1239–1245**. See also *Lameness, canine.*

Canine thyroid tumors, 649–651

Capillary refill time, in assessment of emergency patients, 289

Carbimazole, for feline hyperthyroidism, 176

Cardiogenic shock, in emergency patients, 336

Cardiopulmonary cerebral resuscitation, in young animals, 430–431

Cardiovascular compromise, analgesia and chemical restraint for, 494–498

Cardiovascular disease, in geriatric patients, pharmacology related to, 563

Cardiovascular system
    biochemical testing of geriatric patients effects on, 555
    examination of, in emergency patients, 297–299
    of geriatric patients, physiology of, 572

L-Carnitine supplementation, for feline hepatic lipidosis, 254

Carpal hyperextension, 1370

Carpal luxation, management of, 1178–1180

Carprofen, for osteoarthritic pain in geriatric dogs and cats, 658–659

Carpus, mobilization of, 1301–1303

Cart(s), 1443

Cartilage, LLLT effects on, 1340–1341

Cat(s)
    aging, nutrition for, **713–741**. See also *Geriatric pets, nutrition for.*
    diabetes mellitus in, **211–224**. See also *Diabetes mellitus, in cats.*

Cat(s) *(continued)*
    domestic, tooth resorption in, causes of,
        update on, **913–942.** See also *Feline*
        odontoclastic resorptive lesions (FORL).
    full-mouth extraction in, 982
    ketoacidosis in, 214–215
    liver diseases in, 629–632
        feline infectious peritonitis,
            631–632
        inflammatory liver disease,
            629–631
        neoplasia, 632
        pyogranulomatous hepatitis,
            631–632
        secondary hepatic lipidosis, 632
    malignant musculoskeletal tumors of,
        1159–1172
    oral anatomy of, **763–780**
        bones of cranium, 763–769
        cranial types, 769–770
        dental formulae, 772–773
        muscles, 773–775
        nerves, 775–776
        salivary glands, 775
        teeth and support tissue
            development, 770–772
        temporomandibular joint,
            769
        vascular system, 776–779
    osteosarcoma in, 1161
    permanent teeth of, peculiarities of,
        915–921
    pregnant, analgesia for, 510
Catheter placement
    intra-arterial, analgesia and chemical
        restraint for, 504
    intravenous, analgesia and chemical
        restraint for, 504
    urinary, analgesia and chemical restraint
        for, 504
Catheterization, in pediatric emergencies,
    421–422
Caudal glenoid, incomplete ossification of,
    canine lameness due to,
    1240–1241
Caudal infraorbital nerve blocks, for oral and
    dental procedures, 1045
Caudal mandibulectomy, 1024
Caudal maxillectomy, 1029–1030
CCLR. See *Cranial cruciate ligament disease*
    (CCLR).
CCT injuries. See *Common calcaneal tendon*
    (CCT) injuries.
CED. See *Canine elbow dysplasia (CED).*
Cemented hip replacement systems,
    1221–1225

Central maxillectomy,
    1029–1030
Central nervous system (CNS)
    abnormalities of, in emergency patients,
        343–358
        cerebral blood volume
            optimization for, 351–352
        cerebral edema reduction in,
            350–351
        cerebral hemodynamics regulation
            in, 343–344
        cerebral metabolic rate elevation,
            minimization of, 352
        evaluation of, 345–347
        extracranial stabilization for,
            347–350
        intracranial stabilization for,
            350–352
        monitoring of, 355–356
        pathophysiology of, 344–345
        space-occupying mass elimination
            for, 352
        stabilization of, 352–355
        treatment of, 352–355
    infectious diseases of, **103–128**
        Borna disease virus, 109–113
        causes of, 108–109
        feline spongiform encephalopathy,
            118–121
        increased recognition of, reasons
            for, 104–107
        unusual patterns of seizure
            activity, 117–118
        without inflammatory changes,
            117
    injuries of, pathophysiology of,
        344–345
    of geriatric patients, physiology of,
        573–574
Central venous pressure, monitoring of, for
    perfusion abnormalities in emergency
    patients, 326–327
Cerebral blood volume, optimization of, for
    CNS abnormalities in emergency
    patients, 351–352
Cerebral edema, reduction of, for CNS
    abnormalities in emergency patients,
    350–351
Cerebral hemodynamics, regulation of, for
    CNS abnormalities in emergency
    patients, 343–344
Cerebral metabolic rate, elevation of,
    minimization of, in emergency patients,
    352
Cerebrospinal fluid (CSF)
    antibodies in, in feline infectious
        peritonitis diagnosis, 58

in feline infectious peritonitis
diagnosis, 55
polymerase chain reaction in, in feline
infectious peritonitis, 59

Chemical restraint, in emergency patients,
481–515
for aggression, 484–489
for arrhythmias, 500–501
for cardiovascular compromise,
494–498
for chest trauma, 493
for dehydration, 500
for diaphragmatic hernia, 493
for dilation volvulus, 501–503
for gastric volvulus, 501–503
for gastrointestinal pain, 501
for intra-arterial catheter placement, 504
for intravenous catheter placement, 504
for lower respiratory injury, 492–493
for neurologic compromise, 489
for pancreatitis, 503–504
for peritonitis, 503–504
for respiratory compromise, 489–491
for shock, 498–500
for upper airway obstruction, 491–492
for urinary catheter placement, 504
for visceral pain, 501

Chemotherapy, antiviral, for feline infectious
peritonitis, 63–65

Chest trauma, analgesia and chemical
restraint for, 493

Chondroprotective agents, for osteoarthritic
pain in geriatric dogs and cats, 661–662

Chondrosarcoma, 1162

Chronic infiltrative hepatopathies, in dogs,
622

Chronic inflammatory hepatopathies, in dogs,
617–621

Chronic spinal cord injury, 1399–1402
assessment of, 1400
pathophysiology of, 1399–1400
prognosis of, 1400
recovery from, 1400
rehabilitation for, 1401–1402
active exercises, 1401–1402
goals of, 1401
passive and reflexive exercises,
1401
therapeutic modalities, 1402

Cimetidine, in emergency situations, 521

Circulation, in assessment of emergency
patients, 287

Cirrhosis(es), hepatic, in dogs, 621–622

Cleft palates, in juvenile veterinary dentistry,
791–792

CNS. See *Central nervous system (CNS)*.

Coagulation parameters, in feline infectious
peritonitis diagnosis, 51

Codeine, for oral and dental procedures,
1052–1053

Cognitive decline
β-amyloid and, 690
reactive oxygen species effects on,
690–692
vascular insufficiency and, 692

Cognitive dysfunction syndrome
described, 685–687
in geriatric pets, 685–695
behavioral changes due to,
688–689
diagnosis of, 689
treatment of, 692–695
dietary therapy, 692–693
drug therapy, 693–695
environmental enrichment in, 693
nutritional therapy, 692–693

Cold (cryotherapy), 1317–1321

Cold lasers. See *Low-level laser therapy (LLLT)*.

Cold-packing, in acute spinal cord injury
rehabilitation, 1398–1399

Combination test, in hyperadrenocorticism,
193

Common calcaneal tendon (CCT) injuries
classification of, 1207
diagnosis of, 1207–1208
management of, 1208–1215
conservative, 1208
postoperative, 1213–1214
rehabilitation after, 1214–1215
surgical, 1208–1213
enhancement of tendon
healing in, 1212–1213
primary *vs.* secondary repair,
1209
suture material and size in,
1209
tendon anastomosis,
1209–1212
tendon lengthening, 1212

Companion animal rehabilitation
business communications related to,
1484
equipment and supplies for, 1480–1482
facilities for, 1477–1480
fee structure for, 1482–1484
logistics of, **1473–1484**
personnel for, 1473–1477

Complete blood cell counts, in feline
infectious peritonitis diagnosis, 51

Compulsive disorders, in geriatric pets, 685

Computed tomography (CT), in hyperadrenocorticism, 193

Conditioning
described, 1428
of sporting dogs, **1427–1439**. See also *Sporting dogs, rehabilitation and conditioning of.*

Condylar neck fracture, repair of, 997

Conjunctival grafts, 474

Conjunctivitis, 475–476

Contracture(s)
flexor tendon, rehabilitation for, 1384
infraspinatus, rehabilitation for, 1383

Coordination exercises, in acute spinal cord injury rehabilitation, 1398

Cornea, foreign bodies in, 474–475

Corneal laceration, 473

Corneal perforation, 471–472

Corneal ulcers, 465–471
causes of, 466
clinical signs of, 466–467
corneal laceration, 473
deep, 470
prognosis of, 469
superficial, 469
treatment of, 468–469

Corticotropin stimulation test, in hyperadrenocorticism, 192

Crackles, in heart diseases in aging dogs, 607

Cranial cruciate ligament rupture (CCLR)
gait analysis research in, 1268–1269
rehabilitation after, 1379–1381

Cranial nerve blocks, for oral and dental procedures, 1045

Cranium
bones of, in dogs and cats, 763–769
types of, in dogs and cats, 769–770

Cryotherapy, 1317–1321

CSF. See *Cerebrospinal fluid (CSF).*

CT. See *Computed tomography (CT).*

Cubital joint, osteochondrosis of, 1117

Cyclosporine, for gingivostomatitis, 906–907

Cyst(s), dentigerous, in juvenile veterinary dentistry, 800–801

Cystitis, interstitial/idiopathic, feline, 150–159. See also *Interstitial/idiopathic cystitis, feline.*

Cytauxzoonosis, feline, **89–101**
causes of, 89–90
client education related to, 99–100
clinical features of, 95
diagnostic procedures in, 96–98

epizootiology of, 90–95
laboratory findings in, 95–96
postmortem findings in, 98
prevention of, 99–100
prognosis of, 98–99
treatment of, 98–99

D

Dancing, biomechanics of, 1280–1281

Decubital ulcers, healing of, 1461–1468

Deep digital flexor tendons, rehabilitation for, 1385–1386

Deep pain perception, assessment of, in acute spinal cord injury, 1392–1393

Deformed teeth, in juvenile veterinary dentistry, 808–809

Degrees-of-freedom, analysis of, 1444

Dehydration
analgesia and chemical restraint for, 500
in young animals, 426–428

Dental crowding, in juvenile veterinary dentistry, 802–804

Dental formulae, in dogs and cats, 772–773

Dental morphology, 789

Dental procedures, regional anesthesia and analgesia for, **1041–1058**
α_{-2}-agonists, 1053
analgesia adjuncts, 1054–1057
caudal infraorbital nerve blocks, 1045
cranial nerve blocks, 1045
local anesthetic agents, 1044
mandibular nerve block, 1047–1050
maxillary nerve block, 1046–1047
mental nerve block, 1047
N-methyl-D-aspartate receptor blockers, 1054
multimodal analgesia, 1041–1042
NSAIDs, 1053–1054
opioids, 1050–1053
sites for, 1045–1050
tricyclic antidepressants, 1057

Dentigerous cysts, in juvenile veterinary dentistry, 800–801

Dentistry, for geriatric pets, client compliance in, 749–750

Deracoxib, for osteoarthritic pain in geriatric dogs and cats, 659–660

Descemetocele, 471

Developmental orthopedic diseases (DODs), **1111–1137**
hip dysplasia, 1122–1126
hypertrophic osteodystrophy, 1111–1113
Legg-Calvé-Perthes disease, 1120–1122

osteochondrosis, 1115–1120
panosteitis, 1113–1115
pes varus, 1130–1131
Dexamethasone suppression test
high-dose, in hyperadrenocorticism, 192
low-dose, in hyperadrenocorticism, 191
Diabetes insipidus, feline, 188–189
clinical signs of, 188–189
diagnosis of, 189
pathogenesis of, 188
prognosis of, 189
treatment of, 189
Diabetes mellitus
in cats, **211–224**
causes of, 212–213
clinical signs of, 213–215
concomitant disease with, 215
diagnosis of, 213–215
feeding during, 219–220
remission of, 218–219
therapeutic efficacy in, monitoring of, 217–218
treatment of, 215–217
insulin glargine in, 216–217
urine glucose measurements during, 221
insulin in, 216–217
oral hypoglycemic drugs in, 215–216
water intake during, 220
in geriatric patients, nutrition related to, 728–731
type 2, causes of, 212–213
Diaphragmatic hernia, analgesia and chemical restraint for, 493
Diazepam, for trauma patients, 486, 487
Dietary therapy, for cognitive dysfunction syndrome, 692–693
Digital luxation, management of, 1175–1178, 1196
Dilation volvulus, analgesia and chemical restraint for, 501–503
Disability(ies), in assessment of emergency patients, 288
Dissociative anesthetic agents, for geriatric patients, 577
Distal femoral physeal fractures, rehabilitation for, 1361–1363
Distributive shock, in emergency patients, 334–336
DODs. See *Developmental orthopedic diseases (DODs).*

Dog(s)
aging
mitral regurgitation in, heart diseases related to, 599–603
nutrition for, **713–741.** See also *Geriatric pets, nutrition for.*
appendicular osteosarcoma in, 1159–1161
axial osteosarcoma in, 1162–1163
ESWT in, 1348
geriatric
heart diseases in, **1–19.** See also *Heart diseases, geriatric, in dogs.*
orthopedic problems in, **655–674.** See also *Orthopedic problems, geriatric, in dogs and cats.*
liver diseases in, 617–629
chronic infiltrative hepatopathies, 622
chronic inflammatory hepatopathies, 617–621
hepatic cirrhosis, 621–622
hepatic fibrosis, 621–622
hepatocutaneous syndrome, 622–626
hepatoencephalopathy, 627–628
neoplasia, 628–629
vascular diseases, 626–627
malignant musculoskeletal tumors of, **1159–1172**
oral anatomy of, **763–780**
bones of cranium, 763–769
cranial types, 769–770
dental formulae, 772–773
muscles, 773–775
nerves, 775–776
salivary glands, 775
teeth and support tissue development, 770–772
temporomandibular joint, 769
vascular system, 776–779
pregnant, analgesia for, 510
sporting, rehabilitation and conditioning of, **1427–1439.** See also *Sporting dogs, conditioning of; Sporting dogs, rehabilitation of.*
tooth extraction in, 982
total elbow replacement in, 1233–1234
total joint replacement in, **1219–1238.** See also *Total joint replacement, in dogs.*
Drug metabolism, pain in feline patients and, 131
Drug monitoring, for geriatric pets, client compliance in, 749–750

Drug therapy
    emergency, 521–522
        practical considerations in,
            517–525. See also *Emergency*
            drug therapy.
    for cognitive dysfunction syndrome,
        693–695
    for trauma patients, 486–487
Dysplasia(s)
    elbow, 1126–1130
        rehabilitation for, 1375–1376
    hip, 1122–1126
        gait analysis research in, 1269
        rehabilitation for, 1376–1378
Dyspnea, in heart diseases in aging dogs,
    607–608
Dystocia, 399–406
    causes of, 400–401
    criteria for suspicion of, 402
    defined, 399
    evaluation of, 402–403
    management of, 403–406
    prevalence of, 401
    risk factors for, 401–402

E

ECG. See *Electrocardiography (ECG).*
Echocardiography, in heart diseases in aging
    dogs, 613
Eclampsia, 411–412
Edema, cerebral, reduction of, for CNS
    abnormalities in emergency patients,
    350–351
Edentulous patients, maxillofacial fracture
    repairs in, 999–1001
Edgewise appliances, in small animal
    orthodontics, 880–881
Effusion(s)
    antibodies in, in feline infectious
        peritonitis, 57–58
    feline coronavirus antigen in,
        immunofluorescence staining of,
        60
    in feline infectious peritonitis, tests
        related to, 47–48
    in feline infectious peritonitis diagnosis,
        53–55
    polymerase chain reaction in, in feline
        infectious peritonitis, 59
Elbow, osteochondrosis of
    prognosis of, 1119
    treatment of, 1118
Elbow dysplasia, 1126–1130. See also *Canine*
    elbow dysplasia (CED).
    rehabilitation for, 1375–1376

Elbow incongruity
    rehabilitation for, 1376
Elbow joint, mobilization of, 1299–1301
Elbow luxation, 1369–1370
    management of, 1180–1183
Electrical stimulation, 1327–1331
    in rehabilitation of medical and acute
        care patients, 1421–1422
    in wound healing, 1459
Electrocardiography (ECG), in heart diseases
    in aging dogs, 611–613
Emergency(ies)
    analgesia for, **481–515.** See also
        Analgesia/analgesics, in emergency
        patients.
    anesthesia for, **435–453.** See also
        Anesthesia/anesthetics, for emergencies.
    chemical restraint for, **481–515.** See also
        Chemical restraint, in emergency patients.
    CNS abnormalities after, **343–358.** See
        also *Central nervous system (CNS),*
        abnormalities of, in emergency patients.
    drugs for, **481–515**
    in young animals, **421–434.** See also
        Pediatric emergencies.
    NSAIDs in, 510
    opioids in, 509–510
    perfusion-related, **319–342.** See also
        Perfusion abnormalities, in emergency
        patients.
    reproductive, **397–420.** See also
        Reproductive emergencies.
    sedatives in, 507–509
    urinary tract, **359–373.** See also *Urinary*
        tract emergencies.
Emergency drug therapy
    drug dosages in, 519–520
    drugs used in, 521–522
    guidelines for, 520
    monitoring during, 523–524
    patient factors in, 522–523
    practical considerations in, **517–525**
    resources for, 524
    routes of administration of, 517–519
Emergency patients, global assessment of,
    281–305
    abdomen, 299–300
    airway, 287
    brain stem, 304
    breath sounds, 293–296
    breathing, 287, 293–296
    capillary refill time, 289
    cardiovascular system, 297–299
    circulation, 287
    clarity during, 282
    comprehensive assessment in, 284–286
    critical thinking in, 282

database in, 282
decision making in, 282
disabilities, 288
emergency team in, 281–282
gait, 304
genitourinary system, 300–301
head and neck, 292–293, 303–304
hydration state, 290–291
initial assessment in, 283–284
integument, 301–302
lymph nodes, 302
mental state, 288–289, 303
mucous membrane color, 289, 296
musculoskeletal system, 301
neurologic system, 302–304
pain, 291–292
palpation in, 296–297
percussion in, 297
physical examination in, 286–305
postural response, 304
problem-oriented medical record in, 286
pulse quality in, 290
pulse rate in, 290
pupils, 304
respiratory system, 293–297
seizures, 304–305
shock, 288–289
spine, 304
temperature, 290
tremors, 304–305
triage in, 281
Encephalitides, nonsuppurative, of unknown
    cause, 113–117
Encephalopathy(ies), feline spongiform,
    118–121
Endocrine system, biochemical testing of
    geriatric patients effects on, 552–554
Endocrinopathy(ies), feline, **171–210**
    acromegaly, 181–187
    diabetes insipidus, 188–189
    hyperadrenocorticism, 189–195
    hyperparathyroidism, 200–201
    hyperthroidism, 171–179
    hypoadrenocorticism, 199–200
    hypoparathyroidism, 201–202
    hyposamotropism, 187–187
    hypothyroidism, 179–181
    pheochromocytoma, 197–198
    primary hyperaldosteronism, 196–197
    primary sex hormone–secreting adrenal
        tumors, 195–196
Endodontic(s). See also *Endodontic disease.*
    fundamentals of, **837–868**
Endodontic disease
    causes of, 837–842
    pathophysiology of, 837–842
    treatment of, 842–843

failed, treatment of, 864–865
    follow-up care, 865
nonvital pulp therapy in, 850–865
    described, 850–851
    failure of
        reasons for, 862–863
        signs of, 863–864
    gutta percha application, 859
    master point coating, 859
    softened gutta percha
        techniques, 860–862
    standard root canal therapy,
        851–859
patient preparation for, 843
surgical site preparation in,
    843–844
vital pulp therapy in, 844–850
    described, 844–845
    direct pulp capping, 847–849
    follow-up care, 849–850
    indirect pulp capping,
        846–847
Endogenous corticotropin measurement, in
    hyperadrenocorticism, 193
Endometritis, 410–411
Endurance, in conditioning of sporting dogs,
    1431
Energy, in biomechanics, 1263
Energy needs, aging effects on, 714–716
Enrofloxacin, for ophthalmic emergencies,
    479
Enteric feline coronavirus infection,
    pathogenesis of, 44
Enteric protozoal diseases, **81–88.** See also
    Protozoal diseases, enteric.
Enteric zoonoses, control of, 3–12
Enteritis, feline coronavirus–induced,
    treatment of, 62
Environmental enrichment, for cognitive
    dysfunction syndrome, 693–695
Esophagostomy tube, in feline hepatic
    lipidosis, 246–247, 248
Esophagostomy/endoscopic gastrostomy,
    tube placement in, in feline hepatic
    lipidosis, sedation/anesthesia for, 246
ESWT. See *Extracorporeal shock wave therapy
    (ESWT).*
Etodolac, for osteoarthritic pain in geriatric
    dogs and cats, 660
Etomidate
    for emergencies, 440
    for geriatric patients, 577
Excessive vocalization, in geriatric pets,
    684–685

Excision arthroplasty, for joint disorders, 1367–1368

Exercise(s)
  active
    in acute spinal cord injury rehabilitation, 1396–1398
    in chronic spinal cord injury rehabilitation, 1401–1402
    in peripheral nerve injury rehabilitation, 1404–1405
  aquatic, biomechanics of, 1281–1282
  balance, in acute spinal cord injury rehabilitation, 1398
  coordination, in acute spinal cord injury rehabilitation, 1398
  passive
    in chronic spinal cord injury rehabilitation, 1401
    in peripheral nerve injury rehabilitation, 1404
  passive range-of-motion
    in acute spinal cord injury rehabilitation, 1395–1396
    in peripheral nerve injury rehabilitation, 1404
  reflexive
    in chronic spinal cord injury rehabilitation, 1401
    in peripheral nerve injury rehabilitation, 1404
  sit-to-stand
    in acute spinal cord injury rehabilitation, 1397
    in chronic spinal cord injury rehabilitation, 1402
  therapeutic, biomechanics of, 1277–1282

Exercise modification, biomechanics of, 1274–1277

Exocrine pancreas, biochemical testing of geriatric patients effects on, 549–550

Exodontia, **963–985**
  in infection control, 966
  in pain management, 963–966
  preoperative considerations, 963
  simple and surgical, equipment for, 966–972
    dental elevators, 970
    extraction forceps, 972
    for controlling hemorrhage, 969
    for elevating mucoperiosteum, 966
    for grasping tissue, 969
    for holding mouth open, 970
    for incising tissue, 966
    for removing bone, 969
    for removing soft tissue from bony defects, 969
    for retracting soft tissue, 967–968
    irrigation-related, 970
    scissors, 970
    suturing mucosal incisions, 970
  tooth extraction, 972–984. See also *Tooth extraction.*

Extracorporeal shock wave(s), characteristics of, 1346–1347

Extracorporeal shock wave therapy (ESWT), 1345–1350
  application of, 1348–1350
  biologic effects of, 1347–1348
  in dogs, 1348
  indications for, 1345–1346
  precautions with, 1350

Extraction(s), surgical, **963–985**. See also *Exodontia; Tooth extraction.*

Eye(s), feline infectious peritonitis effects on, 49

F

Facial innervation, 1044–1045

Facilitated standing, in rehabilitation of medical and acute care patients, 1419–1420

Fear, in geriatric pets, 683–684

Fece(s), polymerase chain reaction in, in feline infectious peritonitis, 59

Feline coronavirus antibody–positive cats, healthy, treatment of, 62

Feline coronavirus antigen, in effusion, immunofluorescence staining of, 60

Feline coronavirus infection
  clinical findings in, 46
  endemic, multiple-cat households with, management of, 67
  enteric, pathogenesis of, 44

Feline coronavirus–induced enteritis, treatment of, 62

Feline dental resorptive lesions, **943–962**
  described, 943–944
  diagnosis of, 944–947
  prevention of, 958–960
  radiographic imaging of, 947–952
  treatment of, 952–958

Feline endocrinopathies, **171–210**. See also specific types and *Endocrinopathy(ies), feline.*

Feline hepatic lipidosis (FHL), **225–269**
  amino acid supplementation in, 254–255
  ammonia testing in, 237
  appetite stimulants for, 249–250
  blood tests in, 236–239
  body condition assessment in, 259
  L-carnitine supplementation in, 254

clinical characteristics of, 229–231
clinicopathologic features of, 231–235
diagnostic imaging in, 239–240
drugs to avoid in, 259–261
esophagostomy tube in, 246–247, 248
fat-soluble vitamin supplementation in,
    253–254
feeding regimen in, 248–249
fluid and electrolyte therapy for,
    242–244
gastrostomy tube in, 247–248
liver biopsy in, 240–242
monitoring in, 261, 263
nasogastric tubes in, 246
nutritional recommendations for,
    244–245
nutritional support for, 245–248
oral "force" alimentation in, 245–246
pathomechanisms of, 225–229
refeeding phenomenon in, 258–259
thiamine in, 250–251
thiol antioxidant supplementation in,
    255–258
treatment of
    guidelines for, 262–263
    supplements in, success rate of,
        263–265
trypsin-like immunoreactivity in, 239
UDCA in, 258
urine bile acids in, 236
urine tests in, 236–239
vitamin B$_{12}$ in, 237–239, 251–253
vitamin E in, 253–254
vitamin K$_1$ in, 253
vitamin supplementation in, fat-soluble,
    253–254
vomiting in, management of, 249
water-soluble vitamin supplementation
    in, 250–253
Feline hyperthyroidism, 635–641
    clinical features of, 635–636
    described, 635
    diagnosis of, 636–638
    prognosis of, 641
    treatment of, 639–641
Feline inductive odontogenic tumor, clinical
    presentation of, 1015
Feline infectious peritonitis (FIP), **39–79**,
    631–632
    abdominal changes in, 48–49
    antibody-dependent enhancement in, 46
    causes of, 40–41
    clinical findings in, 46–50
    described, 39
    development of, 45–46
    diagnosis of, 50–61
        antibody antigen complex
            detection in, 59

antibody measurement in, 55–58
antigen detection in, 59–61
antigen in tissue in, 60–61
coagulation parameters in, 51
complete blood cell counts in, 51
CSF tests in, 55
effusion fluid tests in, 53–55
laboratory changes in, 51–55
polymerase chain reaction in,
    58–59
serum chemistry in, 51–53
effusions in, 47–48
epidemiology of, 41–43
histology of, 61
mutation occurrence in, 44–45
neurologic signs in, 50
ocular changes in, 49
pathogenesis of, 43–46
prevalence of, 41–42
prevention of, 66–70
    in breeding catteries, 68–69
    in shelters, 69
    vaccination in, 69–70
public health considerations related to,
    70
thoracic organ changes in, 48–49
transmission of, 42
treatment of, 61–65
    after contact, 66–67
    antiviral chemotherapy in, 63–65
    early weaning and isolation in,
        67–68
    feline interferon-w in, 65
    human interferon-α in, 64–65
    in multiple-cat households with
        endemic feline coronavirus,
        67
    ribavirin in, 63–64
    symptomatic, 62–63
virus shedding in, 43
Feline interferon-w, for feline infectious
    peritonitis, 65
Feline interstitial/idiopathic cystitis, 150–159.
    See also *Interstitial/idiopathic cystitis, feline.*
Feline lower urinary tract disease, recent
    concepts in, **147–171**. See also *Urinary
    tract disease, lower, feline.*
Feline odontoclastic resorptive lesions
    (FORL)
    causes of, update on, **913–942**
    histologic features of, 913–915
    increased vitamin D activity with,
        921–929
    local trauma and, 929–932
    radiologic features of, 913–915
    treatment of
        vitamin D in, 933–936
        vitamin D metabolites in, 933–936

Feline patients, pain in, management of, **129–146.** See also *Pain, in feline patients, management of.*

Feline spongiform encephalopathy, 118–121

Feliway, for interstitial/idiopathic cystitis, 156–157

Femoral capital physeal separations, rehabilitation for, 1363

Fentanyl
  for oral and dental procedures, 1051–1052
  for pain in feline patients, 136
  for trauma patients, 486

Fetal monitoring, 406–407

FHL. See *Feline hepatic lipidosis (FHL).*

Fibrosarcoma, 1161–1162
  clinical presentation of, 1013

Fibrosis(es), hepatic, in dogs, 621–622

FIP. See *Feline infectious peritonitis (FIP).*

Fitness, defined, 1427

Fitness training, of sporting dogs, 1427–1432

Flexor reflex stimulation
  in acute spinal cord injury rehabilitation, 1396
  in chronic spinal cord injury rehabilitation, 1401
  in peripheral nerve injury rehabilitation, 1404

Flexor tendon contracture, rehabilitation for, 1384

Fluid(s)
  abdominal, in acute abdomen, 385–387
    biochemical analysis and culture of, 388–390
    cytologic analysis of, 387–388
  in emergencies, 521
    pediatric, 423

Fluid and electrolyte therapy, for feline hepatic lipidosis, 242–244

Force delivery, in small animal orthodontics, 885

Force plate systems, in lameness evaluation, 1266–1267

Foreign bodies, corneal, 474–475

FORL. See *Feline odontoclastic resorptive lesions (FORL).*

Fracture(s)
  articular, rehabilitation for, 1358–1359
  described, 1148
  in geriatric dogs and cats, 663–673
    management of
      bone grafts in, 665
  surgical approach to, 664–665
  stabilization of, 665–673
    external fixators in, 672–673
    interlocking nails in, 665–668
    plate-rod hybrid in, 668–672
  lateral humeral condylar, rehabilitation for, 1363–1364
  long bone, rehabilitation for, 1364–1365
  management of, **1139–1157,** 1156
    bone biomechanics related to, 1145–1147
    bone grafts in, 1153–1155
    bone healing in, 1147–1148
    decisions in, 1152–1153
    general principles of, 1148–1151
    of problem fractures, 1156
    pain-related, 1143–1144
    postoperative, 1155–1156
      decisions in, 1155–1156
    preoperative patient assessment in, 1139–1142
    prophylactic antibiotics in, 1145
    referral *vs.,* 1151–1152
    temporary preoperative stabilization in, 1144–1145
  mandibular
    bilateral, repair of, 994–1006
    with maxillary fracture, repair of, 999
  mandibular body, repair of, 990–994
  mandibular condylar, repair of, 997
  mandibular ramus, repair of, 995–996
  maxillary, repair of, 997–999
  maxillofacial, in juvenile veterinary dentistry, 814–815
  multiple limb, rehabilitation for, 1365
  of lateral fabella, canine lameness due to, 1245
  pelvic
    bilateral, rehabilitation for, 1365
    rehabilitation for, 1365
  physeal, rehabilitation for, 1359–1364. See also *Physeal fractures.*
  referral for *vs.* repair of, 1151–1152
  rehabilitation for, 1357–1365
    articular fractures, 1358–1359
    described, 1357–1358
    physeal fractures, 1359–1364. See also *Physeal fractures.*

Fractured primary teeth, in juvenile veterinary dentistry, 795–796

Fractured teeth, 711

Fragmented medial coronoid process, 1128

Friction, anchorage and, in control of tooth movement in small animal orthodontics, 874–876

Fungal osteomyelitis, 1101–1102

Fungus(i), zoonoses due to, control of, 14–15

G

Gabapentin
 for oral and dental procedures, 1054, 1057
 in emergency patients, 511–512

Gait
 assessment of
  in acute spinal cord injury, 1392
  kinematic, 1265–1266
   research on, 1267–1269
  kinetic, 1263–1265
   research on, 1267–1269
  CCLR effects on, research in, 1268–1269
 examination of, in emergency patients, 304
 normal, 1267–1268

Gas exchange, 307–308

Gastric volvulus, analgesia and chemical restraint for, 501–503

Gastrointestinal pain, analgesia and chemical restraint for, 501

Gastrointestinal system, in geriatric patients, biochemical testing effects on, 550–552

Gastrostomy tube, in feline hepatic lipidosis, 247–248

General anesthesia
 defined, 437
 for emergencies, 436–441

General nursing care, in rehabilitation of medical and acute care patients, 1413–1414

Genital zoonoses, control of, 16–17

Genitourinary system, examination of, in emergency patients, 300–301

Geriatric care programs
 benefits of, 753
 client compliance for, 748–749
 defining of, 747–748
 financial benefits of, 752–753
 for veterinarians, **743–753**
  benefits of, 753
  Metzger Animal Hospital five-step program, 750–752

Geriatric pets. See also *Aging.*
 anesthesia for, **571–580**. See also *Anesthesia/anesthetics, for geriatric patients.*
 behavior problems in, **675–698**. See also *Behavior problems, in geriatric pets.*
 biochemical testing of, **537–556**

blood substitutes in, 543
 cardiovascular system–related, 555
 endocrine system–related, 552–554
 gastrointestinal system–related, 550–552
 group-specific variables in, 540
 hemolysis in, 541–542
 hepatic system–related, 546–549
 hyperbilirubinemia in, 542
 icterus in, 542
 interfering substances in, solutions to, 543–544
 laboratory methodology and substance interference in, 540–541
 laboratory-specific variables in, 539
 lipemia in, 541–542
 musculoskeletal system–related, 554–555
 organ system–oriented biochemical profiling in, 544
 oxyglobin in, 543
 pancreas-related, 549–550
 reference intervals in, establishment of, 538–539
 urinary system–related, 544–546
clinical pathology in, **537–556**
defining of, 744–745
dentistry for, client compliance in, 749–750
diet-sensitive conditions in, 721–734
 diabetes mellitus, 728–731
 obesity, 724–728
 osteoarthritis, 731–734
 weight loss, 721–724
diseases of, systemic, 746–747
drug monitoring screens for, 749
heart diseases in, dogs, **597–615**. See also *Heart diseases, geriatric, in dogs.*
liver disease in, **617–634**
medical conditions in, behavior effects of, 678–679
nutrition for, **713–741**
 evaluation of, 718–721
  dietary-related, 719–721
  feeding management–related, 721
  patient-related, 719
orthopedic problems in, dogs and cats, **655–674**. See also *Orthopedic problems, geriatric, in dogs and cats.*
pharmacology related to, **557–569**. See also *Pharmacology, geriatric.*
physiology of, 571–574
 cardiovascular system, 572
 CNS, 573–574
 hepatic system, 573

Geriatric pets (*continued*)
    pulmonary system, 572
    renal system, 573
    preanesthetic sedation of, 574–576
    preanesthetic testing for, 749
    preoperative assessment of, 574
    thyroid disorders in, **635–653.** See also
        Thyroid disorders, in geriatric patients.
    vaccines for, for client compliance, 750
    veterinary dentistry in, **699–712.** See
        also *Veterinary dentistry, in geriatric*
        patients.

Gingiva, functions of, 821–822

Gingival contouring, in small animal
    orthodontics, 884

Gingivostomatitis, **891–911**
    evaluation of, 895–896
    pathogenesis of, 896–899
    pathologic findings in, 891–895
    treatment of, 899–907
        anti-inflammatory medications in,
            904–905
        antimicrobials in, 902–904
        cyclosporine in, 906–907
        human immunoglobulin in, 906
        laser thermoablation in, 901–902
        oral surgery in, 901
        plasmapheresis in, 905
        tonsillectomy in, 901

Gland(s), salivary, in dogs and cats, 775

Glaucoma, 458–461
    causes of, 458
    prognosis of, 461
    secondary, causes of, 458
    treatment of, 459–461

Glucocorticoid(s)
    for feline hepatic lipidosis, avoidance of,
        259–260
    for osteoarthritic pain in geriatric dogs
        and cats, 661

Graft(s), conjunctival, 474

Group-specific variables, in biochemical
    testing of geriatric patients, 540

Growth factors, in wound healing, 1460–1461

Gutta percha application, for endodontic
    disease, 859

H

H blockers, in emergency situations, 521

Halothane, in anesthesia maintenance in
    geriatric patients, 578

Head, examination of, in emergency patients,
    292–293, 303–304

Head trauma, in young animals, 431–432

Heart diseases, geriatric, in dogs, **597–615**
    approach to, 604–605
    auscultation in, 605–607
    blood chemistry in, 613–614
    bronchial breath sounds in, 607
    causes of, 598–599
    crackles in, 607
    dyspnea in, 607–608
    ECG in, 611–613
    echocardiography in, 613
    mitral regurgitation and, 599–603
    percussion in, 608
    pharmacologic classification of, 603–604
    prevalence of, 598
    radiography in, 608–611
    tachypnea in, 607–608

Heat, 1321–1327

Hemangiosarcoma, 1167–1168

Hemodynamic monitoring, for perfusion
    abnormalities in emergency patients,
    325, 327

Hemolysis, in biochemical testing of geriatric
    patients, 541–542

Hemorrhage
    after oral tumor excision, 1033
    as reproductive emergency, 407
    in emergency patients, 332–334

Hepatic cirrhosis, in dogs, 621–622

Hepatic diseases. See *Liver diseases.*

Hepatic failure, in geriatric patients,
    pharmacology related to, 561–562

Hepatic fibrosis, in dogs, 621–622

Hepatic insufficiency, in geriatric patients,
    pharmacology related to, 561–562

Hepatic system
    biochemical testing of geriatric patients
        effects on, 546–549
    of geriatric patients, physiology of, 573

Hepatitis, pyogranulomatous, in cats,
    631–632

Hepatocutaneous syndrome, in dogs,
    622–626

Hepatoencephalopathy, in dogs, 627–628

Hepatopathy(ies)
    chronic infiltrative, in dogs, 622
    chronic inflammatory, in dogs, 617–621

Hernia(s), diaphragmatic, analgesia and
    chemical restraint for, 493

High-dose dexamethasone suppression test, in
    hyperadrenocorticism, 192

Hip dysplasia, 1122–1126
    causes of, 1122

clinical signs of, 1123
diagnosis of, 1123–1124
gait analysis research in, 1269
pathogenesis of, 1122
prognosis of, 1126
rehabilitation for, 1376–1378
signalment of, 1122
treatment of, 1124–1126
Hip joint, mobilization of, 1304–1308
Hip luxation, 1369–1370
management of, 1184–1188
Hock, osteochondrosis of
prognosis of, 1120
treatment of, 1119
Hock luxation, management of, 1193–1196
Hock shear injuries, 1371
House soiling, by geriatric pets, 683
Human immunoglobulin, for
gingivostomatitis, 906
Human interferon-α, for feline infectious
peritonitis, 64–65
Hydration state, in assessment of emergency
patients, 290–291
Hydromorphone
for oral and dental procedures, 1052
for trauma patients, 486, 487
Hyperadrenocorticism, feline, 189–195
clinical signs of, 190
diagnosis of, 190–193
combination test in, 193
corticotropin stimulation test in,
192
CT in, 193
endogenous corticotropin
measurement in, 193
high-dose dexamethasone
suppression test in, 192
low-dose dexamethasone
suppression test in, 191
MRI in, 193
ultrasonography in, 193
urine cortisol-to-creatinine ratio in,
191
pathogenesis of, 189–190
prognosis of, 195
treatment of, 194–195
Hyperaldosteronism, primary, feline,
196–197
Hyperbilirubinemia, in biochemical testing of
geriatric patients, 542
Hyperextension, carpal, 1370
Hyperparathyroidism, feline, 200–201
Hyperthyroidism, feline, 171–179, 635–641.
See also *Feline hyperthyroidism.*

clinical signs of, 171–172
diagnosis of, 172–175
retesting in, 174
thyroid-stimulating hormone
response test in, 175
thyrotropin-releasing hormone
stimulation test in, 174
trial course of antithyroid therapy
in, 175
triiodothyronine suppression test
in, 174
pathogenesis of, 171
prognosis of, 179
treatment of, 175–179
medical, 175–177
percutaneous intrathyroid ethanol
injections in, 178
percutaneous ultrasound-guided
radiofrequency heat ablation
in, 178–179
radioiodine in, 178
thyroidectomy in, 177–178
Hypertrophic osteodystrophy, 1111–1113
Hyphema
causes of, 465
prognosis of, 465
treatment of, 464–465
Hypoadrenocorticism, feline, 199–200
Hypoglycemia, in young animals, 426
Hypoparathyroidism, feline, 201–202
Hypoperfusion
classification of, 320
consequences of, 320–321
in emergency patients, treatment of,
331
local, assessment of, in emergency
patients, 330–331
Hyposamotropism, feline, 187–188
clinical signs of, 187–188
diagnosis of, 188
pathogenesis of, 187
prognosis of, 188
treatment of, 188
Hypothyroidism
canine, 641–649. See also *Canine
hypothyroidism.*
feline, 179–181
clinical signs of, 179–180
diagnosis of, 180–181
pathogenesis of, 179
prognosis of, 181
treatment of, 181
Hypovolemia
in emergency patients, treatment of,
331–332
in young animals, 426–428

Hypovolemic shock, nonhemorrhagic, in emergency patients, 334

Hypoxemia, causes of, 308–309

I

Icterus, in biochemical testing of geriatric patients, 542

Immunofluorescence staining, of feline coronavirus antigen in effusion, 60

Immunoglobulin(s), human, for gingivostomatitis, 906

Immunoreactivity, trypsin-like, in feline hepatic lipidosis, 239

Impaction, soft tissue, in juvenile veterinary dentistry, 801–802

Impulse, 1260–1261

Incisivectomy, 1027

Incline capping, in small animal orthodontics, 882–884

Infant(s), analgesia for, 506–507

Infection(s)
  of skeletal system, **1093–1110**. See also *Skeletal system, infections of.*
  oral, control of, exodontia in, 966
  periodontal, 823–824

Infectious diseases
  feline, in shelters
    described, 21–22
    prevention of, **21–37**
      air quality in, 29
      disease recognition in, 28–29
      disinfection in, 25–27
      environmental management in, 22
      host factors in, 30–34
      nutrition in, 33–34
      population density in, 22–25
      principles of, 22–34
      sanitation in, 25–27
      segregation and animal flow in, 27–28
      vaccination in, 32–33
  of CNS, **103–128**. See also *Central nervous system (CNS), infectious diseases of.*

Inflammatory liver disease, in cats, 629–631

Infraspinatus contracture, rehabilitation for, 1383

Infrasponatus bursal ossification, canine lameness due to, 1239–1240

Inhalant(s), for geriatric patients, 577

Injection site sarcomas, 1167

Insulin, for diabetes mellitus in cats, 216–217

Insulin glargine, for diabetes mellitus in cats, 216–217
  urine glucose measurements during, 221

Integument, examination of, in emergency patients, 301–302

Interferon-α, human, for feline infectious peritonitis, 64–65

Interstitial/idiopathic cystitis, feline, 150–159
  diagnosis of, 152–154
  pathophysiology of, 150–152
  treatment of, 154–159
    amitriptyline in, 158–159
    dietary modifications in, 156–157
    environmental modification in, 156
    Feliway in, 156–157
    oral GAG replacement in, 159

Intra-arterial catheter placement, analgesia and chemical restraint for, 504

Intravenous catheter placement, analgesia and chemical restraint for, 504

Iodine, for feline hyperthyroidism, 177

Isoflurane, in anesthesia maintenance in geriatric patients, 578

J

Joint(s). See specific type, e.g., *Shoulder joint;* specific types, e.g., *Cubital joint.*
  conditions involving
    rehabilitation for, 1366–1381
    surgery for
      amputation, 1368–1369
      arthrodesis, 1368
      excision arthroplasty, 1367–1368
      general guidelines, 1366–1369
  tumors of, 1166–1167

Joint diseases, 1372–1381
  in geriatric dogs and cats, 655–663. See also specific disorder, e.g., *Osteoarthritis.*
  rehabilitation for, 1372–1381
    CCLR, 1379–1381
    elbow dysplasia, 1375–1376
    hip dysplasia, 1376–1378
    Legg-Calvé-Perthes disease, 1378
    osteoarthritis, 1372–1373
    osteochondritis dissecans, 1373–1375
    patellar luxation, 1378–1379

Joint disruption, 1369–1371

Joint luxations, 1369–1370

Joint mobilization, **1287–1316**
  basic principles of, 1289–1291

clinical environment for, 1292–1295
contraindications to, 1289
described, 1287–1288
indications for, 1288
of carpus, 1301–1303
of elbow joint, 1299–1301
of hip joint, 1304–1308
of shoulder joint, 1295–1299
of spine, 1311–1315
of stifle joint, 1308–1311
precautions with, 1289

Joint motion, biomechanics of, 1270–1271

Juvenile veterinary dentistry, **789–817.** See also *Veterinary dentistry, juvenile.*

K

Ketamine
for pain in feline patients, 140–141
for trauma patients, 487
in emergency patients, 440, 511

Ketoacidosis, in cats, 214–215

Kinetic(s)
angular, 1261–1262
linear, 1259–1261

L

Laboratory-specific variables, in biochemical testing of geriatric patients, 539

Laceration(s), corneal, 473

Lactate, measurement of, for perfusion abnormalities in emergency patients, 327–329

Lameness
canine
abductor pollicis longus tenosynovitis and, 1241–1243
causes of, **1239–1245**
incomplete ossification of caudal glenoid and, 1240–1241
infrasponatus bursal ossification and, 1239–1240
lateral fabella fracture and, 1245
proximal long digital extensor tendon displacement and, 1243–1244
evaluation of
force plate systems, 1266–1267
kinematic assessment, 1265–1266
kinetic assessment, 1263–1265
motion analysis systems, 1266–1267

Laser(s)
cold. See *Low-level laser therapy (LLLT).*
described, 1335–1336
low-level, biologic effects of, 1338

properties of, 1336–1337

Laser therapy, low-level, 1335–1345. See *Low-level laser therapy (LLLT).*

Laser thermoablation, for gingivostomatitis, 901–902

Lateral fabella fracture, canine lameness due to, 1245

Lateral humeral condylar fractures, rehabilitation for, 1363–1364

Legg-Calvé-Perthes disease, 1120–1122
rehabilitation for, 1378

Lesion(s), resorptive, dental, feline, **943–962.** See also *Feline dental resorptive lesions.*

Levers, in biomechanics, 1258–1259

Lidocaine, in emergency patients, 511

Ligament(s), periodontal, 873

Linear kinetics, 1259–1261

Lipemia, in biochemical testing of geriatric patients, 541–542

Lipidosis
feline hepatic, **225–269.** See also *Feline hepatic lipidosis (FHL).*
secondary hepatic, in cats, 632

Liver. See also under *Hepatic.*

Liver biopsy, in feline hepatic lipidosis, 240–242

Liver diseases
in cats. See also specific disease and *Cat(s), liver diseases in.*
in dogs. See also specific disease and *Dog(s), liver diseases in.*
in geriatric pets, **617–634.** See also *Geriatric pets, liver disease in.*

Liver failure, in geriatric patients, pharmacology related to, 561–562

Long bone fractures, rehabilitation for, 1364–1365

Long digital extensor muscle, tendon of, avulsion of, rehabilitation for, 1383–1384

Low-dose dexamethasone suppression test, in hyperadrenocorticism, 191

Lower respiratory injury, analgesia and chemical restraint for, 492–493

Lower urinary tract disease, feline, recent concepts in, **147–171.** See also *Urinary tract disease, lower, feline.*

Low-level laser(s), biologic effects of, 1338

Low-level laser therapy (LLLT), 1335–1345
application of, 1343–1345
bone and cartilage effects of, 1340–1341

Low-level laser (*continued*)
  described, 1335–1336
  for osteoarthritis, 1342–1343
  in analgesia and pain management,
      1341–1342
  in wound healing, 1338–1339
  spinal cord–related, 1343

Lung(s), diseases affecting, 313–315

Lymph nodes, examination of, in emergency
    patients, 302

M

Magnetic resonance imaging (MRI), in
    hyperadrenocorticism, 193

Malignant melanoma, clinical presentation of,
    1012

Malocclusion, in juvenile veterinary dentistry,
    792–795, 804–808

Mandibular body fracture, repair of, 990–994

Mandibular condylar fracture, repair of, 997

Mandibular fracture
  bilateral, repair of, 994–1006
  with maxillary fracture, repair of, 999

Mandibular nerve block, for oral and dental
    procedures, 1047–1050

Mandibular ramus fracture, repair of,
    995–996

Mandibulectomy, 1018–1026
  bilateral rostral, 1021–1023
  caudal, 1024
  classification of, 1019
  described, 1018
  rim excision in, 1019–1020
  segmental, 1023–1024
  total unilateral, 1024–1026
  unilateral rostral, 1021

Manual therapy, **1287–1316.** See also *Joint
    mobilization.*

Massage, in rehabilitation of medical and
    acute care patients, 1420–1421

Master point coating, for endodontic disease,
    859

Mastitis, 409–410

Maxillary fracture
  repair of, 997–999
  with mandibular fracture, repair of, 999

Maxillary nerve block, for oral and dental
    procedures, 1046–1047

Maxillectomy, 1026–1030
  bilateral rostral, 1027–1029
  caudal, 1029–1030
  central, 1029–1030
  classification of, 1026–1027

  described, 1026
  incisivectomy, 1027
  total unilateral, 1029–1030
  unilateral rostral, 1027–1029

Maxillofacial fracture(s), in juvenile
    veterinary dentistry, 814–815

Maxillofacial fracture repairs, **985–1007**
  before dentistry, 985–987
  complications of, 1001–1004
  emergency procedures in, 985
  for bilateral mandibular fracture,
      994–1006
  for condylar neck fracture, 997
  for mandibular body fracture, 990–994
  for mandibular condylar fracture, 997
  for mandibular ramus fracture, 995–996
  for maxillary and mandibular fractures,
      999
  for maxillary fracture, 997–999
  for symphyseal separation, 988–990
  in edentulous patients, 999–1001
  planning for, 985
  since dentistry, 987–988
  stabilization prior to, 985
  symphyseal separation, 988–990

Medetomidine, for trauma patients, 486, 487

Medial coronoid process, fragmented,
    rehabilitation for, 1375

Medical patients
  general nursing care for, 1413–1414
  rehabilitation in, **1411–1426.** See also
      Rehabilitation, in medical patients.
  systemic illness in, metabolic and tissue
      changes associated with, 1413

Melanoma(s), malignant, clinical presentation
    of, 1012

Meloxicam, for osteoarthritic pain in geriatric
    dogs and cats, 660

Mental nerve block, for oral and dental
    procedures, 1047

Mental state, examination of, in emergency
    patients, 288–289, 303

Meperidine
  for pain in feline patients, 134
  for trauma patients, 486

Metacarpal luxation, management of,
    1178–1180

Metacarpophalangeal luxation, 1371

Metastatic bone tumors, 1165–1166

Metatarsal luxation, management of, 1196

Metatarsophalangeal luxation, 1371

Methadone, for oral and dental procedures,
    1051

Methimazole, for feline hyperthyroidism, 176

N-Methyl-D-aspartate receptor blockers, for oral and dental procedures, 1054

Methylprednisolone, for gingivostomatitis, 905

Metzger Animal Hospital five-step program, 750–752

Microalbuminuria, in dogs and cats, 590–594
 causes of, 591–593

Microglossia, 790–791

Midazolam, for trauma patients, 486, 487

Mitral regurgitation, in aging dogs, heart diseases related to, 599–603

Mobilization, in rehabilitation of medical and acute care patients, 1418–1420

Moments, in biomechanics, 1255–1258

Monochromatic near-infrared photo energy, in wound healing, 1460

Morphine
 for oral and dental procedures, 1051
 for pain in feline patients, 134

Motion analysis systems, in lameness evaluation, 1266–1267

MRI. See *Magnetic resonance imaging (MRI)*.

Mucous membrane, color of, in assessment of emergency patients, 289, 296

Multilobular osteochondrosarcoma, 1163–1164

Multiple myeloma, 1164–1165

Muscle(s), in dogs and cats, 773–775

Musculoskeletal system
 biochemical testing of geriatric patients effects on, 554–555
 examination of, in emergency patients, 301

Musculoskeletal tumors, malignant, of dogs and cats, **1159–1172**
 appendicular osteosarcoma, 1159–1161
 axial osteosarcoma, 1162–1163
 chondrosarcoma, 1162
 fibrosarcoma, 1161–1162
 hemangiosarcoma, 1167–1168
 injection site sarcomas, 1167
 joint tumors, 1166–1167
 metastatic bone tumors, 1165–1166
 multilobular tumor of bone, 1163–1164
 multiple myeloma, 1164–1165
 osteosarcoma, 1161
 pelvic tumors, 1164
 plasma cell tumors, 1164
 rib tumors, 1164
 soft tissue tumors, 1167–1168
 solitary osseous plasmacytoma, 1165

 synovial cell sarcoma, 1166
 vertebral tumors, 1164

Myeloma, multiple, 1164–1165

N

Naloxone, for oral and dental procedures, 1053

Nasogastric tubes, in feline hepatic lipidosis, 246

Neck, examination of, in emergency patients, 292–293, 303–304

Negative pressure wound therapy, in wound healing, 1459–1460

Neonatal resuscitation, 406

Neonate(s)
 analgesia for, 506–507
 respiratory distress of, 429–430

Neoplasia
 in cats, 632
 in dogs, 628–629

Nerve(s), in dogs and cats, 775–776

Nerve blocks
 for oral and dental procedures
  caudal infraorbital, 1045
  cranial, 1045
  mandibular, for oral and dental procedures, 1047–1050
  maxillary, for oral and dental procedures, 1046–1047
  mental, for oral and dental procedures, 1047

Neuritis, optic, 478–479

Neurologic compromise, analgesia and chemical restraint for, 489

Neurologic diseases, in cats, prevalence of, 103–104

Neurologic patients, rehabilitation for, **1389–1409**
 acute spinal cord injury, 1394–1399
 chronic spinal cord injury, 1401–1402
 neuromuscular disease, 1406–1407
 peripheral nerve injury, 1403–1405

Neurologic signs, in feline infectious peritonitis, 50

Neurologic system, examination of, in emergency patients, 302–304

Neuromuscular disease
 assessment of, 1405–1406
 pathophysiology of, 1405
 prognosis of, 1406
 recovery from, 1406
 rehabilitation for, 1406–1407

Neuromuscular stimulation
  in acute spinal cord injury rehabilitation, 1399
  in peripheral nerve injury rehabilitation, 1405
Newborn(s). See *Neonate(s)*.
Nocturnal restlessness, in geriatric pets, 684–685
Noncemented hip replacement systems, 1225–1227
Nonhemorrhagic hypovolemic shock, in emergency patients, 334
Nonsuppurative encephalitides of unknown cause, 113–117
Nonvital pulp therapy, for endodontic disease, 850–865
NSAIDs. See *Anti-inflammatory drugs, nonsteroidal*.
Nursing care, analgesia in, 512
Nursing mothers, analgesia for, 505–506
Nutraceutical(s), for osteoarthritic pain in geriatric dogs and cats, 662–663
Nutrient(s), aging effects on, 714–718
Nutrition
  aging effects on, 714–718
  for aging cats and dogs, **713–741**. See also *Geriatric pets, nutrition for*.
  for feline hepatic lipidosis, 244–245
  in feline infectious disease control in shelters, 33–34
Nutritional support
  for cognitive dysfunction syndrome, 692–693
  for feline hepatic lipidosis, 245–248

O

Obesity, in geriatric patients, nutrition related to, 724–728
Occlusal pits, deep, in juvenile veterinary dentistry, 811
Odontoma
  clinical presentation of, 1015
  in juvenile veterinary dentistry, 809–811
Ophthalmic emergencies, **455–480**. See also specific disorders, e.g., *Anterior uveitis*.
  anterior uveitis, 456–458
  blindness, sudden, 476
  conjunctival grafts for, 474
  conjunctivitis, 475–476
  corneal foreign bodies, 474–475
  corneal laceration, 473
  corneal perforation, 471–472
  corneal ulcers, 465–471
  descemetocele, 471

  enrofloxacin for, 479
  glaucoma, 458–461
  hyphema, 464–465
  optic neuritis, 478–479
  retinal separation, 476–478
  SARDS, 478
  traumatic proptosis, 462–464
Opioid(s)
  for oral and dental procedures, 1050–1053
  for pain in feline patients, 132–137
  for trauma patients, 486, 487
  in emergency patients, 509–510
  in preanesthetic sedation of geriatric patients, 575
Optic neuritis, 478–479
Oral "force" alimentation, in feline hepatic lipidosis, 245–246
Oral hypoglycemic drugs, for diabetes mellitus in cats, 215–216
Oral neoplasia, 711
Oral procedures, regional anesthesia and analgesia for, **1041–1058**. See also *Dental procedures, regional anesthesia and analgesia for*.
Oral tumors, **1009–1039**
  biopsy of, 1011–1012
  clinical presentation of
    ameloblastoma, 1014
    feline inductive odontogenic tumor, 1015
    fibrosarcoma, 1013
    malignant melanoma, 1012
    odontoma, 1015
    osteosarcoma, 1013
    peripheral odontogenic fibroma, 1014
    squamous cell carcinoma, 1012–1013
  clinical staging of, 1009–1010
  diagnostic imaging of, 1010
  in juvenile veterinary dentistry, 815
  nonodontogenic, clinical presentation of, 1012–1013
  odontogenic, clinical presentation of, 1014–1015
  treatment of
    anesthetic management in, 1017
    appearance after, 1030–1033
    aseptic preparation in, 1018
    complications of, 1033–1036
    decision making in, 1015
    function following, 1030–1033
    mandibulectomy in, 1018–1026. See also *Mandibulectomy*.
    maxillectomy in, 1026–1030. See also *Maxillectomy*.

outcome following, 1030–1033
patient positioning in, 1018
postoperative care, 1030
preoperative considerations in,
1017–1018
prophylactic antibiotics in, 1017
surgical principles in, 1015–1017
Organ system–oriented biochemical profiling,
in biochemical testing of geriatric
patients, 544
Orthodontic(s), small animal
ancillary services related to, 887–888
appliances in current use, 879–884
force delivery in, 885
fundamentals of, **869–889**
gingival contouring in, 884
periodontal ligament, 873
periodontitis, 869–871
retainers in, 887
surgical intervention in, 885–887
tooth movement in
bodily movement or translation,
878
control of, 871–878
absolute anchorage in, 874
anchorage in, 873
friction and anchorage in,
874–876
reinforced anchorage in,
873
extrusion, 879
intrusion, 879
rate of, 877–878
rotation or torsion movement,
878–879
tipping, 878
types of, 878–879
Orthopedic patients, rehabilitation for,
1357–1388
fracture-related, 1357–1365. See also
Fracture(s), rehabilitation for.
joint-related, 1366–1381. See also *Joint
diseases, rehabilitation for.*
tendon-related, 1381–1386
Orthopedic problems, geriatric, in dogs and
cats, **655–674**
fractures, 663–673. See also *Fracture(s), in
geriatric dogs and cats.*
in postoperative period, 673
joint-related disorders, 655–663. See
also specific disorder and *Joint
disorders, in geriatric dogs and cats.*
Orthotic devices, 1443–1446
achieving desired outcomes through,
1444
degrees-of-freedom analysis for, 1444
prescriptions for, functional
considerations for, 1444

Osteoarthritis
diagnosis of, 1081
in geriatric dogs and cats, 655
diagnosis of, 655–656
treatment of, 656–663
carprofen in, 658–659
chondroprotective agents in,
661–662
deracoxib in, 659–660
etodolac in, 660
glucocorticoids in, 661
goals for, 656
meloxicam in, 660
NSAIDs in, 658–660
nutraceuticals in, 662–663
nutrition in, 731–734
steps in, 656
tepoxalin in, 660
LLLT for, 1342–1343
management of, 1082–1086
pathophysiology of, 1073–1080
rehabilitation for, 1372–1381
Osteochondritis dissecans,
1129–1130
rehabilitation for, 1373–1375
Osteochondrosarcoma, multilobular,
1163–1164
Osteochondrosis, 1115–1120
causes of, 1116
clinical signs of, 1117
described, 1115
diagnosis of, 1117
of cubital joint, 1117
of elbow
prognosis of, 1119
treatment of, 1118
of hock
prognosis of, 1120
treatment of, 1119
of scapulohumeral joint, 1117
of shoulder
prognosis of, 1119
treatment of, 1118
of stifle joint, 1117
prognosis of, 1119
treatment of, 1118–1119
of tibiotarsal joint, 1117–1118
pathogenesis of, 1116
prognosis of, 1119–1120
signalment of, 1115
treatment of, 1118–1119
Osteodystrophy, hypertrophic,
1111–1113
Osteomyelitis
acute, 1098–1099
acute hematogenous, 1096–1097
chronic, 1099–1101
fungal, 1101–1102

Osteosarcoma
  appendicular, in dogs, 1159–1161
  axial, in dogs, 1162–1163
  clinical presentation of, 1013
  in cats, 1161
Oxalate urolithiasis, feline, 164–166
Oxygen therapy, for respiratory distress,
    309–310
Oxygenation, systemic parameters of, in
    emergency patients, 329–330
Oxyglobin, in biochemical testing of geriatric
    patients, 543
Oxymorphone
  for oral and dental procedures, 1051
  for pain in feline patients, 134–135
  for trauma patients, 486

P

Pain
  abdominal, perception of, 375–376
  fracture-related, management of,
      1143–1144
  gastrointestinal, analgesia and chemical
      restraint for, 501
  generation of, process of, 1042–1044
  in assessment of emergency patients,
      291–292
  in feline patients
    assessment of, 129–131
    management of, **129–146**
        α-adrenoceptor agonists in,
            140
        analgesics in, 131–137
        buprenorphine in, 135–136
        butorphanol in, 133–134
        drug metabolism in, 131
        fentanyl in, 136
        ketamine in, 140–141
        local anesthetics in, 139–140
        meperidine in, 134
        morphine in, 134
        NSAIDs in, 137–139
        opioids in, 132–137
        oxymorphone in, 134–135
        tricyclic antidepressants in,
            141
  level of, in emergency conditions,
      481–484
  range of motion effects of, 1290–1291
  visceral, analgesia and chemical restraint
      for, 501
Pain management
  adjunct, in rehabilitation of medical and
      acute care patients, 1422–1424
  anesthesia/anesthetics in, 441–442
  exodontia in, 963–966
  LLLT in, 1341–1342

Palate(s), cleft, in juvenile veterinary
    dentistry, 791–792
Pancreas
  biochemical testing of geriatric patients
      effects on, 549–550
  exocrine, biochemical testing of geriatric
      patients effects on, 549–550
Pancreatitis
  analgesia and chemical restraint for,
      503–504
  biochemical testing of geriatric patients
      and, 549–550
Panosteitis, 1113–1115
Paraparesis, acute spinal cord injury and,
    prognosis and recovery, 1393–1394
Parturition, normal, 397–399
Passive exercises
  in chronic spinal cord injury
      rehabilitation, 1401
  in peripheral nerve injury rehabilitation,
      1404
Passive range-of-motion exercises
  in acute spinal cord injury rehabilitation,
      1395–1396
  in peripheral nerve injury rehabilitation,
      1404
Patellar luxation
  management of, 1188–1189
  rehabilitation for, 1378–1379
Patellar reflex stimulation
  in acute spinal cord injury rehabilitation,
      1396
  in chronic spinal cord injury
      rehabilitation, 1401
  in peripheral nerve injury rehabilitation,
      1404
Patient positioning, in rehabilitation of
    medical and acute care patients,
    1414–1415
Peak force, 1260
Peak vertical force, 1261
Pediatric emergencies, **421–434**
  cardiopulmonary cerebral resuscitation,
      430–431
  catheterization in, 421–422
  defined, 421
  dehydration, 426–428
  fluid requirements in, 423
  head trauma, 431–432
  hypoglycemia, 426
  hypovolemia, 426–428
  imaging in, 424–426
  initial examination in, 421–422
  laboratory values in, 423–424
  pharmacology in, 424–426

respiratory distress of the newborn, 429–430
sepsis, 428–429
Pediatric patients, analgesia for, 506–507
Pelvic fractures, bilateral, rehabilitation for, 1365
Pelvic limb, tendon conditions of, 1206–1207
Pelvis, tumors of, 1164
Pentoxifylline, for gingivostomatitis, 905
Percussion, in heart diseases in aging dogs, 608
Percutaneous intrathyroid ethanol injections, for feline hyperthyroidism, 178
Percutaneous ultrasound-guided radiofrequency heat ablation, for feline hyperthyroidism, 178–179
Perforation(s), corneal, 471–472
Perfusion
    clinical assessment of, in emergency patients, 321–324
    defined, 319
Perfusion abnormalities, in emergency patients, **319–342**
    arterial blood pressure monitoring for, 325–326
    cardiogenic shock, 336
    central venous pressure monitoring for, 326–327
    distributive shock, 334–336
    hemodynamic monitoring of, 325, 327
    hemorrhage, 332–334
    hypoperfusion
        classification of, 320
        consequences of, 320–321
        treatment of, 331
    hypovolemia, treatment of, 331–332
    lactate measurement for, 327–329
    local hypoperfusion assessment for, 330–331
    nonhemorrhagic hypovolemic shock, 334
    systemic oxygenation parameters, 329–330
Periodontal disease
    clinical effects of, 825–827
    environment for, 822–824
    pathologic effects of, 825–827
    prevention of, 831
    treatment of, 709–711, **819–836**
        described, 831–832
        prioritization in, 832–834
Periodontal infection, 823–824
Periodontal ligament, 873
Periodontal tissues, functions of, 820–822

Periodontic(s), in gold standard of veterinary oral health care, 784–786
Periodontitis, orthodontics and, 869–871
Periodontopathogen(s), described, 824–825
Peripheral nerve injury, 1402–1405
    assessment of, 1403
    pathophysiology of, 1402
    prognosis of, 1403
    recovery from, 1403
    rehabilitation for, 1403–1405
        active exercises, 1404–1405
        goals of, 1403–1404
        neuromuscular stimulation, 1405
        passive and reflexive exercises, 1404
        therapeutic modalities, 1405
Peripheral odontogenic fibroma, clinical presentation of, 1014
Peritonitis
    analgesia and chemical restraint for, 503–504
    feline infectious, **39–79**. See also *Feline infectious peritonitis (FIP)*.
    infectious, feline, 631–632
Persistent primary teeth, in juvenile veterinary dentistry, 798–800
Pes varus, 1130–1131
Phalangeal luxation, 1371
Pharmacology, geriatric, **557–569**
    cardiovascular disease and, 563
    dosage adjustments, 563–566
    hepatic insufficiency and, 561–562
    renal failure and, 560–561
    renal insufficiency and, 558–561
Pheochromocytoma, feline, 197–198
Phobia(s), in geriatric pets, 683–684
Physeal fractures, rehabilitation for, 1359–1364
    distal femoral physeal fractures, 1361–1363
Physical agent modalities, **1317–1333**
    cold (cryotherapy), 1317–1321
    electrical stimulation, 1327–1331
    heat, 1321–1327
Physical rehabilitation
    candidates for, 1249
    delivery of, 1253
    evaluation for, 1249
    introduction to, **1247–1254**
    philosophy of, 1248–1249
    plan of care in, development of, 1249–1253
Physical therapy, described, 1247–1248
Plasma cell tumors, 1164

Plasmapheresis, for gingivostomatitis, 905

Pleural space, diseases of, 315–316

Polymerase chain reaction, in feline infectious peritonitis diagnosis, 58–59

Postural response, examination of, in emergency patients, 304

Power, in biomechanics, 1263

Preanesthetic testing, for geriatric pets, client compliance in, 749

Prednisone, for gingivostomatitis, 905

Pregnancy, in dogs and cats, analgesia during, 510

Pressure sores, healing of, 1461–1468

Primary dental formulas, normal, 789

Primary hyperaldosteronism, feline, 196–197

Primary sex hormone–secreting adrenal tumors, feline, 195–196

Primary teeth
    delayed eruption of, in juvenile veterinary dentistry, 796–798
    fractured, in juvenile veterinary dentistry, 795–796
    persistent, in juvenile veterinary dentistry, 798–800

Problem-oriented medical record, in global assessment of emergency patients, 286

Prolapse, uterine, as reproductive emergency, 408–409

Propofol
    for emergencies, 438–439
    for feline hepatic lipidosis, avoidance of, 260
    for geriatric patients, 577–578

Proprioception, in conditioning of sporting dogs, 1430–1431

Proptosis, traumatic, 462–464
    enucleation of, 464
    long-term complications of, 463–464
    prognosis of, 464
    surgical procedure for, 462–463

Prosthetics, 1445–1446

Protein needs, aging effects on, 716–718

Proteinuria
    as diagnostic marker of early chronic renal disease, 589–590
    implications of, 593–594

Protozoal diseases, enteric, **81–88**
    clinical complaints associated with, 82–83
    diagnosis of, 83–84
    distribution of, 81–82
    pathogenesis of, 82

prevention of, 86
transmission of, 81–82
treatment of, 84–86
zoonotic considerations in, 86

Proximal long digital extensor tendon, displacement of, canine lameness due to, 1243–1244

Pulmonary system, of geriatric patients, physiology of, 572

Pulse quality, in assessment of emergency patients, 290

Pulse rate, in assessment of emergency patients, 290

Pupil(s), examination of, in emergency patients, 304

Pyogranulomatous hepatitis, in cats, 631–632

Pyometra, 412–417

R

Radial nerve stimulation, in peripheral nerve injury rehabilitation, 1404

Radiography
    in heart diseases in aging dogs, 608–611
    in tooth extraction, 973
    of feline dental resorptive lesions, 947–952

Radioiodine, for feline hyperthyroidism, 178

Radiology, in gold standard of veterinary oral health care, 783–784

Range of motion
    in rehabilitation of medical and acute care patients, 1418–1419
    pain effects on, 1290–1291

Ranitidine, in emergency situations, 521

Reactive oxygen species, in cognitive decline, 690–692

Rechecks, in gold standard of veterinary oral health care, 787

Reconditioning, in rehabilitation of sporting dogs, 1436–1437

Refeeding phenomenon, in feline hepatic lipidosis, 258–259

Reflexive exercises
    in chronic spinal cord injury rehabilitation, 1401
    in peripheral nerve injury rehabilitation, 1404

Regurgitation, mitral, in aging dogs, heart diseases related to, 599–603

Rehabilitation
    after CCT injuries, 1214–1215

biomechanics of, **1255–1285.** See also
  Biomechanics.
    applicable mechanical theory,
      1255–1263. See also
      *Applicable mechanical theory, in
      biomechanics of rehabilitation.*
    gait
      kinematic, 1265–1256
      kinetic, 1263–1265
companion animal, **1473–1484.** See also
  Companion animal rehabilitation.
defined, 1255
emerging modalities in, **1335–1355**
ESWT, 1345–1350
for neurologic patients, **1389–1409.** See
  also specific disorder, e.g., *Chronic
  spinal cord injury, rehabilitation for.*
for orthopedic patients, **1357–1388.** See
  also *Orthopedic patients, rehabilitation
  for.*
for peripheral nerve injury, 1403–1405
in acute care patients, **1411–1426**
    adjunct pain management in,
      1422–1424
    applications of, 1411–1412
    assisted walking in, 1419–1420
    electrical stimulation in,
      1421–1422
    facilitated standing in, 1419–1420
    general nursing care in, 1413–1414
    mobilization in, 1418–1420
    patient positioning in, 1414–1415
    range of motion in, 1418–1419
    suction in, 1417–1418
    thoracic percussion and vibration
      in, 1416–1417
    thoracic postural drainage
      techniques in, 1415–1416
in medical patients, **1411–1426**
    adjunct pain management in,
      1422–1424
    applications of, 1411–1412
    assisted walking in, 1419–1420
    electrical stimulation in,
      1421–1422
    facilitated standing in, 1419–1420
    general nursing care in, 1413–1414
    massage in, 1420–1421
    mobilization in, 1418–1420
    patient positioning in, 1414–1415
    range of motion in, 1418–1419
    suction in, 1417–1418
    thoracic percussion and vibration
      in, 1416–1417
    thoracic postural drainage
      techniques in, 1415–1416
LLLT, 1335–1345
of sporting dogs, **1427–1439.** See also
  Sporting dogs, rehabilitation of.

physical. See *Physical rehabilitation.*
static magnet field therapy, 1351–1352
wound healing in, **1453–1471.** See also
  *Wound healing, in veterinary
  rehabilitation patients.*
Renal damage
  acute, in dogs and cats
    described, 581–583
    early detection of, 581–587
    early recognition of, 585–587
    risk factors for, 583–585
  early detection of, in dogs and cats,
    581–596
Renal disease
  chronic
    early, diagnostic markers of,
      proteinuria as, 589–590
    in dogs and cats, 587–590
      described, 587–588
      early detection of,
        588–589
  in dogs and cats
    albuminuria, 590–594
    early detection of, **581–596**
    microalbuminuria, 590–594
Renal failure
  acute, 366–371. See also *Acute renal
    failure.*
  in geriatric patients
    hepatic metabolism in, 560
    metabolic balance in, 560–561
Renal insufficiency, in geriatric patients,
  558–561
    absorption in, 559
    bioavailability in, 559
    drug distribution and, 559–560
    renal clearance of drugs in, 558–559
Renal system, of geriatric patients, physiology
  of, 573
Repetitive disorders, in geriatric pets, 685
Reproductive emergencies, **397–420**
    dystocia, 399–406
    eclampsia, 411–412
    endometritis, 410–411
    fetal monitoring, 406–407
    hemorrhage, 407
    mastitis, 409–410
    neonatal resuscitation, 406
    pyometra, 412–417
    uterine monitoring, 406–407
    uterine prolapse, 408–409
    uterine torsion, 409
Resorptive lesions, dental, feline, **943–962.**
  See also *Feline dental resorptive lesions.*
Respiratory compromise, analgesia and
  chemical restraint for, 489–491

Respiratory distress
    approach to patient with, **307–317**
    assessment of, 310
    diseases affecting lungs, 313–315
    diseases of pleural space, 315–316
    gas exchange and, 307–308
    of lower airway, 312–313
    of upper airway, 310–312
    oxygen therapy for, 309–310
Respiratory distress of the newborn, 429–430
Respiratory function, assessment of, in acute
    spinal cord injury, 1393
Respiratory system
    examination of, in emergency patients,
        293–297
    lower, injury of, analgesia and chemical
        restraint for, 492–493
Respiratory zoonoses, control of, 15–16
Restlessness, nocturnal, in geriatric pets,
    684–685
Restraint, chemical, in emergency patients,
    481–515. See also *Chemical restraint, in
    emergency patients.*
Resuscitation
    cardiopulmonary cerebral, in young
        animals, 430–431
    neonatal, 406
Retainer(s), in small animal orthodontics, 887
Retinal separation, 476–478
Rheumatoid arthritis, 1086–1088
Rib, tumors of, 1164
Ribavirin, for feline infectious peritonitis,
    63–64
Root canal therapy, standard, for endodontic
    disease, 851–859
Rupture(s)
    Achilles, rehabilitation for, 1384–1385
    cranial cruciate ligament, rehabilitation
        for, 1379–1381

S
Salivary glands, in dogs and cats, 775
Sarcoma(s)
    injection site, 1167
    synovial cell, 1166
SARDS. See *Sudden acquired retinal degeneration
    syndrome (SARDS).*
Scapulohumeral joint, osteochondrosis of,
    1117
Secondary hepatic lipidosis, in cats, 632
Sedation
    defined, 436

for emergencies, 436, 507–509
for esophagostomy/endoscopic
    gastrostomy tube placement, in
    feline hepatic lipidosis, 246
Sedative(s)
    for trauma patients, 486
    in emergency patients, 436, 507–509
    in preanesthetic sedation of geriatric
        patients, 575–576
Segmental mandibulectomy, 1023–1024
Seizure(s)
    in emergency patients, 304–305
    unusual patterns of, in infectious
        diseases, 117–118
Senior pets. See *Geriatric pets.*
Separation anxiety, in geriatric pets, 683–684
Sepsis, in young animals, 428–429
Septic arthritis, 1102–1105
    clinical findings in, 1102
    described, 1102
    diagnosis of, 1103
    pathophysiology of, 1102–1103
    treatment of, 1103–1105
Serum chemistry, in feline infectious
    peritonitis diagnosis, 51–53
Sevoflurane, in anesthesia maintenance in
    geriatric patients, 579
Shared environment zoonoses, control of,
    17
Shared vector zoonoses, control of, 17
Shelters, feline infectious disease control in,
    21–37. See also *Infectious diseases, feline, in
    shelters, prevention of.*
Shock
    analgesia and chemical restraint for,
        498–500
    cardiogenic, in emergency patients, 336
    distributive, in emergency patients,
        334–336
    hypovolemic, nonhemorrhagic, in
        emergency patients, 334
    in assessment of emergency patients,
        288–289
Shock waves, characteristics of, 1346–1347
Shoulder(s), osteochondrosis of
    prognosis of, 1119
    treatment of, 1118
Shoulder joint, mobilization of, 1295–1299
Shoulder luxation, 1369–1370
    management of, 1183–1184
Sit-to-stand exercises
    in acute spinal cord injury rehabilitation,
        1397

in chronic spinal cord injury rehabilitation, 1402

Six-month spaying or neutering visit, in juvenile veterinary dentistry, 800–811

Skeletal muscle, biomechanics of, 1271–1274

Skeletal system, infections of, **1093–1110**
  acute hematogenous osteomyelitis, 1096–1097
  antimicrobial therapy for, 1094–1095
  imaging of, 1095–1096
  microbiology of, 1093–1094
  osteomyelitis
    acute, 1098–1099
    chronic, 1099–1101
    fungal, 1101–1102
  osteomyelitis from exogenous sources, 1097–1101
  septic arthritis, 1102–1105

SLE. See *Systemic lupus erythematosus (SLE)*.

Slings, 1442–1443

Sodium ipodate, for feline hyperthyroidism, 176–177

Soft tissue impaction, in juvenile veterinary dentistry, 801–802

Soft tissue tumors, of musculoskeletal system, 1167–1168

Softened gutta percha techniques, for endodontic disease, 860–862

Solitary osseous plasmacytoma, 1165

Sore(s), pressure, healing of, 1461–1468

Sound(s), breath, bronchial, in heart diseases in aging dogs, 607

Space-occupying masses, elimination of, in emergency patients, 352

Spinal cord, LLLT effects on, 1343

Spinal cord injuries
  acute, in neurologic patients, 1389–1399
  chronic, in neurologic patients, 1399–1402
  in neurologic patients, 1389–1402

"Spinal walking," 1394

Spine
  examination of, in emergency patients, 304
  mobilization of, 1311–1315

Sporting dogs
  activities of, physical skills in, 1428
  conditioning of
    balance and proprioception in, 1431–1432
    endurance in, 1431
    strengthening, 1430–1431
  injuries in, 1432–1433

rehabilitation of, **1427–1439**
  acute, 1434–1435
  fitness training, 1427–1432
  reconditioning in, 1436–1437
  subacute, 1436

Sports injuries, in sporting dogs, 1432–1433

Squamous cell carcinoma, clinical presentation of, 1012–1013

Standing, facilitated, in rehabilitation of medical and acute care patients, 1419–1420

Stanozolol, for feline hepatic lipidosis, avoidance of, 259

Static magnet(s)
  studies of, 1351
  use of, 1352

Static magnet field therapy, 1351–1352

Steroid(s), topical, for gingivostomatitis, 905

Stifle joint
  mobilization of, 1308–1311
  osteochondrosis of, 1117
    prognosis of, 1119
    treatment of, 1118–1119

Stifle luxation, 1370–1371
  management of, 1189–1193

Strengthening, in conditioning of sporting dogs, 1430–1431

Stretching
  in chronic spinal cord injury rehabilitation, 1401
  in peripheral nerve injury rehabilitation, 1404

Stromal ulcers, infected, 470–471

Struvite urolithiasis, feline, 163–164

Suction, in rehabilitation of medical and acute care patients, 1417–1418

Sudden acquired retinal degeneration syndrome (SARDS), 478

Sudden blindness, 476

Superficial digital flexor tendon(s), rehabilitation for, 1385–1386

Superficial digital flexor tendon luxation, rehabilitation for, 1385

Supernumerary teeth, in juvenile veterinary dentistry, 802

Supraspinatus tendon mineralization, rehabilitation for, 1383

Swimming, in acute spinal cord injury rehabilitation, 1397–1398

Symphyseal separation, repair of, 988–990

Synovial cell sarcoma, 1166

Systemic illness, metabolic and tissue changes associated with, in medical and acute care patients, 1413

Systemic lupus erythematosus (SLE), 1088

T

Tachypnea, in heart diseases in aging dogs, 607–608

Temperature, in assessment of emergency patients, 290

Temporomandibular joint, in dogs and cats, 769

Tendon conditions, **1201–1218**
  common calcaneal injuries, 1207–1214. See also *Common calcaneal tendon (CCT) injuries.*
  of pelvic limb, 1206–1207
  of thoracic limb, 1203

Tendon healing, 1201–1203

Tendon injuries, rehabilitation for, 1381–1386
  Achilles rupture, 1384–1385
  avulsion of tendon of long digital extensor muscle, 1383–1384
  biceps tenosynovitis, 1382
  deep digital flexor tendons, 1385–1386
  flexor tendon contracture, 1384
  infraspinatus contracture, 1383
  superficial digital flexor tendon luxation, 1385
  superficial digital flexor tendons, 1385–1386
  supraspinatus tendon mineralization, 1383

Tenosynovitis
  abductor pollicis longus, canine lameness due to, 1241–1243
  biceps, rehabilitation for, 1382
  bicipital, 1203–1206. See also *Bicipital tenosynovitis.*

Tepoxalin, for osteoarthritic pain in geriatric dogs and cats, 660

Tetracycline(s), for feline hepatic lipidosis, avoidance of, 260

Tetraparesis, acute spinal cord injury and, prognosis and recovery, 1394

Therapeutic exercises, biomechanics of, 1277–1282

Therapeutic modalities, in peripheral nerve injury rehabilitation, 1405

Therapeutic ultrasound, in acute spinal cord injury rehabilitation, 1399

Thermoablation, laser, for gingivostomatitis, 901–902

Thiamine (vitamin B$_1$), in feline hepatic lipidosis, 250–251

Thiol antioxidant supplementation, in feline hepatic lipidosis, 255–258

Thiopental, for emergencies, 439–440

Thoracic limb, tendon conditions of, 1203

Thoracic organs, feline infectious peritonitis effects on, 48–49

Thoracic percussion and vibration, in rehabilitation of medical and acute care patients, 1416–1417

Thoracic postural drainage techniques, in rehabilitation of medical and acute care patients, 1415–1416

Thyroid disorders, in geriatric patients, **635–653**. See also specific disorder, e.g., *Feline hyperthyroidism.*
  canine hypothyroidism, 641–649
  canine thyroid tumors, 649–651
  feline hyperthyroidism, 635–641

Thyroid tumors, canine, 649–651

Thyroidectomy, for feline hyperthyroidism, 177–178

Thyroid-stimulating hormone response test, in feline hyperthyroidism, 175

Thyrotropin-releasing hormone stimulation test, in feline hyperthyroidism, 174

Tibiotarsal joint, osteochondrosis of, 1117–1118

Tissue(s)
  antigen in, in feline infectious peritonitis diagnosis, 60–61
  periodontal, functions of, 820–822

Tongue, bird, 790–791

Tonsillectomy, for gingivostomatitis, 901

Tooth (teeth)
  deformed, in juvenile veterinary dentistry, 808–809
  development of, in dogs and cats, 770–772
  fractured, 711
  functions of, 820–821
  movement of, in small animal orthodontics, 871–878. See also *Orthodontic(s), small animal, tooth movement in.*
  permanent, of cats, peculiarities of, 915–921
  primary
    delayed eruption of, in juvenile veterinary dentistry, 796–798
    fractured, in juvenile veterinary dentistry, 795–796

persistent, in juvenile veterinary
dentistry, 798–800
supernumerary, in juvenile veterinary
dentistry, 802
Tooth (teeth) eruption, timing of, 789
Tooth (teeth) extraction
canine teeth, 981–982
complications of, 982–983
coronal gingiva incised from tooth in,
973
described, 972–973
elevating, luxating, and removing tooth
in, 979–980
flaps in, 974
home care follow-up, 984
in cats, 982
in dogs, 981–982
precautions in, 982–983
radiographs in, 973
roots and root pieces, 982
sectioning tooth and alveolar bone
removal in, 975–978
smoothing alveolar bone in, 980
steps in, 973–981
suturing flap in, 981
Tooth (teeth) resorption, in domestic cats,
causes of, update on, **913–942**. See also
Feline odontoclastic resorptive lesions (FORL).
Torsion, uterine, as reproductive emergency,
409
Total elbow replacement, in dogs,
1233–1234
Total joint replacement
history of, 1219
in dogs, **1219–1238**
atypical cases, 1233
cemented hip replacement
systems, 1221–1225
complications of, 1228–1233
contraindications to, 1220–1221
indications for, 1219–1220
noncemented hip replacement
systems, 1225–1227
perioperative care, 1227–1228
Total unilateral mandibulectomy, 1024–1026
Total unilateral maxillectomy, 1029–1030
Tramadol, for oral and dental procedures,
1053
Tranquilizer(s), in preanesthetic sedation of
geriatric patients, 575–576
Trauma
acute abdomen in, causes of, 379, 384
chest, analgesia and chemical restraint
for, 493
head, in young animals, 431–432
local, FORL and, 929–932

Traumatic luxations, of appendicular
skeleton, management of, 1175–1196.
See also specific luxation and
*Appendicular skeleton, traumatic luxations of,
management of.*
Traumatic proptosis, 462–464
Treadmill walking, biomechanics of,
1277–1278
Tremor(s), in emergency patients, 304–305
Tricyclic antidepressants, for oral and dental
procedures, 1057
Triiodothyronine suppression test, in feline
hyperthyroidism, 174
Trypsin-like immunoreactivity, in feline
hepatic lipidosis, 239
Tumor(s). See also Pelvis, tumors of; *specific
types, e.g.,* Musculoskeletal tumors.
musculoskeletal, malignant, of dogs and
cats, **1159–1172**
of long bones of appendicular skeleton,
1159–1162
oral, **1009–1039**. See also *Oral tumors.*
primary sex hormone–secreting adrenal,
feline, 195–196
thyroid, canine, 649–651

U

UDCA. See *Ursodeoxycholic acid (UDCA).*
Ulcer(s)
corneal, 465–471. See also *Corneal ulcers.*
decubital, healing of, 1461–1468
stromal, infected, 470–471
Ultrasound
in hyperadrenocorticism, 193
in wound healing, 1458–1459
therapeutic, in acute spinal cord injury
rehabilitation, 1399
Unilateral rostral mandibulectomy, 1021
Unilateral rostral maxillectomy, 1027–1029
Ununited anconeal process, 1129
Upper airway obstruction, analgesia and
chemical restraint for, 491–492
Urate urolithiasis, feline, 162–163
Urethral obstructions, 166–169, 359–364
clinical signs of, 361
described, 359–361
initial database for, 361
treatment of, 361–364
goal of, 361
Urinary catheter placement, analgesia and
chemical restraint for, 504
Urinary system, biochemical testing of
geriatric patients effects on, 544–546

Urinary tract disease, lower, feline
  described, 147–148
  diagnosis of, 161
  diagnostic workup for, 148–150
  prevalence of, 159–161
  recent concepts in, **147–171**
  treatment of, 161
Urinary tract emergencies, **359–373**. See also
    specific type, e.g., *Urethral obstructions.*
  acute renal failure, 366–371
  urethral obstructions, 359–364
  uroperitoneum, 364–366
Urine bile acids, in feline hepatic lipidosis,
    236
Urine cortisol-to-creatinine ratio, in
    hyperadrenocorticism, 191
Urine tests, in feline hepatic lipidosis,
    236–239
Urolithiasis
  feline, 162–169
  oxalate, feline, 164–166
  struvite, feline, 163–164
  urate, feline, 162–163
Uroperitoneum, 364–366
  described, 364–365
  laboratory parameters in, 365–366
  physical examination of, 365–366
  treatment of, 366
Ursodeoxycholic acid (UDCA), in feline
    hepatic lipidosis, 258
Uterine monitoring, 406–407
Uterine prolapse, as reproductive emergency,
    408–409
Uterine torsion, as reproductive emergency,
    409
Uveitis
  anterior, 456–458. See also *Anterior
      uveitis.*
  causes of, 457

V

Vaccination
  in feline infectious disease control in
      shelters, 32–33
  in feline infectious peritonitis
      prevention, 69–70
Vaccine(s), for client compliance in geriatric
    pets, 750
Variable(s)
  group-specific, in biochemical testing of
      geriatric patients, 540
  laboratory-specific, in biochemical
      testing of geriatric patients, 539
Vascular diseases, in dogs, 606–607

Vascular insufficiency, in cognitive decline,
    692
Vascular system, in dogs and cats, 776–779
Velocity, 1260
Vertebra(ae), tumors of, 1164
Veterinarian(s), geriatric care programs for,
    743–753. See also *Geriatric care programs,
    for veterinarians.*
Veterinary dentistry
  in geriatric patients, **699–712**
    client education related to,
        701–702
    complete prophylaxis in, 705–709
    dental procedure in, 704–705
    fractured teeth, 711
    introducing of, 699–701
    oral neoplasia, 711
    periodontal disease treatment,
        709–711
    preprocedure evaluation in,
        702–704
  juvenile, **789–817**
    cleft palates, 791–792
    conditions that occur at any time,
        814–815
    deep occlusal pits, 811
    deformed teeth, 808–809
    delayed eruption of primary teeth,
        796–798
    dental crowding, 802–804
    dentigerous cysts, 800–801
    first visits (8-week and 12-week
        checkups), 792–798
    fracture of immature permanent
        teeth, 813–814
    malocclusions, 792–795, 804–808
    maxillofacial fractures, 814–815
    microglossia, 790–791
    odontomas, 809–811
    oral tumors, 815
    persistent primary teeth, 798–800
    problems recognized in first weeks
        of life, 790–792
    six months to 1 year, 811–814
    six-month spaying or neutering
        visit, 800–811
    soft tissue impaction, 801–802
    supernumerary teeth, 802
    third visit (4-month checkup),
        798–800
Veterinary oral health care, gold standard of,
    781–787
  anesthesia and preoperative workup in,
      782–783
  periodontics in, 784–786
  radiology in, 783–784
  rechecks in, 787

Virus(es), zoonoses due to, control of, 15

Visceral pain, analgesia and chemical restraint for, 501

Vital pulp therapy, for endodontic disease, 844–850

Vitamin(s)
fat-soluble, in feline hepatic lipidosis, 253–254
water-soluble, in feline hepatic lipidosis, 250–253

Vitamin B_1, in feline hepatic lipidosis, 250–251

Vitamin B_{12}, in feline hepatic lipidosis, 251–253

Vitamin B_{12} status, in feline hepatic lipidosis, 237–239

Vitamin D
activity of, FORL effects on, 921–929
for FORL, 933–936

Vitamin D metabolites, for FORL, 933–936

Vitamin E, in feline hepatic lipidosis, 253–254

Vitamin K_1, in feline hepatic lipidosis, 253
avoidance of, 260–261

Vocalization, excessive, in geriatric pets, 684–685

Volvulus
dilation, analgesia and chemical restraint for, 501–503
gastric, analgesia and chemical restraint for, 501–503

W

Walking
assisted
for medical and acute care patients, 1419–1420
in acute spinal cord injury rehabilitation, 1397
"spinal," 1394
treadmill, biomechanics of, 1277–1278

Water-soluble vitamin supplementation, in feline hepatic lipidosis, 250–253

Weanling(s), analgesia for, 506–507

Weight loss, in geriatric patients, nutrition related to, 721–724

Wheelbarrowing, biomechanics of, 1278–1280

Work, in biomechanics, 1262–1263

Wound(s), nonhealing, causes of, 1456–1458

Wound dehiscence, after oral tumor excision, 1034–1035

Wound healing
in veterinary rehabilitation patients, **1453–1471**
decubital ulcers, 1461–1468
electrical stimulation in, 1459
emerging modalities in, 1 459–1461
growth factors in, 1460–1461
monochromatic near-infrared photo energy in, 1460
negative pressure wound therapy in, 1459–1460
pressure sores and, 1461–1468
ultrasound in, 1458–1459
inflammatory phase of, 1453–1455
physiology of, 1453–1456
proliferative phase of, 1455
remodeling phase of, 1455–1456

Y

Young animals, emergencies in, **421–434.** See also *Pediatric emergencies.*

Z

Zoonotic diseases
control of
bacteria-related, 12–14
bite-, scratch-, or exudate exposure–related, 12–15
enteric-related, 3–12
for direct contact zoonoses, 3–17
for enteric zoonoses, 3–12
for genital zoonoses, 16–17
for respiratory zoonoses, 15–16
for shared environment zoonoses, 17
for shared vector zoonoses, 17
fungi-related, 14–15
general concepts in, **1–20**
genital-related, 16–17
guidelines for, 2–3
respiratory-related, 15–16
shared environment–related, 17
shared vector–related, 17
viral-related, 15
described, 1

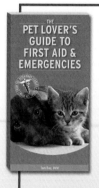
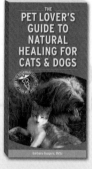
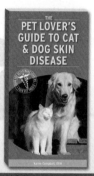
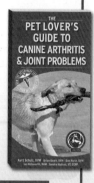
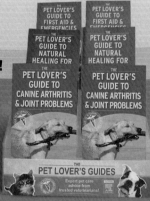

Changing Your Address?

Make sure your subscription changes too! When you notify us of your new address, you can help make our job easier by including an exact copy of your Clinics label number with your old address (see illustration below.) This number identifies you to our computer system and will speed the processing of your address change. Please be sure this label number accompanies your old address and your corrected address—you can send an old Clinics label with your number on it or just copy it exactly and send it to the address listed below.

We appreciate your help in our attempt to give you continuous coverage. Thank you.

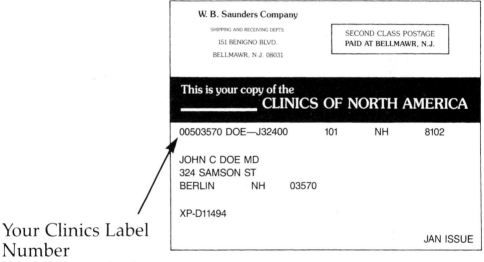

W. B. Saunders Company

SHIPPING AND RECEIVING DEPTS

151 BENIGNO BLVD.

BELLMAWR, N.J. 08031

SECOND CLASS POSTAGE
PAID AT BELLMAWR, N.J.

This is your copy of the
_____ **CLINICS OF NORTH AMERICA**

00503570 DOE—J32400   101   NH   8102

JOHN C DOE MD
324 SAMSON ST
BERLIN   NH   03570

XP-D11494

JAN ISSUE

Your Clinics Label Number

Copy it exactly or send your label
along with your address to:
W.B. Saunders Company, Customer Service
Orlando, FL 32887-4800
Call Toll Free 1-800-654-2452

Please allow four to six weeks for delivery of new subscriptions and for processing address changes.

United States Postal Service
Statement of Ownership, Management, and Circulation

1. Publication Title	2. Publication Number	3. Filing Date
Veterinary Clinics of North America: Small Animal Practice	0 1 9 5 - 5 6 1 6	9/15/05

4. Issue Frequency	5. Number of Issues Published Annually	6. Annual Subscription Price
Jan, Mar, May, Jul, Sep, Nov	6	$170.00

7. Complete Mailing Address of Known Office of Publication (Not printer) (Street, city, county, state, and ZIP+4)	Contact Person
Elsevier Inc. 6277 Sea Harbor Drive Orlando, FL 32887-4800	Gwen C. Campbell
	Telephone
	215-239-3685

8. Complete Mailing Address of Headquarters or General Business Office of Publisher (Not printer)

Elsevier Inc., 360 Park Avenue South, New York, NY 10010-1710

9. Full Names and Complete Mailing Addresses of Publisher, Editor, and Managing Editor (Do not leave blank)

Publisher (Name and complete mailing address)

Tim Griswold, Elsevier Inc., 1600 John F. Kennedy Blvd., Suite 1800, Philadelphia, PA 19103-2899

Editor (Name and complete mailing address)

John Vassallo, Elsevier Inc., 1600 John F. Kennedy Blvd., Suite 1800, Philadelphia, PA 19103-2899

Managing Editor (Name and complete mailing address)

Heather Cullen, Elsevier Inc., 1600 John F. Kennedy Blvd., Suite 1800, Philadelphia, PA 19103-2899

10. Owner (Do not leave blank. If the publication is owned by a corporation, give the name and address of the corporation immediately followed by the names and addresses of all stockholders owning or holding 1 percent or more of the total amount of stock. If not owned by a corporation, give the names and addresses of the individual owners. If owned by a partnership or other unincorporated firm, give its name and address as well as those of each individual owner. If the publication is published by a nonprofit organization, give its name and address.)

Full Name	Complete Mailing Address
Wholly owned subsidiary of	4520 East-West Highway
Reed/Elsevier Inc., US holdings	Bethesda, MD 20814

11. Known Bondholders, Mortgagees, and Other Security Holders Owning or Holding 1 Percent or More of Total Amount of Bonds, Mortgages, or Other Securities. If none, check box   ☐ None

Full Name	Complete Mailing Address
N/A	

12. Tax Status (For completion by nonprofit organizations authorized to mail at nonprofit rates) (Check one)
The purpose, function, and nonprofit status of this organization and the exempt status for federal income tax purposes:
☐ Has Not Changed During Preceding 12 Months
☐ Has Changed During Preceding 12 Months (Publisher must submit explanation of change with this statement)
(See Instructions on Reverse)

PS Form 3526, October 1999

---

13. Publication Title	14. Issue Date for Circulation Data Below
Veterinary Clinics of North America: Small Animal Practice	July 2005

15.	Extent and Nature of Circulation		Average No. Copies Each Issue During Preceding 12 Months	No. Copies of Single Issue Published Nearest to Filing Date
a.	Total Number of Copies (Net press run)		4700	4400
b. Paid and/or Requested Circulation	(1)	Paid/Requested Outside-County Mail Subscriptions Stated on Form 3541. (Include advertiser's proof and exchange copies)	2874	2799
	(2)	Paid In-County Subscriptions Stated on Form 3541 (Include advertiser's proof and exchange copies)		
	(3)	Sales Through Dealers and Carriers, Street Vendors, Counter Sales, and Other Non-USPS Paid Distribution	572	591
	(4)	Other Classes Mailed Through the USPS		
c.	Total Paid and/or Requested Circulation [Sum of 15b. (1), (2), (3), and (4)]	▲	3446	3390
d. Free Distribution by Mail (Samples, complementary, and other free)	(1)	Outside-County as Stated on Form 3541	123	113
	(2)	In-County as Stated on Form 3541		
	(3)	Other Classes Mailed Through the USPS		
e.	Free Distribution Outside the Mail (Carriers or other means)	▲		
f.	Total Free Distribution (Sum of 15d. and 15e.)	▲	123	113
g.	Total Distribution (Sum of 15c. and 15f.)	▲	3569	3503
h.	Copies not Distributed		1131	897
i.	Total (Sum of 15g. and h.)	▲	4700	4400
j.	Percent Paid and/or Requested Circulation (15c. divided by 15g. times 100)		97%	97%

16. Publication of Statement of Ownership
☐ Publication required. Will be printed in the **November 2005** issue of this publication.   ☐ Publication not required

17. Signature and Title of Editor, Publisher, Business Manager, or Owner   Date

[signature] Joel Milliot – Executive Director of Subscription Services   9/15/05

I certify that all information furnished on this form is true and complete. I understand that anyone who furnishes false or misleading information on this form or who omits material or information requested on the form may be subject to criminal sanctions (including fines and imprisonment) and/or civil sanctions (including civil penalties).

Instructions to Publishers

1. Complete and file one copy of this form with your postmaster annually on or before October 1. Keep a copy of the completed form for your records.
2. In cases where the stockholder or security holder is a trustee, include in items 10 and 11 the name of the person or corporation for whom the trustee is acting. Also include the names and addresses of individuals who are stockholders who own or hold 1 percent or more of the total amount of bonds, mortgages, or other securities of the publishing corporation. In item 11, if none, check the box. Use blank sheets if more space is required.
3. Be sure to furnish all circulation information called for in item 15. Free circulation must be shown in items 15d, e, and f.
4. Item 15h. Copies not Distributed, must include (1) newsstand copies originally stated on Form 3541, and returned to the publisher, (2) estimated returns from news agents, and (3), copies for office use, leftovers, spoiled, and all other copies not distributed.
5. If the publication had Periodicals authorization as a general or requester publication, this Statement of Ownership, Management, and Circulation must be published; it must be printed in any issue in October or, if the publication is not published during October, the first issue printed after October.
6. In item 16, indicate the date of the issue in which this Statement of Ownership will be published.
7. Item 17 must be signed.
   Failure to file or publish a statement of ownership may lead to suspension of Periodicals authorization.

PS Form 3526, October 1999 (Reverse)

8 Ways To Expand Your Practice
Step 1: Return this card.

Elsevier Clinics and Journals offer you that rare combination of up-to-date scholarly data, step-by-step techniques and authoritative insights...information you can easily apply to the situations you encounter in daily practice. You'll be better able to diagnose and treat a wider range of veterinary problems and broaden your client base.

Just indicate your choice(s) on the card below, fill out the rest of the card and drop it in the mail.

Your satisfaction is guaranteed. If you do not find that the periodical meets your expectations, write *cancel* on the invoice and return it within 30 days. You are under no further obligation.

SUBSCRIBE TODAY!
DETACH AND MAIL THIS NO-RISK CARD TODAY!

YES! Please start my subscription to the periodicals checked below with the ❑ first issue of the calendar year or ❑ current issues. If not completely satisfied with my first issue, I may write "cancel" on the invoice and return it within 30 days at no further obligation

Please Print:

Name_____

Address_____

_____

City_____ State_____

ZIP _____

Method of Payment

❑ Check (payable to **Elsevier**; add the applicable sales tax for your area)

❑ VISA   ❑ MasterCard   ❑ AmEx   ❑ Bill me

Card number _____

Exp. date _____

Signature _____

Staple this to your purchase order to expedite delivery

*To receive in-training rate, orders must be accompanied by the name of affiliated institution, dates of residency and signature of coordinator on institution letterhead. Orders will be billed at the individual rate until proof of resident status is received.

This is not a renewal notice. Professional references may be tax-deductible.
© Elsevier 2005. Offer valid in U.S. only. Prices subject to change without notice. **MO 10806 DF4169**

❑ **Clinical Techniques in Equine Practice**
Volume 4 (4 issues)
Individuals $124; Institutions $209; In-training $62*

❑ **Clinical Techniques in Small Animal Practice**
Volume 10 (4 issues)
Individuals $134; Institutions $220; In-training $67*

❑ **Journal of Equine Veterinary Science**
Volume 22 (12 issues)
Individuals $171; Institutions $242; In-training $54*

❑ **Seminars in Avian and Exotic Pet Medicine**
Volume 4 (4 issues)
Individuals $116; Institutions $220; In-training $54*

❑ **Veterinary Clinics-Equine Practice**
Volume 21 (3 issues)
Individuals $145; Institutions $230

❑ **Veterinary Clinics-Exotic Animal Practice**
Volume 8 (3 issues)
Individuals $130; Institutions $215

❑ **Veterinary Clinics-Food Animal Practice**
Volume 21 (3 issues)
Individuals $115; Institutions $182

❑ **Veterinary Clinics-Small Animal Practice**
Volume 35 (6 issues)
Individuals $170; Institutions $260

Elsevier, the premier publisher in veterinary medicine, keeps you current with the latest developments in your field to help you achieve optimal patient care. Subscribe today to any of the publications listed below and save considerably over the single issue price.

Clinical Techniques in Equine Practice
Clinical Techniques in Small Animal Practice
Journal of Equine Veterinary Science
Seminars in Avian and Exotic Pet Medicine
Veterinary Clinics – Equine Practice
Veterinary Clinics – Exotic Animal Practice
Veterinary Clinics – Food Animal Practice
Veterinary Clinics – Small Animal Practice

Just fill out the card on the reverse and drop it in the mail.
YOUR SATISFACTION IS GUARANTEED.

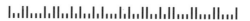